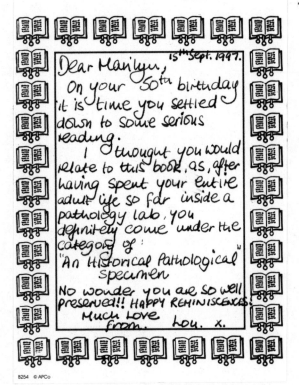

Dear Marilyn,                    15th Sept. 1997.

On your 50th birthday it is time you settled down to some serious reading.

I thought you would relate to this book, as, after having spent your entire adult life so far inside a pathology lab, you definitely come under the category of:

"An Historical Pathological specimen"

No wonder you are so well preserved!! HAPPY REMINISCENCES!

Much Love from. Lou. x.

8254  © APCo

# THE HISTORY OF
# British Pathology

## George J. Cunningham MBE.MD.FRCPath

Sometime Professor of Pathology at the
Royal College of Surgeons, England, and at
the Medical College of Virginia, Richmond,
USA.

## Edited by G. Kemp McGowan, BM.BCH.FRCPath

Sometime Consultant Chemical Pathologist
at the British Royal Infirmary

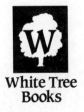

White Tree
Books

First published in 1992
by White Tree Books
an imprint of Redcliffe Press Ltd
49 Park St, Bristol

© *George J. Cunningham and G. Kemp
McGowan*

ISBN 1 872971 57 1

Typeset by Mayhew Typesetting, Rhayader,
Powys
Printed by The Longdunn Press Ltd, Bristol

# Contents

Author's Preface      vi

Editor's Foreword      vii

1   Beginnings in London and Paris 1750–1836      1

2   Medical developments and training 1823–46      10

3   Pathology in the 1820s      26

4   The Clinician-Pathologists 1820–50      42

5   Microscopy, Museums and the Birth of Public Health 1840–55      52

6   Advancs of Pathology 1830–1900      59

7   The continential background 1700–1870      74

8   Developments at Oxford and Cambridge 1830–1920      96

9   The other early British medical schools 1700–1830      116

10   English and Welsh provincial medical schools 1824–93      143

11   The first Pathologists from 1830      170

12   The birth of Physiology and Experimental Medicine 1820–90      195

13   John Simon and Public Health 1840–71      204

14   Army Medicine and Pathology 1742–1907      227

15   Growth of Physiology in France, Germany and Britain 1813–78      237

16   The Research Establishments 1871–98      251

17   Parasitology 1835–1900      271

18   The development of Bacteriology 1850–90      277

19   The growth of Clinical Pathology 1910–48      303

20   Problems of training and qualification 1947–52      322

21   College or Faculty? 1952–58      335

22   How the College was formed 1958–64      345

23   Pathology in the 1960s      362

Appendix I Document accompanying voting paper      369

Appendix II Letter to Branch Secretaries      371

Index      372

# Author's Preface

This project began about 1965 when C. G. Signy and G. J. Cunningham decided to write a history of the Association of Clinical Pathologists. Signy was to deal with the earlier years and Cunningham the later ones. In 1968 Signy died without having written any of his part. As a result Cunningham decided not to proceed any further.

About 1975 G. K. McGowan asked me to collaborate with him in writing a history of Pathology and this I readily agreed to do. We had several meetings but as time went on McGowan felt it would be better if I did the writing while he offered to supply me with any information which was not readily available in the USA. During this period he wrote a short account of some of the events which led up to the voting as to whether there should be a College or Faculty of Pathology. I had also written a similar chapter. I suggested that as I had written a few chapters I should amalgamate our chapters into one and this I called College or Faculty?

In 1968 Dr. W. D. Foster was appointed librarian to the College of Pathologists, and it subsequently became known that he had been commissioned to write the early history of the College. Therefore I decided to broaden the scope of the work and I provisionally called it 'The History of British Pathology'. I worked on it while in Richmond, Virginia and it was completed in its present form when I returned to England in December 1983. Foster's book (undated) was published by the College in the early 1980s and a copy was sent to every member. It turned out that approx 20% was devoted to a history of British Pathology prior to the founding of The Association of Clinical Pathologists.

My lists of references were complete but not standardised, and some of the chapters needed renaming and rearranging. From what has been said it will be clear that I take full responsibility for all the text and I should say that much of it had never been seen by McGowan. As I was in America most of the time we had very few meetings in the years 1976–1983 before he undertook the editing.

**George J. Cunningham**
**St Leonards**
**Sussex**

# Editor's Foreword

In 1990 I asked George Cunningham what progress he had made in the publication of his book. He told me that he had not been able to find a commercial publisher, that he was not in good health, and that the typescript had been deposited with the Royal College. It seemed to me a tragedy that his book should not see the light of day, and I offered to find a private publisher and to edit his typescript and see it through the press. To this he readily agreed. The editing has involved, as the author indicated in his Preface, the rearrangement and renaming of chapters, the standardisation of references, and the correction of minor errors. The text remains essentially as George Cunningham wrote it, but I am responsible for editorial mistakes.

**G. K. McGowan**
**Morfa Nefyn**
**Gwynedd**

# ONE
# Beginnings in London and Paris
# 1750–1836

Although in retrospect it can be seen that the seeds of pathology were being sown in the 17th century, it was not until the 18th that substantial growth occurred. By the second half of that century there had been contributions from several European countries, the earliest being from Italy where Morgagni of the University of Padua published his famous book, 'The Bases and Causes of Disease', in 1761. As Morgagni himself was a professor of anatomy it is not surprising that his pathology took the form of pathological anatomy.

These descriptions of diseased organs came mostly from autopsies, for surgical operations were very limited at the time. Collections of diseased organs led to the formation of museums and it was in this field that England made her first real contribution. The Hunter brothers from Glasgow had settled in London, and William collected specimens for the courses in his anatomy school in Great Windmill Street. His younger brother John, who assisted him, later made a collection which in variety and number of specimens has never been surpassed and which eventually found its way into the Royal College of Surgeons. Its diversity was such that it should be termed 'biological' rather than 'medical' and it revealed John Hunter as a naturalist as well as a surgeon.

There is some evidence that lesser collections were started at an earlier date. In the Treasurer and Almoner's Order Book of St. Bartholomew's Hospital, London, there is an order dated 23rd June 1726 which states [1]

'Two convenient rooms being prepared under the Cutting Ward, one for the more decent laying the dead Patients before the buryale, the other a Repository for anatomical or chyrurgical Preparations'

These preparations were to be collected and recorded by the Assistant Surgeon who at that time was John Freke.[2] They must have been rather limited because the main operations then were 'cutting the stone', 'couching for cataract' and occasionally amputations. In fact most of Freke's specimens were probably urinary calculi, and they were to form the nucleus of a very much larger collection in the 19th century. It is interesting to note that although there was a 'dead room' provided in 1726 it was not until 1750[3] that permission to perform post-mortem examinations was given, thus indicating that the study of pathology at Bart's had not yet really started.

John Hunter became well-known in his lifetime both for his surgical ability and for his large collection of museum specimens. After Pott's death he became generally recognised as the foremost surgeon in the country. His industry was enormous and it is hard to believe that so

1

much could have been achieved by one man in a lifetime. The full worth of his contribution to surgery was not appreciated for many years. Although there were many publications on diverse subjects his complete works were not collected until 42 years after his death when Palmer (1935) edited them in five volumes[4]. Hunter showed his collection to the medical profession in 1783 and in the following year to 'those noblemen and gentlemen who felt an interest in such subjects.' But again the full extent of his ideas could not be recognised because a proper catalogue was lacking. Lastly the extraordinary destruction of many of his manuscripts by Sir Everard Home was a further deterrent to a full appreciation of the work and ideas of this remarkable man.

John Hunter gave much encouragement to younger men including his nephew, Matthew Baillie, who had come from Scotland to join him. There seems little doubt that a study of John Hunter's pathological specimens greatly assisted Baillie in the production of his famous book in 1793 entitled 'The Morbid Anatomy of some of the Most Important Parts of the Human Body', and was followed in 1799 by his beautifully illustrated 'Atlas of Diseases'. The popularity of Baillie's Morbid Anatomy is indicated by the fact that it went through eight English and three American editions, and was translated into Italian, French,[5] German and Russian.[5] In it he attempted to establish clinicopathological correlation between symptoms during life and disease as evidenced by post-mortem lesions, as indeed had Morgagni in preceding years. Baillie, however, went further and attempted to study the pathogenesis of disease as well. He published much other work which passed unrecognised until Wardrop collected and published it in 1825[5] two years after Baillie's death. Baillie had done much to establish British pathological anatomy and he might even have done more had he not been at the same time a very accomplished physician with a decided flair for diagnosis. This caused him to go into private practice for the rest of his life. This happenned in 1799 when he was only 38, and he rapidly became one of the most renowned physicians in London. In his earlier years he had collected 1,281 specimens of which 50% were pathological and these he gave to the Royal College of Physicians. They were subsequently given to the Royal College of Surgeons but unfortunately were destroyed in a bombing raid in May 1941.

Between 1799 and the era of the great physicians at Guy's some 30 years later, there is little of pathological interest in the British literature with the exception of an erudite work entitled, 'Treatise on the Diseases of Arteries and Veins'[6] published in 1815 by Joseph Hodgson (1788–1869) who was surgeon to the General Hospital at Birmingham for 30 years. It would be a mistake to think that pathology lay stagnant during this time for in reality it was a period of great activity. This was centred in France but its influence was wide and extended to Great Britain amongst other countries.

After the death of Morgagni, the Italian school, which had really launched Pathological Anatomy, declined and the School of Paris took over the initiative. This may come as a surprise for between the years 1792 and 1815 France was torn asunder by civil and foreign wars. Yet during this period Paris became the leading school in pathological anatomy in Europe. It became known for a number of distinguished physicians and surgeons who naturally attracted many students from foreign countries including Great Britain. It is for this reason that no account of British pathology would be complete without a brief account of some of the events in France and particularly in Paris.

Eighteenth century medicine in France was at a low ebb and in 1788 Tenon gave a report revealing the appalling conditions in the Paris hospitals. By contrast the French military hospitals were much better, for attention had been given earlier to improvements in hygiene largely due to a work by Sir John Pringle, a leading officer in the British Army (see Chapter 14). But the improvement in the French military hospitals was not maintained and after 1780 they deteriorated chiefly owing to financial stringency. Also the training of military doctors was affected by the need for economy. In 1775 training schools known as 'ampitheatres' were opened at the regional hospitals in Lille, Metz and Strasbourg – and later at Brest and Toulon.[7] Five years later these were closed as an economy measure, though following an outcry from military medical circles they were reopened on a reduced scale a year later.[8]

The main aim of the Revolution of 1789 was to destroy once and for all the Old Regime with all its privileges, unequalities and injustices. This was to affect the medical profession very widely in the following ways.

Prior to the Revolution most hospitals depended for their financing on charitable institutions often connected with the Church, charity from individuals, land endowments and government supplements. It was now suggested that hospitals be abolished but in the end the National Assembly embarked on a policy of reorganisation. As the general plan included confiscation of church and other lands, the income of the hospitals fell from 30 million livres in 1789 to 3–4 million livres a few years later. Thus the State which had also confiscated all hospital properties suddenly found itself completely responsible for financing the hospitals. As a result it was forced to give subsidies of up to 10 million livres in order to maintain them in their sad and reduced state. A further responsibility facing the Assembly was the support of the indigent poor.

The University of Paris and various Medical Societies, being products of the Old Regime, also came under fire. They certainly had monopolies distasteful to the revolutionaries, for the Faculty of Medicine at the University alone could grant the degree of 'docteur regent', a requisite for a teaching appointment in the Paris medical schools. In a similar way the College of Surgery of St. Come could alone authorise anyone to practice surgery in Paris.[9] Because of these privileges, the University, the Colleges and the Medical Societies were abolished in February 1791 as were all examinations for entry into Medicine. In their eagerness to make the medical profession available to all, the National Assembly went to the absurd extreme of decreeing that anyone could practise medicine on payment of a small fee. He needed no experience nor did he have to pass any examination.[10] It is therefore not difficult to see why in the spring of 1792 the medical profession was in disarray and the hospitals in a serious plight due to shortage of beds, skill, medical staff, and materials.

This would seem to have been trouble enough, but in April 1792 the National Assembly, sensitive of criticism from other countries and fearful of the possibility of invasion, declared war on Austria and Prussia. Plans for building up a volunteer army had not fully materialised, and it was soon realised that the military hospitals, chaotic as they were, could not provide an adequate service in time of peace, let alone in time of war. By July 1792 the situation was growing desperate and the Assembly decided that a medical military service must be improvised. To bring this about J. F. Coste, a distinguished medical veteran, was given very wide powers and was assisted by Sabatier, a well-known surgeon, and Parmentier, a pharmacist.[11] They surveyed the medical scene with great rapidity and, unhampered by administrators (the so-called 'war commissioners'), completed a report for the Committee of Health some four months later. Thus by the end of 1792 there was a standardised plan for organisation of the army medical services. This was encouraging but the year 1793 opened disastrously and by the spring the French armies were in full retreat and the improvised medical service had already collapsed. Casualties had been heavy and epidemics of typhus and cholera had taken their toll. Worst of all, three-quarters of the medical men enrolled since 1792 had been lost either by war or disease in addition to a number of desertions.[12] The National Convention, which had replaced the legislative Assembly in September 1792, responded to this disaster by appointing a Committee of Public Safety headed by Danton in April 1793. Later in the year this committee took complete control of the military medical service and effected substantial improvements by providing badly needed money and additional hospital beds. The latter were obtained by such measures as moving veterans out of the Invalides, by converting the old monastery of Val de Grace into a hospital and by expanding other civilian hospitals such as the Midi, the Hotel Dieu and the Charité[13]. 'Representatives on mission' were appointed to ensure that the Army carried out the recommendations of the Committee. Although these men were not popular with the Army officers, who felt that they were simply 'interfering', their presence resulted in a welcome tightening up of discipline which had become lamentably lax during the early revolutionary years. The net result was great improvement in the efficiency of the Army and its services. At the same time the fortunes of the armies improved decidedly and, aided by the strategy of Carnot, the enemy invaders were hurled back.

The military medical services had come a long way, but there were still

4

some striking deficiencies. One great problem was the shortage of skilled medical staff resulting from the suspension of training in 1791. There had been no organised attempt to train doctors and the only unofficial training was given by men such as Larrey who had started a school of anatomy and military surgery in the field. Thus the Committee of Public Safety realised that training of doctors had to be resumed. In August 1793 it was decided to create an independent military medical service, and authorisation was given for medical training in the military hospitals at Strasbourg, Lille, Metz and Toulon. This decision came at a very inopportune time as three of the above towns were being threatened by the enemy and at the end of August Toulon was captured by the British. Following an improvement in the fortunes of the armies the Committee conducted many discussions during 1794 on the question of resumption of medical training. There was much delay and indecision because any proposal which in any way resembled education under the Old Regime was immediately vetoed. At last, late in the year, a committee of six commissioners presented a plan to the National Convention and it was accepted with some modifications. The Old Academy of Surgery became the Paris School of Health and the other centres were established in Strasbourg and Montpellier. These three schools could accommodate 550 students and they were opened in January 1795.[14] A further extension of this movement occurred in March 1795 when the committee of Public Safety authorised the resumption of medical training at some private medical schools such as Caen, and provided financial assistance.

In the course of seven years the medical profession had been dis-mantled and reorganised and it is necessary to examine some of the most important changes which took place. In the first instance it seems remarkable that the revolutionaries who set out to abolish the hospitals and disrupt medical training should in the end have produced such remarkable improvements in both. Undoubtedly, the doctors had their say, for many were in sympathy with the revolution and thus were well represented on the ruling bodies. On the National Assembly they had seventeen representatives, on the Legislative Assembly twenty-eight and on the National Convention forty-nine.[15]

One of the main changes which occurred was in the status of the hospital. Care of patients was greatly improved and hygienic measures were installed to check infectious disease in the absence of any knowledge as to its exact nature. Attention was given to more rapid evacuation of wounded from the battlefield and it was at this time that Larrey invented his 'flying ambulance'. The doctors obtained a large amount of clinical experience, and the statistics of the military hospitals revealed the importance of medical diseases which were three or even five times as common as battle wounds. In the absence of any set training medical officers learned while working on the job. In fact, there was nowhere else to learn, except in the hospital and it became realised that this might be the ideal centre for training. Indeed, when training was

5

resumed in 1795 the students attended in the hospital wards from the first day.

In pre-revolutionary days the physicians and surgeons were trained separately and tended to stand aloof from one another, the physician having the higher social status. As the war went on and the physicians stood by helpless in the epidemics of dysentery, typhus and cholera their status declined and that of the surgeon advanced. As they worked side by side in the hospitals they became more closely associated and both became known as 'health officers'. As the surgeons studied autopsies and looked for localised lesions so the physicians followed their example. Thus the study of pathological anatomy with clinical correlation was perhaps the most important factor in drawing physicians and surgeons closer together. The importance of Pathology at this time is emphasised by a glance at the staff of the new medical schools opened in 1795. At Paris where there were twelve Professors with assistants, there was a Professor of Surgical Pathology as well as one for Medical Pathology; at Montpellier there were ten Professors including one for Pathology, Drugs, and Meteorology; at Strasbourg eight Professors including one of Pathology, Hygiene and Prophylaxis.[16].

Lastly, the physicians realised that a knowledge of anatomy was essential for them as well as for surgeons, and at this time there was no shortage of bodies for the purpose.

While these important advances were occurring in the military hospitals there was also progress in the civilian institutions. The top physicians and surgeons had tended to stay at their posts during wartime as, for example, the surgeon Dessault at the Hotel Dieu, and the physician Pinel at the Bicetre, and Corvisart at the Charité. All three men who were the leading doctors in Paris, were great admirers of Morgagni and as such were devoted to the study of pathological anatomy. Desault studied and improved the methods of treating fractures, while Pinel advanced the treatment of mental illness in addition to having a lifelong interest in the classification of disease. Corvisart developed the use of percussion as discovered by the Austrian physician, Auenbrugger, and aimed at correlating physical signs elicited during life with lesions discovered at autopsy. He wrote only one book, 'Maladies du coeur' (1806) which illustrates his method for it contains many excellent case histories and autopsy records. He also planned but never wrote a work which was to have been entitled, 'On the Bases and Causes of Diseases Investigated by Diagnostic Signs and Confirmed by Autopsy'.[17]

The development of medicine in Paris is a complex story and one which has been excellently told by Ackerknecht[17] who covers the period 1794–1848. Only a few of the surprisingly large numbers of eminent men will be referred to here.

The importance of pathological anatomy in stimulating medical thought has already been emphasised. Much of this work was originally done by surgeons and Wunderlich, the Leipzig physician, was right when he stated that 'the whole new trend in medicine has come out of the surgical school'.[18] Interestingly enough, many leaders of internal medicine, namely Bichat, Recamier, Laennec, Broussais and Cruveilhier, were all trained as surgeons.

The tradition of the earlier workers, and the further development of pathological anatomy were carried on by several pupils. Bichat (1771–1802) greatly respected Pinet, and was trained by the surgeon Desault whose works he subsequently edited. As an early pioneer of pathology Bichat is remembered as the first one who separated organs into tissues, though it is surprising that he and later Laennec did not believe in the use of the microscope. In his short life of 31 years he achieved a remarkable amount. He performed a large number of autopsies, an experience which enabled him to give a course in pathological anatomy. The only record of this comes from Beclard's 1801 lecture notes which were published in 1825[19]. In spite of this Bichat's influence at the time was considerable and extended to later workers such as Laennec, Broussais, and Cruveilhier.

Gaspar Laurent Bayle (1774–1816) was a pupil of Corvisart whom he succeeded at the Charité. He was interested in the classification of disease and, being an advocate of pathological anatomy, believed that it should be based on lesions and not on symptoms. He is chiefly remembered for his work, 'Studies on Pulmonary Phthisis' (1810). This involved a study of 900 autopsies and included 54 excellent selected case histories with autopsy reports. As a result he divided the disease into six types[20] but he was really observing different stages of the disease.

Laennec (1781–1816) commenced his studies at Nantes, and proceded to Paris where he came under the influence of Corvisart, Bichat, Dupuytren, and G .L. Bayle. He was appointed physician to the Hospital Necker in 1816 and in that year invented the stethoscope. Three years later he published his famous work, 'De l'auscultation mediate ou taite du diagnostic des maladies des poumons et du coeur'.[21] His name is so closely bound up with the stethoscope that it is sometimes forgotten that on the basis of his training his main interest was in pathological anatomy. When only 22 he gave a course on the subject and announced a forthcoming text-book as well. This never materialised, possibly because for economic reasons he was compelled to go into private practice in 1804 and was thus diverted from his first love.

With the passing of Pinel and Laennec a different school of thought was initiated by Broussais (1772–1838). Taught by Pinet and Bichat his earlier work on fevers followed traditional lines. Much of his experience was in the army or navy and he served during the Napoleonic wars. Suddenly he changed his philosophy and introduced his 'physiological concept' that disease was inflammatory and caused by irritation. In most cases he believed that there was gastrointestinal irritation either at the beginning or end of the disease, and this concept might have arisen from

7

the number of typhoid cases which he must have seen. With such aetiology, the universal treatment was 'anti-phlogistic' and consisted of special diet and bleeding, mostly by application of leeches. This theory became very popular, possibly because of Broussais's strong personality, and he attracted many students. The demand for leeches became enormous and whereas in 1823 only 320,000 had been imported into France, the number had reached over 21 million by 1834.[22] In his later years his theory became discredited and nowadays he is almost forgotten. He made a final attempt to regain prominence when he became a pioneer of Phrenology and was a founder member of the Phrenological Society.

Amongst the critics of Broussais's theory was Andral (1797–1876) who published in 1829 a five-volume work entitled, 'Precis d'anatomie pathologigue'. It had been described by Ackerknecht[23] as 'the culminating point in the classic macroscopic pathological anatomy of the school'.

The end of this period saw the appearance of a five volume work on pathological anatomy by Cruveilhier (1791–1873) between 1848 and 1861. Although there had been so much activity in the study of pathological anatomy by almost every Paris clinician, the subject had not so far been recognised as a discipline. Cabanis as early as 1799 had advocated a Chair of Pathological Anatomy but this had not come about until 1836 when Dupuytren willed the money for such a purpose. In the event the State paid for the Chair, and the legacy of Dupuytren was used for supporting a Museé Dupuytren. Cruveilhier, a pupil of Dupuytren, was appointed to the Chair and held it for the next 30 years. Although 1836 is a landmark in the history of pathology there are two points which should be borne in mind namely

(1) that Cruveilhier although occupying a Chair of Pathological Anatomy remained a clinician.
(2) that recognition of the subject had occurred earlier in some other Universities on the Continent, namely Caen in 1756 and Strasbourg in 1819.

In reviewing this 50 year period of growth of pathological anatomy at the Paris School, it should be remembered that France was at war for just over 20 years. In spite of this, medicine and surgery had steadily advanced and Paris had become the centre of pathological anatomy in Europe.

Even in the 18th century Paris proved an attraction to foreign medical men who were mostly surgeons and anatomists. With the peace of 1815 there was a tremendous influx of students of medicine, at all stages of their careers. They came from several different countries and thus the influence of Parisian medicine came to be felt all over Europe. Great Britain sent many students of quality and, stimulated by their French teachers, they returned home to establish outstanding medical schools such as those of Guy's Hospital in London and the Dublin school in

Ireland. An outline of some of these men's lives and their achievements will be dealt with later. Before attempting this it will be necessary to examine the state of medicine in Britain prior to another landmark in the history of pathology, namely the founding of the Pathological Society of London in 1846.

REFERENCES

1  Medvei, V.C. and Thornton, J.L., 'The Royal Hospital of St. Bartholomew 1123–1973'. St. Bartholomew's Hospital, London 1974, p. 47.
2  Chalstrey, J., (1757) 'St. Bartholomew's Hospital Journal'. March 1957, p. 86.
3  Whitteridge, Gweneth and Stokes, Veronica, 'A Brief History of the Hospital of St. Bartholomew'. Hospital of St. Bartholomew, 1961, p. 37.
4  Palmer, J.F., 'The Surgical Works of John Hunter, F.R.S. London'. Rees, Orme, Brown, Green and Longman, London 1835. Vol. 1, p. 107.
5  Wardrop, J., 'The works of Matthew Baillie, M.D.' in 2 vols. Longman, Rees Orme, Brown and Green. London 1835 (quoted by A.E. Rodin. The Influence of Matthew Baillie's Morbid Anatomy. Charles C. Thomas, Springfield, Illinois 1973, p. 36).
6  Long, E.R., 'A History of Pathology'. The Williams and Wilkins Company, Baltimore 1928, p. 155.
7  Vess, D. M., 'Medical Revolution in France 1789–1796'. University Presses of Florida, Gainesville 1975, p. 27.
8  Ibid p. 34.
9  Ibid p. 17.
10  Ibid p. 58.
11  Ibid p. 72.
12  Ibid p. 88.
13  Ibid p. 137.
14  Ibid p. 162.
15  Ibid p. 45.
16  Ibid pp. 170–1.
17  Ackerknecht, E. H., 'Medicine at the Paris Hospital 1794–1848'. The Johns Hopkins Press, Baltimore 1967, p. 84.
18  Ibid p. 25.
19  Ibid p. 165.
20  Ibid p. 87.
21  Ibid p. 90.
22  Ibid p. 62.
23  Ibid p. 168.

# TWO
# Medical developments and training
# 1823–46

The dominance of the Paris School in medicine and in pathological anatomy in the post-revolutionary years was followed by a progressive movement in Great Britain, which was to bear fruit during the first half of the 19th century. Many of those responsible for this movement had attended the Paris School, or had studied the publications of its outstanding medical men. There followed the foundation of famous medical schools at Guy's Hospital, London and at Dublin, Ireland. It will now be necessary to study this movement in some detail, for it led to the consolidation of pathology and culminated in the foundation of the Pathological Society of London in October 1846. This society was to have a long life and was to be eventually incorporated together with a number of other medical associations into the Royal Society of Medicine in 1907.

In this brief review an attempt will be made to portray the state of the medical profession, medical education and the growth of pathology between the years 1823 and 1846. The appearance of a weekly medical publication, the 'Lancet', in 1823 made this possible, and what follows has been mostly derived from a study of this journal.

In 1823 Thomas Wakley founded the 'Lancet', a journal which has maintained its influence on the medical profession until the present day. Wakley came from a Devon farming family and was a reformer at heart. He trained at Guy's Hospital and became a member of the Royal College of Surgeons, in addition to obtaining his MD degree at Aberdeen. Later he was returned to Parliament as a Radical in the election of 1835 when Lord Melbourne, who disliked Radicals, was Prime Minister. In 1839 he was made Coroner for West Middlesex.[1] Remarkably outspoken in his zeal for reform, he was in constant conflict with the London Teaching Hospitals and certain members of their staffs, the Royal Colleges, and the Apothecaries Company. These activities were to involve him in many lawsuits in the first 10 years of the 'Lancet', and his very colourful life is attractively described by Squire Sprigge.[2]

Perhaps the most surprising thing about the first issue of the 'Lancet' was the publishing date of 5th October 1823, which was a Sunday. The first volume covered the last 3 months of that year, and was noteworthy for the diversity of its contents. In addition to medical articles there were reports of drama at Covent Garden, and the Birmingham Musical Festival. Wakley's enthusiasm for chess was indicated by a history of the game and a number of chess problems. His antagonism towards quackery was illustrated by publication of the contents of such quack remedies as Dalby's Carminative, Daffy's Elixir, Spilsbury's Antiscorbutic Drops, and

10

many others[3]. There was even a note of the convictions under the Vagrant Act, to say nothing of a short note on 'Acupuncturation'. During the next year the Lancet took the form which was to be maintained for the next 20 years. The publication day was changed to Saturday, general articles were discontinued, and the journal became purely medical and scientific.

Medical education was at this time far from being stereotyped. In fact, before 1815 it was not illegal for any unqualified person to practise medicine. The little control that existed came from the two Royal Colleges in London and the Apothecaries Company.[4] The surgeons had started as a guild in 1540 and had been given a Royal College Charter in 1800. It was at this time in the process of formulating rules and regulations for effective control of its members, but this was to be in future years. The Royal College of Physicians by its charter of 1518 was given virtual control of Medicine as a whole, though it really confined its authority to an area within seven miles of the City of London. A further function was the control of the apothecaries with whom there was frequent conflict. By 1800 the Apothecaries Company had obtained a certain amount of independence, and once they had been granted permission to give medical advice, for which they could not charge, and to dispense medicines for which they could charge, they had evolved into general practitioners. This position became consolidated when the Apothecaries Act of 1815 was passed. It stated that to become an apothecary an individual had to serve an apprenticeship, to have some dispensary experience, and to pass an examination. He was then made a Licentiate of the Apothecaries Company (LSA) and without this was not allowed to practise medicine. The Royal College of Physicians retained some limited control because anyone wishing to practise medicine or surgery within a seven-mile radius of London had to obtain its Licentiateship. They examined the applications of individuals, who were required to pay a fee.[5] In the succeeding years it became the custom for general practitioners to obtain the Diploma of the Royal College of Surgeons (MRCS) as well as the LSA. This was a logical step for the LSA did not include any training in Surgery, whereas the MRCS required the taking of approved courses mostly related to Surgery, Anatomy and Physiology, and the submission of Certificates of Attendance. This was the procedure for what might be called the rank and file of the profession. For those who wished to become hospital physicians or surgeons it was quite different.

Physicians for hospital appointments were chosen from Fellows of the Royal College of Physicians, who were relatively few in number. The Fellowship was only awarded to persons who possessed a degree from the Universities of Oxford or Cambridge, and no one could become a student there unless he was a member of the Established Church of England; hence no Dissenter could become a Fellow of the Royal College of Physicians of London. As a result many Dissenters obtained degrees at the Scottish Universities, of which Edinburgh was predominant at this time.

The would-be surgeon was faced with a different obstacle, namely one of finance. He had to be apprenticed to a hospital surgeon and this cost as much as £500. In return, it was assumed that he would either succeed his master, or have some similar appointment found for him. This was usually possible in spite of the fact that a Hospital Committee made the appointments, for the master was frequently very influential. The large fee for apprenticeship was sometimes waived in the case of a relative or friend of a famous surgeon. This procedure smacked of monopoly, privilege, and even nepotism and was calculated to attract the attention of a reformer such as Wakley. An excellent example of this existed at the United Borough Hospitals of Guy's and of St. Thomas's, while the elder Henry Cline was lecturer in Anatomy and Surgery. Astley Cooper was his apprentice and later became a colleague of his master. When Cline resigned his son succeeded him, and there then followed the appointment of three of Astley Cooper's nephews to various posts. The next surgical vacancies were filled by Astley Cooper's apprentice, Benjamin Travers, and J. H. Green who was Henry Cline's cousin. It has been pointed out that although all these men possessed undoubted ability they 'owed their elections to claims other than their merit'.[6] Thus, to summarise the position, the medical profession at the time consisted of a few Fellows and Licentiates of the Royal College of Physicians, rather more Members of the Royal College of Surgeons, and a large number of Licentiates of the Society of Apothecaries.

The difficulties facing the student of this period were well known to Wakley from personal experience, for he came to London in 1815, the year in which the Apothecaries' Act was passed. He decided that he would study for the Diploma of the Royal College of Surgeons. Such a student customarily selected a number of courses given by various teachers in London. At that time there were only three hospitals with acknowledged medical schools, namely St. Bartholomew's, the United Borough Hospitals (Guy's and St. Thomas's) and the London.[7] In effect, this meant that these institutions provided a complete course in all subjects related to Medicine. Some courses were also provided at the three other hospitals, namely the Middlesex, St. George's and the Westminster.[8] After due consideration and having attended some lectures, Wakley decided to join the medical school of the United Borough Hospitals, and this gave him the advantage of attending courses at both Guy's and St. Thomas's. He was certainly influenced in his choice by the personality of Sir Astley Cooper at Guy's.

If a student decided to enrol at a particular medical school he could do so on payment of his fees. If he wished ultimately to obtain the Diploma of the Royal College of Surgeons, he had to enrol at the College at the outset of his studies and pay a fee. To be eligible for admission to the examination he had to produce evidence of having taken certain courses of instruction, namely 'Certificates of Attendance'. If a course attended was given at an acknowledged medical school, there was no difficulty about obtaining such a Certificate. Wakley soon grew to dislike the Royal College of Surgeons and its various regulations. In subsequent years he openly accused them of money-making and referred to the 'Certificate Trade', of which more will be said later.

The London hospitals thus provided a programme of lectures on a number of subjects, and also tuition on the hospital wards. Inevitably the quality of teaching varied a good deal from hospital to hospital, and many students complained that having paid their fees they were not given the tuition to which they felt themselves entitled. The 'Lancet' set out to assist students in their choice of hospital by giving a survey at the commencement of the winter term, usually in September or October. Details of each hospital included the number of beds, the lecturers and teachers, and a timetable of the hospital's activities. For the further assistance of the prospective student there were comments on the hospital and certain members of the staff. It might be added that the candour of some of the remarks was literally astounding. Of one hospital, which was identified, it was said that it 'contains about 180 beds, but we look upon the practice of this institution as entirely worthless'.[9] At yet another 'there is an impressive hours of attendance list, which looks like punctuality *par excellence*. Yet, it is assuredly a fact that irregularity more gross exists in no establishment however ill-arranged and slovenly its system in all London'[10]. The individual lecturer fared no better for one 'declines lecturing on the cases', another is 'not less dumb', while a third is described as 'silent'.[11]

At this time the student could supplement his training by taking additional courses, which were given at private schools and dispensaries on payment of a fee. The idea of the private school seems to have originated with William Smellie, who in the previous century gave courses in obstetrics at his private house. William Hunter, following Smellie's example, started private courses in Anatomy and Operative Surgery in 1746 and built his famous Anatomical Theatre and Museum in Great Windmill Street in 1768.[12] This private school was still in existence in 1829 but the range of subjects taught had widened considerably and included Pathology, Physiology, Materia Medica, Physic, Surgery and Midwifery. Many other similar schools had sprung up and these were located near the teaching hospitals. The one in Great Windmill Street was relatively close to St. George's and the Middlesex hospitals, while the Webb Street school in the Borough (where Wakley enrolled to take the Grainger Course in Anatomy) was within easy reach of Guy's and St. Thomas's. Also, as might be anticipated, the staff at these private schools included some lecturers from the neighbouring teaching hospital. Many such schools were recognised by the Royal College of Surgeons, especially as their teachers were often members of the council or of the Court of Examiners. Thus their Certificates of Attendance were readily accepted for the College Diploma examination. The question of recognition at times caused trouble and there was occasionally blatant unfairness. A case in point was that of the Royal Western Hospital in Bryanstone Square, and the 'Lancet' hurried to lend its support. This hospital, which was small and in a way similar to a private school, had developed a fairly extensive teaching programme including lectures on Anatomy, Physiology, Medicine, Surgery, Materia Medica, Chemistry, Natural Philosophy, Botany and Midwifery. Its teachers were reputable yet the Royal College of Surgeons refused to accept its Certificates of Attendance. The rivalry of the age becomes apparent when we read that the Royal College of Surgeons of Edinburgh hastened to give them recognition and at the same time pointed out that the fee for the Edinburgh Diploma was only six guineas whereas that for the London Diploma was twenty-two.[13]

The Dispensary system commenced in 1696 when 53 leading doctors from the Royal College of Physicians agreed to contribute £10 each to provide medicines for the indigent poor of London.[14] This lasted for about 30 years but later during the 18th century a number of 'voluntary dispensaries' appeared. They were charitable institutions and one of the earliest was the Aldersgate Dispensary, founded by the Quaker philanthropist physician, Lettsom, in 1770. During the next 20 years a number of others sprang up and it was estimated that by the end of the century about 50,000 poor were receiving relief. By this time these dispensaries were doing a great deal more than merely supplying medicines. The distinctive features now were that physicians were in attendance and gave their services free, while patients too ill to come to the Dispensary were visited in their homes.[15] The doctors took turns in their hours of duty, and the apothecary was resident and thus easily available for supplying medicines. As the dispensaries developed they attracted more sick persons, though the numbers were limited because attendance was conditional on obtaining a card from a subscriber. It should be pointed out, however, that at the time a similar system of admission cards was in existence at all the hospitals. Fully developed, the voluntary dispensary functioned like a modern Out-Patient Department. It was usually located near a large hospital, and the Aldersgate Dispensary was within a few minutes walk of St. Bartholomew's.

In 1815 the passing of the Apothecaries' Act led to a new development for the dispensaries. By this Act, the Apothecaries' Company had agreed to accept Certificates of Attendance at these dispensaries for entry into the Licentiate examination. At this time the larger hospitals were not enthusiastic about training students for the LSA and this was where men like Henry Clutterbuck saw their opportunity and seized on it. Clutterbuck was a physician who had joined the staff of the Aldersgate Dispensary in 1807. Seeing the importance of this action by the Apothecaries, he started the 'Aldersgate School of Physic' with the help of his friends Dr. Birkbeck, Dr. Lambe, Mr. Norris, and Mr. Young.[16] For this purpose they must have acquired additional premises, for both establishments were in Aldersgate Street, the Dispensary at No. 36 and the school at No. 58.[18] The School was a great success, attracting many students to its courses on Medicine and Materia Medica, which were held three times annually over a period of twenty-five years. At one time it even posed a threat to its illustrious neighbour, St. Bartholomew's. This is only one example of similar instances in other parts of London. The movement lost its momentum about the middle of the 19th century, possibly because of improvements in teaching at the larger medical schools. The dispensaries were gradually merged with the local teaching hospital, though it was not until 1932 that the Aldersgate Dispensary was finally absorbed by St. Bartholomew's Hospital.[17]

Thus the medical student of the early 19th century was faced with a choice of courses and lectures. In 1825, in addition to those given at Medical Schools, Private Schools and Dispensaries, there were 14 individual doctors in London running courses at private addresses. If there was no shortage of lectures in the Metropolitan area, the same could not be said of the provinces. One of Wakley's original aims was to make available to 'distant Practitioners as well as to Students in Medicine and Surgery, reports of the Metropolitan lectures'. Consequently the earliest issues of the 'Lancet' published evening lectures on surgery given by Sir Astley Cooper,[19] and were followed in 1824–25 by some lectures by Benjamin Travers and John Abernethy. This was the signal for an outburst of indignation from the latter and having expressed his strong disapproval, Abernethy adopted an unusual countermeasure by giving one of his Monday evening lectures at St. Bartholomew's 'in the dark'.[20] In this way any representatives from the 'Lancet' would be prevented from taking notes. It proved to be ineffective because Mr. Abernethy's lectures had remained the same for many years. Consequently, the 'Lancet' was able to obtain the material and to publish it as usual. Pandemonium had followed the lecture, and there was a meeting of the students to discuss whether there should be no lights, some lights or all the lights during future lectures, and as can be imagined no conclusions were reached. Wakley was not a man to pour oil on troubled waters, and before long articles attacking and ridiculing Abernethy appeared in the 'Lancet'. Abernethy, in reply, attempted to obtain a Court Injunction to restrain the 'Lancet' from publishing his lectures and was unsuccessful.

The matter might have ended there had not Abernethy made some remarks about the 'Lancet' during his lectures and, true to form, Wakley returned to the attack. Abernethy sought an injunction for the second time and on this occasion was successful. He had contended that his lectures were under copyright and that he would suffer pecuniary loss, as it would be cheaper for the students to buy the 'Lancet' and read the lectures, rather than pay the fee for attending the course. Wakley had counter-attacked by maintaining that the lecture material was not original, and had indeed been given by others for the past years. The question of student attendance he ridiculed, and at the same time seized upon the opportunity of attacking the Royal College of Surgeons. This body had recently ruled that it would only recognise for examination purposes Certificates of Attendance from schools in London, Dublin, Aberdeen, Glasgow and Edinburgh.[21] Wakley rightly maintained that this ruling was very unfair to schools outside these towns, and that in London the Court of Examiners was simply looking after its own vested interests. In the case of Surgery, the members of the Court of Examiners (of which Abernethy was one) gave the courses which were approved. The students were bound to attend one of these in order to obtain a Certificate of Attendance, and could not do so if they had simply read the lectures in the 'Lancet'. Shortly afterwards, Wakley's lawyer applied to the Lord Chancellor to dissolve the injunction and this was allowed, there having been no opposition from Abernethy. With this the whole matter closed, as three days prior to the appeal Abernethy had resigned from the staff of St. Bartholomew's.

The above may sound trouble enough, but there was more to come because the 'Lancet' had succeeded in making many other enemies in a remarkably short space of time. Reports of the proceedings of bodies such as the Westminster Medical Society and the Medico-Chirurgical Society had also been published. The latter had attempted to prevent this practice[22] and had urged its members to preserve the utmost secrecy about its meetings. Lastly, the Apothecaries Company had taken exception to the publication of the names of four students who had been successful in one of its recent examinations.[23] In this hostile atmosphere a chance remark by one of the surgeons resulted in a debate by the St. Thomas's students on 'The propriety of suppressing the "Lancet"'.[24]

But if the Lancet had made enemies, it had also collected a number of friends, chiefly amongst students and provincial practitioners, who probably enjoyed the fearless attacks, from week to week, on official bodies and their vested interests. So Wakley battled on, publishing more and more lectures, encouraged by the circulation rate of his journal which had reached 4,000 at the end of its second year of publication.

Perhaps the most impressive feature of the lectures which were published was their variety. At first they related to Surgery and Medicine and came from eminent figures such as Astley Cooper, Abernethy, Travers, Clutterbuck, and others. It was customary to open the new Academic year at the teaching hospitals with an introductory lecture by one of the more eminent teachers, and these found a place in Wakley's 'Lancet'. Special subjects were included, often at great length, as for example when Mr. Lawrence of St. Bartholomew's gave over twenty lectures on the Anatomy, Physiology, and Diseases of the Eye. One of the more surprising inclusions was a lecture by Joshua Brookes, a foremost anatomist and founder of the private Blenheim Street School, on the 'Anatomy of the Ostrich'.[25] The enterprise shown by the journal was praiseworthy for there were also translations from eminent lecturers in the School of Paris. Amongst many others there may be mentioned lectures on Surgery by Baron Dupuytren and on Human Embryology by M. Flourens. Evidently the association between British doctors and their colleagues on the Continent, which had followed the end of the Napoleonic wars, was still very much in existence. In 1827 the 'Lancet' commented on numerous foreigners who had been seen at St. Bartholomew's. Also we find that in September 1826 Baron Dupuytren visited the United Borough Hospitals. At St. Thomas's he saw Mr. Travers perform some operations.[26] A day or so later he went to Guy's where Mr. Aston Key performed a lithotomy, and Sir Astley Cooper showed the Museum and the new buildings to the Baron.[27] This must have been a return visit for Sir Astley had been received by the Baron at the Hotel Dieu in Paris in the previous year. In September 1826 Napoleon's surgeon, Larrey, paid a rapid visit to the Dublin hospitals, the United Borough Hospitals and St. Bartholomew's. Larrey's visit was not very successful, partly because of its rapidity and partly because of his frequent recommendation of treatment by a 'moxa', a remedy which had been long discarded in London. The students at Guy's, activated more by curiosity rather than a desire to learn, asked Larrey to perform a moxa, which he did to their eminent satisfaction.[28] A moxa consisted of some lint or cotton held in a simple apparatus known as a 'porte-moxa', which when ignited produced a burn on the skin. It was really a form of counter-irritation often used in inflammatory conditions such as gout.

A good idea of the medicine and surgery of the period can be obtained by a survey of the hospital reports, which in 1824 became a regular feature of the 'Lancet'. Initially, these came from the London teaching hospitals, but in the succeeding years reports from hospitals in Birmingham, Colchester, Winchester, and others were included. In some instances the case report was serialised and followed the course of the illness of a particular patient from week to week. Again, it is interesting to see further evidence of a relationship with the Continent, for case reports came from many countries, chiefly France, Germany, and Italy.

It is easy to look back on these hospital reports and think of them for their educational value, but in reality they were also used as a means of attacking some undesirable practices. With his reforming zeal at fever pitch, Wakley was to turn his attention to the Constitution of the Royal College of Surgeons, and the administration of the Metropolitan Hospitals. For this purpose he chose to direct his attack on individuals rather than on the bodies themselves. In the case of the College it was criticism of the Certificates of Attendance, which have already been mentioned. Wakley attacked the members of the Court of Examiners (of whom Abernethy was one), who were confining their recognition of courses in Anatomy and Surgery to those given by themselves or their relatives and friends. They had thus created a monopoly to their financial advantage, at the expense of the students. In the case of the

Metropolitan Hospitals, he attacked members of the staff through his hospital reports. These reports included clinical and frequently operative details together with, at times, very frank criticism of the line of treatment and of the operative procedures. Such reports posed a threat to the career of any physician or surgeon and excited understandable concern amongst the staff of the larger hospitals. What was worse was the fact that the situation could not be controlled because Wakley obtained his information from agents whom he employed, including senior students, who were often dissatisfied with the educational facilities provided at the hospital and therefore only too willing to supply ammunition for criticism of the staff. So serious did it become that announcements were made that any student found providing such information would be immediately expelled. This anxiety was not confined to London and is indicated by the fact that a medical student from Glasgow Royal Infirmary was expelled for writing two letters to the 'Lancet' criticising the treatment of a nurse, who was suffering from a hip disease and died after being treated for a fracture.[29]

To those of us who regard the contemporary rash of malpraxis suits as a kind of modern epidemic, it is surprising to learn that similar cases occurred at the time under discussion. It was stated in the 'Lancet'[30] that 'if a surgeon commit an error in the practice of his profession, from a deficient knowledge of Anatomy, by the common law of the land, the patient or sufferer may recover heavy damages'. It goes on to cite a case where a shoulder dislocation was mistaken for a sprain and £700 damages were awarded against the surgeon. In subsequent correspondence relating to the case,[31] the danger to the profession is indicated by the surgeon who commented in a letter to the 'Lancet' 'were the perusal of your publication confined to my professional brethren, to most of whom the case is already known, I should not have trespassed upon your attention; but, as I find it is read by a large portion of the "reading public", it will be but an act of justice to me to insert this letter'.

Doubtless there were many shortcomings in diagnosis and treatment which passed unnoticed, but some at St. Bartholomew's which did not might be mentioned. There was a fatal case of severe comminuted fracture of the femur which was missed by the surgeons and diagnosed by the ward sister.[32] Another example was that of a boy aged 12 suffering from a head injury, who was found at autopsy to have a perforation of the bowel caused by a clyster pipe used for the administration of an enema.[33]

To return to the importance of the hospital reports, the crux of the matter was reached when a case of lithotomy was reported from Guy's Hospital, in which the operation took about an hour and resulted in the death of the patient some 29 hours later. This case is of great interest for it records the value of the opinion of a pathologist at autopsy. The 'Lancet' reported the case[34] and the surgeon, Mr. Bransby Cooper, was accused of incompetence for having taken an hour to do an operation which in the best hands should only have taken 4–5 minutes. As a result the surgeon felt himself obliged to bring a libel suit against Wakley in an attempt to defend his reputation. This was Wakley's opportunity to prove his contention of privilege, monopoly, and nepotism in hospital staff appointments. Mr. Bransby Cooper was a surgeon at Guy's Hospital, and a nephew of Sir Astley Cooper. It was therefore plausible, but not necessarily true, to suggest that he was lacking in skill, and that he owed his appointment to the influence of, and his relationship to, his eminent predecessor. The case excited tremendous interest and in the end Bransby Cooper won, but it was a Pyrrhic victory, for instead of being awarded the £2,000 damages which he had claimed, the jury only awarded £100.[35] During the trial, evidence on the post-mortem findings was given by Dr. Thomas Hodgkin, Lecturer in Morbid Anatomy, who had carried out the autopsy and was later to become a famous pathologist. Mr. Lambert, an agent of Wakley, who had written the report on the case for the 'Lancet', attended the post-mortem examination and asked Dr. Hodgkin whether he might examine the bladder himself. This he did when Dr. Hodgkin had temporarily left the room. On Hodgkin's return, Lambert showed him a rent in the bladder wall which he said had been made at the time of operation. Hodgkin at once 'taxed Mr. Lambert with having made the rent, it being his firm conviction that it had been made after death'.[36] In the end, it was Mr. Lambert who came out of it badly for he was expelled from the Westminster Medical Society[37] and the London Medical Society[38] in January 1829.

A repercussion of the libel trial occurred at St. Bartholomew's shortly after. Here, a man was taken to the operating theatre to have a hydrocoele tapped but when he saw the crowd of students and the surgeon with the trocar in his hand, he suddenly bolted from the room, saying that he had heard of Bransby Cooper's operation for the stone and that they would take no stone away from him. He was rapidly followed by a chimney sweep who was about to have a cancer of the scrotum removed.

The Norfolk and Norwich Hospital was founded in 1771 and by the early 19th century had obtained a European reputation as a centre for treatment for bladder stone.[39] The condition was thought to be particularly prevalent in this area because of the chalky soil of the district. It is of interest that in the Bransby Cooper libel suit his competence had been defended because he had spent some time as a pupil at the Norwich Hospital. In addition one of the lithotomists from the Hospital had been called as an expert witness. It had been noted in Norwich that bladder stone often occurred in young boys and this age incidence is noticeable in the cases reported in the 'Lancet' in the period at present under review. Fortunately many calculi had been kept in the museum of the Norwich Hospital and a recent examination showed that those occurring in young boys were composed of calcium oxalate or ammonium acid urate, whilst those in elderly men with urinary infections were made up calcium phosphate or ammonium magnesium phosphate. Although this incidence in children has disappeared in the modern Western world it still occurs in the Third World and a possible nutritional aetiology has been suggested.[40]

In an era without anaesthetics any surgical procedure was formidable, but lithotomy would seem to have been one of the worst. Even in the best hands the mortality was high either from shock, haemorrhage, or infection. Speed was essential and in the reports the time taken in minutes and seconds is usually recorded. The best operators took 4–5 minutes, but there does not appear to have been anyone to approach Cheselden's record of 56 seconds. Mention should be made of the famous lithotomist Professor Giltebrandt of Moscow. He was said to have performed over 1,000 lithotomies and that his 'coolness, dexterity, and neatness' astonished every beholder. He smoked a pipe continuously, even in bed, and of course throughout every operation.[41] Perhaps the most remarkable case ever recorded was that of a military surgeon, who had been cut for the stone five times by the age of twenty-two. Two years later he had a further stone and on this occasion performed the operation on himself, suggesting that he had lived up to his name which was M. Clever de Maldigny. By the time he had a seventh stone a new operation was in vogue. This had been invented in France, being named 'lithotritie' and used an instrument to crush the stone. This technique was taken up by a French surgeon, M. Civiale, who performed the operation on M. C. De Maldigny, who stated that he had suffered very little compared with the awful ordeal of lithotomy.[42] Subsequently a doctor of the Faculty in Paris, namely Baron Heurteloup, invented some new instruments[43] and wrote a treatise on the art of extracting the stone without incision.[44] The Baron visited England, gave a demonstration of his method before the leading surgeons, and performed a number of operations including one at his private house in Vere Street, Cavendish Square.

Considering the difficulties which were involved, many of the operations attempted were decidedly heroic. Amputations were not infrequent. In cases of strangulated hernias the operation was often unduly delayed and thus carried a high mortality. Many cases of aneurysm were reported for which arteries such as the femoral, carotid and innominate were tied. In one case at a provincial hospital the aorta was ligatured for an aneurysm of the external iliac artery, and not surprisingly the patient died some 3 hours later. Some carcinomas of the breast were removed and there was one remarkable case of a removal of part of the lower jaw for a tumour. The patient was a 16 year old girl, who most bravely bore this ordeal of over an hour, having been given substantial doses of opium prior to operation. One of the most sensational cases was that of a Chinaman, Hoo Loo aged 32, who came from Canton. He had a large scrotal 'tumour', obviously an example of elephantiasis, and he came to

Guy's Hospital because none of the doctors in his native country would attempt to remove it. The case excited a lot of interest and the operation had to be postponed because the operating room was too small to accommodate all the onlookers. Eventually it was carried out in the Anatomical Theatre, which would hold 680 persons. The operation took 1 hour and 44 minutes and a mass weighing 56 pounds was removed. The patient bore this terrible ordeal with the greatest fortitude.[45] There was much discussion about this operation, which many felt should never have been attempted. However, soon afterwards a letter appeared in the 'Lancet' from a surgeon who claimed that the operation was fully justified because he had successfully removed a similar mass of tissue weighing 70 pounds from a native of the island of St. Kitts.[46] Hoo Loo died soon after the operation, but had suffered several attacks of syncope in the later stages of it. It is of some interest to learn that it was decided to give him a blood transfusion, and six ounces were taken from a student's arm for the purpose, there having been several volunteers. Although transfusions were not introduced as a routine procedure for almost a century, a number of attempts were made at this time. Between 1825 and 1829 there were six successful cases recorded in the 'Lancet'. In only one was there any reaction, but there was no other untoward effect, presumably because only four ounces were given. Two cases had fifteen[47] and fourteen ounces[48] respectively, and in each case there was a striking improvement. All cases were obstetrical and had suffered a post-partum haemorrhage after either a full-term delivery or an abortion. The subject was evidently one of great interest at the time for a debate on it was held at the Hunterial Society of London.[49] During the discussion, one eminent obstetrician said that transfusion was unnecessary because women did not die from post-partum haemorrhage. Other cases of obstetrical interest at the time included a Caesarian section in Florence, Italy, which was reported as successful although the foetus was dead before the operation was commenced.[50] There was also a case of locked twins[51] and one of a lithopedion at the Salpetriere Hospital in Paris[52].

Surgical cases recorded in the 'Lancet' at this time far outnumbered medical, though this may be due to a selection on Wakley's part because of his greater interest in surgery. There is also the possibility that ill-effects due to treatment were more easily recognised in surgical rather than in medical cases, and thus 'better material' for criticising the hospital staff. However at one stage lists of all surgical cases admitted during the week at St. Bartholomew's were published, but no corresponding medical lists appeared. Our information about medical conditions seen at the time comes from clinical lectures by physicians which were freely illustrated by studies from current cases. There were cases of acute rheumatism and chorea, but in neither is there any indication of cardiac abnormality, not even at a post-mortem examination on a fatal case of chorea. There were a number of chest cases including phthisis, lung abscess, empyema and emphysema. Foreign bodies in the respiratory tract were not infrequent and one case of fatal asphyxia was caused by inhalation of a sixpenny coin. Calcific aortic stenosis was referred to as 'ossification of the aortic valve'. Heart failure with cardiomegaly presumably due to hypertension was encountered, though not recognised as such. Accidental poisoning was caused by a variety of agents such as arsenic, lead, belladonna, and mushrooms. Fevers presented a great difficulty in the absence of any knowledge of the aetiology of typhus, typhoid, and malaria, and the difficulty was compounded with the appearance of cholera for the first time in 1831. Enlarged lymph nodes in the necks of young people were probably due to tuberculosis or less commonly Hodgkin's disease. Smoking was thought by some to be injurious, but in a remarkable way. It was stated that in smokers the 'pancreas was in a scirrhous state'.

It can therefore be seen that the student of the early 19th century had a wide variety of clinical material of study even if the basic understanding of it was rather fragmentary. That there was no shortage of case material in the larger hospitals is seen from a report given to the Lord Mayor of London in 1824.[53] It states that during the past year St. Bartholomew's Hospital treated 10,312 patients and St. Thomas's 10,984. Many of these especially at St. Thomas's were out-patients, but it appears that each hospital had slightly less than 500 beds. At a time when surgery presented so many problems, it is surprising to find that about two-thirds of the beds were surgical. At St. Bartholomew's there were many accident cases, either occurring from traffic in the streets or from falls on building sites. But surgery, for all the terrors which it held for the patients, had a certain amount of glamour for the students. In these hospitals a majority of students enrolled for the surgical courses and were entitled to attend operations. The fee for such a surgical course was at least twice that charged for a similar medical course. The operations were carried out under very unhygienic conditions, and the crowd of students in attendance often hampered the movements of the surgeon, besides creating an atmosphere in which it was difficult for the patient to breathe. Some recorded events seem hard to believe. There was a pauper boy aged 16 in a Poor Law Institution just outside London, who was forcibly taken by the surgeons and their assistants and made to have an unsuccessful lithotomy against his will.[54] We are again reminded of the cruelty of the age by the case of a marine who was whipped with the cat-o-nine tails and died from his wounds about two weeks later.[55]

At such a time, one might well be curious to enquire just what the trained doctor might be expected to know. We can gain some idea of this from a list of examination questions given to a candidate for the degree of MD at Edinburgh in 1828[56] and those for the MB degree at Trinity College, Dublin in 1834.[57] Things had certainly advanced since the days of Smollett who, on being examined at Surgeon's Hall, London was asked 'If during an engagement at sea, a man should be brought to you with his head shot off, how would you behave?' In reply Smollett said that he did not remember having read of any method of cure proposed for such an accident.[58] The reference to the Dublin examination for M.B. is probably not reliable as it has been written by a disgruntled student. The first question reminds one of the earlier period already referred to and runs as follows, 'What supports the brain and hinders it from falling into a confused mass?' When the student could not answer this the Professor stated that he could not have attended his lectures, even though he had presented his Certificate of Attendance. Following the end of the examination there was much delay before the student was told that he had been rejected. However, he was admitted to a Latin examination the next day when the examiners changed their minds and passed him. The questions for the Edinburgh M.D. were totally different. They were arranged in groups and included Anatomy, Medicine, Pharmacy, and Chemistry. In anatomy the first question is 'What is a muscle?', and this is followed by progressively more difficult questions. Examples of other questions are:

(1)  Are there any valves in the arteries?
(2)  Are there any valves in the veins?
(3)  Are there any symptoms denoting the approach of an epileptic fit?
(4)  Why does he breathe more easily in the erect posture? (in reference to a case of hydrothorax)

Two cases were given for diagnosis and the history was in Latin. Finally, the student had to defend in public his 'Inaugural Dissertation'. All in all this would appear a very reasonable examination for the time.

One gains the impression that the hospitals were not happy places, for in addition to the suffering of the patients, which has been outlined, there was a good deal of jealousy and quarrelling amongst members of the staff. Much of this was probably related to unjust systems of appointment including nepotism, and the practice of selling one's post on retirement only added to the dissatisfaction. It would be a mistake to think that student discontent is a modern disease, for it seems to have existed in plenty during the 1820s and 1830s. The evils of the 'Certificate Trade' have already been mentioned. Having paid their fees, the students often found that the hours when they were allowed in the wards were very limited, and the Case books, meant to inform them of the location of cases in the hospital, were often not available. There was lack of punctuality on the part of the staff in arriving for ward rounds and lectures and, when they did turn up, the quality of the teaching was frequently sub-standard. Yet there is a likelihood that this has been exaggerated, for it must be remembered that Wakley was an ardent reformer and therefore eager to seize upon any grievance and to make the most of it. All the London hospital staffs were criticised in turn, and without mercy, except those of the new University of London Hospital. Events which need not have come to light were publicised. A case in point happened at St. Bartholomew's where two dressers disputed which of them should treat a patient, and ended up by having a fight in one of the wards. This was duly reported in the 'Lancet'[60] and also reached the daily newspapers.

REFERENCES

1 McMenemey, W. H., (1973) 'British Medical Journal' ii, 681.
2 Sprigge, S. Squire, 'The life and times of Thomas Wakley'. Facsimile of 1899 edition with introduction by Charles G. Roland. Robert E. Krieger Publishing Company 1974.
3 'Lancet', London, (1823) i, 30.
4 Cope, Zachary, 'The history of the Royal College of Surgeons of England'. Anthony Blond, London, 1859 p. 35.
5 'Medicine in 17th Century England. Ed. by Allen G. Debus. University of California Press 1974. Article on Quackery by L. R. C. Agnew p. 320.
6 Sprigge, S. Squire, 'The Life and times of Thomas Wakley'. Robert E. Grieger Publishing Company 1974. p. 15.
7 Ibid p. 13.
8 'Lancet', London, (1825–6) *10*, 724–5.
9 Ibid (1829–30) i, 49.
10 Ibid (1833–4) i, 9.
11 Ibid (1839–40) i, 28.
12 Garrison, F. H., 'History of Medicine'. W. B. Saunders Company, Philadelphia & London, 4th ed. reprinted 1966. pp. 338–9.
13 'Lancet', London, (1829) i, 11.
14 Davis, Michael M. Jr. & Warner, Andrew R., 'Dispensaries; their management and development'. The Macmillan Company, New York, 1918 p. 2.
15 Johnston, Abraham J., 'Lettsom'. William Heinemann 1933, p. 109.
16 Ibid p. 166.
17 Ibid p. 166.
18 'Lancet', London (1829–30) i, 13–15.
19 Ibid (1823) *1*, 37.
20 Ibid (1824) *5*, 141–43.
21 Ibid (1824) *3*, 116–17.
22 Ibid (1824) *2*, 51–54.
23 Ibid (1823) *1*, 416.
24 Ibid (1824) *2*, 329–31.
25 Ibid (1827) *12*, 132–4.
26 Ibid (1825–26) *10*, 791.
27 Ibid (1825–26) *10*, 861.
28 Ibid (1825–26) *10*, 849.
29 Ibid (1828–29) i, 486–9.
30 Ibid (1824) *2*, 136.
31 Ibid (1824) *2*, 228.
32 Ibid (1828–9) i, 282–3.
33 Ibid (1827–8) ii, 444–5.
34 Ibid (1827–8) i, 959.
35 Ibid (1828–9) i, 353–81.

36  Sprigge, S. Squire., 'The life and times of Thomas Wakley,' Robert E. Krieger Publishing Company 1974. p. 149.
37  'Lancet', London, (1828-9) i, 468-76.
38  Ibid (1828-9) i, 540.
39  Shaw, A. Batty, (1971), 'British Medical Journal' ii, 698:
40  Noordin, B.E.C., (1978) Ibid 1610-11. 'Review of idiopathic urinary bladder stone disease.' Fogarty International Center Proceedings No. 37) Edited by Robert van Reen 1977.
41  'Lancet', London, (1825-6), 9, 457-60.
42  Ibid (1826-7) 12, 556.
43  Ibid (1828-29) ii, 568-70.
44  Ibid (1831-32) i, 169-73.
45  Ibid (1830-1) ii, 87-9.
46  Ibid (1831-2) ii, 171-2.
47  Ibid (1827-8) i, 662.
48  Ibid (1825-6) 10, 58-62.
49  Ibid (1825-6) 10, 279-80.
50  Ibid (1828-9) i, 253.
51  Ibid (1823) 1, 158-62.
52  Ibid (1828-9) i, 317-18.
53  Ibid (1828-9), ii, 177.
54  Ibid (1824) 3, 121.
55  Ibid (1834-5) i, 897: 933.
56  Ibid (1828-9) i, 874-6.
57  Ibid (1828-9) i, 340-2.
58  Ibid (1834-5) ii, 513-15.
59  Roscoe. T., 'The complete works of Tobias Smollett'. George Bell & Sons, London 1881. p. 33 in 'Roderick Random'.
60  'Lancet', London, (1832-3), ii, 667.

# THREE
# Pathology in the 1820s

The commonest complaint by the students brings us to the most important part of our survey, namely the state of Pathology at the time. The complaint was related to the fact that students saw very few post-mortem examinations in the 'dead house'.[1] This applied to all the London hospitals and also to some in the provinces. The reasons for this deficiency were quite complex. In some cases, of course, the relatives would not grant permission for the examination. When a patient died it was the responsibility of the beadles to arrange for the disposal of the body to the undertakers. If a post-mortem examination was to be performed, the body was taken to the dead house by the 'box carriers', who were really porters. There were instances when the box carriers refused to do this and at times the beadles left the body in the ward (sometimes for a whole day) and then handed it directly to the undertakers. This not only saved them the trouble of moving the body to the dead house, but also eliminated the delay caused by the post-mortem examination. Frequently the post-mortem examinations were not announced and thus went on without the knowledge of the students. As indeed one student said 'How are we to learn Pathology if we cannot attend the dead house?'. Again, it appears that no specific person or persons were assigned the duty of performing the autopsy, and in most reports this individual is not named. In some cases it was one of the dressers[2], and they were accused of deliberately keeping such dissections from the students. A further source of discontent was the practice of some beadles who charged the students sixpence for every attendance at the dead house. A lot obviously depended on the attitude of the physician or surgeon in charge of the case. One student complained that he had only seen his surgeon teacher enter the dead house twice in six months. Mr. Joberns of the Middlesex Hospital was quoted as having said 'There is no use in pulling dead bodies about'.[3] Dr. Pelham Warren, a physician at St. George's, went even farther. He boasted that in his 12 years on the staff of the hospital, he had never once been in the dead house, and went on to say 'this damned morbid anatomy will spoil the practice of Physic'.[4] If this indicated the state of affairs at the Middlesex and St. George's, the same could not be said of Guy's, St. Bartholomew's, or St. Thomas's, where many post-mortems were carried out and some relatively good reports issued. In spite of some exceptions it appears that the majority of leading physicians and surgeons were following the example of Corvisart, Laennec, Pinel and others in Paris, who were attempting to correlate clinical observations with pathological findings. At St. Bartholomew's there were Mr. Lawrence and Mr. Stanley, who

26

often carried out post-mortems in the presence of their pupils. The dead house must have provided limited accommodation, for on some occasions the examination was carried out in the larger operating theatre after the operations for the day had been concluded. On one occasion Mr. Lawrence performed an autopsy on a case of strangulated hernia and took some parts to the museum for 'more minute' examination.[5] At Guy's Hospital some excellent dissections were carried out by the surgeon, Mr. Aston Key, and by Dr. Thomas Hodgkin, Lecturer in Morbid Anatomy. Hodgkin probably had an added incentive as he wished to obtain specimens for the Museum at Guy's Hospital of which he was the Curator.

National museums were a product of more modern times, but at the period under consideration many individuals made private collections of varying kinds. Biological and anatomical museums were possible once William Croone had shown to the Royal Society in 1662 that soft tissues could be preserved in alcohol ('spirits of wine'). The Hunter brothers, who made their collections almost a hundred years later, used this same method of preservation. At this time there was a great shortage of bodies for dissection, and the Hunters therefore used many preserved specimens for tuition in their Anatomical and Surgical Courses. Other surgeons running private schools were not slow to accumulate their own private collections. Many celebrated medical museums existed in Europe, such as those of Sandifort and Burgman in Leiden, Bonn in Amsterdam, Walther in Berlin, Meckel in Halle, and of course, in Paris at the School of Medicine.[6] Matthew Baillie, the nephew and pupil of John Hunter, had done the grand tour of Europe in the spring and summer of 1788. He visited many hospitals and examined specimens from the museums at the Ecole Veterinaire in Paris, and others at Strasbourg, Frankfurt, Mannheim, Rotterdam, and Amsterdam. He was dissatisfied with the technique of mounting and seems to have found it much inferior to that of John Hunter's museum in London.[7] The large London hospitals all had museums and the one at St. Thomas's was used to illustrate lectures in Anatomy and Surgery. It had been started by Mr. Cline Senior and Sir Astley Cooper. As appointed lecturers they literally owned the museum, for on the appointment of a new lecturer he was requested to pay £1,000 to the retiring lecturer for use of the museum. In 1825 there was a bitter dispute amongst the surgeons over the right to use this museum.[8] Private schools with similar collections were the Grainger School in Webb Street, and Sir Joshua Brooke's School in Blenheim Street. Specimens were collected by the surgeons who were frequently also members of the staff of the teaching hospital in the vicinity. The 'Lancet', in one of its tirades against the Middlesex Hospital, had said 'If bodies are ever pulled at this hospital, it is not so much for the sake of affording professional information to the pupils, as of supplying Mr. Bell's Museum'[3] (in Great Windmill Street).

Some provincial hospitals also had museums, for we read that in 1833 some gall stones were given to the museum of the Bristol Royal Infirmary,[9] and reference has been made already to the collection of bladder stones at the Norfolk and Norwich Hospital. Amongst others there was the museum of Dr. Gideon Mantell, a general practitioner with a great interest in Geology; this was opened in 1836 but was unfortunately a failure, the contents being sold to the British Museum in 1839.[10]

An unusual event occurred at the beginning of 1830 when the Duke of Northumberland made a donation to the Royal College of Surgeons of Ireland to set up a waxworks museum of anatomical and pathological specimens.[11] It is tempting to wonder whether this idea had come from seeing the famous wax figures of Madame Tussaud. This lady had come to England from Paris at the commencement of the 19th century, and had exhibited her work in England, Scotland, and Ireland, prior to setting up her renowned museum in London.[12] Although waxworks museums did not exist in England at this time, Florence, Pavia, Vienna, and Paris were boasting of their wax preparations, which were mostly anatomical.[6] Museums were sometimes located in strange places, as for example that of Dupuytren, which consisted of 1500 specimens and was housed in a small disused Gothic church formerly attached to the Covent des Cordeliers in Paris.[13] There was a catalogue of the specimens, probably made by M. Orfila, a lecturer in Medical Chemistry and one of the earlier workers on Toxicology. Many of the specimens had been made by Dupuytren's Anatomy students. The high quality of this type of work in France is illustrated by some preparations made by M. Dumontier of Paris. They included a cranium showing the internal ear, and a heart mounted on a metallic globe which could be rotated so that all parts of it could be seen. It was said that the specimen of the cranium had a quality unequalled in any museum either in Paris or London.[14] From what has been said it appears that there was considerable enthusiasm for the collection of pathological specimens at this time. They were frequently exhibited at the meetings of medical societies and we read that, at the inaugural meeting of the Anatomical Society of Paris on the 12th January 1826, M. Cruveilhier displayed some pathological specimens.[15] Specimens were also used for teaching medical students, and how well this was done depended, as ever, on the teacher. Pride of place for enthusiasm should probably go to Mr. Stanley of St. Bartholomew's for holding a special session at 7 o'clock on Saturday evenings to study specimens from surgical operations or from autopsies.[16]

In 1823 an article entitled 'Anatomical Investigations' lamented the difficulty of learning Anatomy when bodies for dissection were so difficult to obtain. It emphasised that pictures were no good and that the body had to be dissected. It went on to regret that more attention was not paid to Morbid Anatomy, for 'without it the nature of disease can never be understood'.[17] In spite of the progress in correlating clinical findings with pathological anatomy, there had been cases in which no lesions could be found to account for the symptoms. Such instances, in an era when the Vitalistic Theory was still believed by many, led to the suggestion that there had been injury of the vital functions and this, of course, could not be seen. The concern that this caused is illustrated by the announcement in 1823 by the Royal Society of Medicine at a meeting in Bordeaux. A price of 300 francs was offered for the best essay on 'Do any diseases exist, in which the vital functions are alone injured, without any alterations of the organic tissues? Can these diseases be recognised and demonstrated by positive characters, and subsequently confirmed by examinations after death?'[18] Twelve years later a similar article appeared on Pathological Anatomy. By this time the supply of bodies had been improved by the passage of the Anatomy Act in 1832 and so this problem was not mentioned. The article pointed out however that in the practices of medicine, next to a careful examination at the bedside, pathological anatomy was the most important branch. It maintained that 'Pathological Anatomy' is treated with a degree of neglect which can be explained only on the supposition that the importance of its study is generally unknown.[19] This undesirable situation was produced not so much because there was an absence of good works on pathological anatomy as 'the want of a system instruction, and a constant and efficient attendance in the dead houses of the hospitals'. It was implied that England was lagging behind Continental countries. This may well have been so, because many doctors and students went to Paris where it was said that there were greater facilities for the study of Pathology than in any other school in Europe. A greater proportion of the population went into hospital than in England and by law the body of any person dying in hospital could be opened and examined. The width of pathological experience can well be imagined when we learn that in a single year there were 7,089 deaths in the civil hospitals in Paris.[20] Also, in some of the Continental hospitals there were young men expressly appointed to perform the autopsies. They were lodged in the hospitals and not distracted from their duties by the cares of a large private practice. This certainly contrasts strongly with the position in England where no set person was appointed for this very necessary duty.

This survey of the medical scene in the early 19th century prompts the question why, in Pathology, Great Britain lagged behind some of the Continental countries. It should not have been on account of geographical isolation, for we have already seen that there were frequent contacts between Great Britain and Europe. The value of the subject was realised and the method of clinico-pathological correlation was being used by the best teachers. Its importance must have been a frequent matter of comment, for we find students constantly demanding more Pathology. There was no shortage of material. The rapid expansion of hospitals in the 18th century provided clinical material and pathological specimens so essential for teaching and the latter were already being assembled into museums. Although the word 'Pathology' was in frequent use, the term 'Pathologist' was much less common. The subject was taught by the clinicians as a sideline to their subject, and there were no specific persons assigned to carry out autopsies or examine surgical specimens, tasks which comprised the very heart of the subject at the time. There was in fact no organisation. This could have been remedied by the recognition of Pathology as an academic subject, if a University had established a Chair. But in England the universities lagged behind, particularly in London where for many years the hospitals rather than the universities dominated undergraduate medical teaching. By contrast, in many Continental countries the University and its Hospital stood side by side at a comparatively early time.

At this stage it might be of interest to see what was available on Pathological Anatomy in the literature of the time. Some books were devoted to Pathology, and others on general Medicine included a considerable amount of Morbid Anatomy.

Morgagni's great work had done much to stimulate interest in Pathology and the contribution of Bichat on Tissues, during his short life, had been considerable. Between 1800 and 1850 the two texts most widely read were those of Baillie and Carl Rokitanski. Morgagni had produced a clinical text with anatomical explanations of disease symptoms. Some of his observations were surprising, as for instance the association of anencephaly with the small size of the adrenals.[21] Baillie was much influenced by Morgagni and had a copy of his great work in his library. His work, 'The Morbid Anatomy of some of the most important parts of the Human Body' appeared in 1793, and went through eight editions in all, five of them during his lifetime. As already mentioned it was translated into several foreign languages and appears to have been the outstanding text between 1793 and 1842. It was the first work on systematic pathology, dealing with organs and their diseases rather than employing the case report format. His pathological descriptions were succinct and remarkably good. In his section on 'Diseased appearances of the Stomach', the prevalence of carcinoma at the pylorus was noted, as was also the characteristic ulceration seen in leiomyoma, which was described by him as 'circumscribed scirrhous tumour'.[22] He also gave the first description of cirrhosis which he called 'tubercle of the liver and scirrhous liver'. It has been said that Baillie's book has received little historical recognition, and this may be correct. However, this is certainly true of his other writings. Fortunately an eminent surgeon of the time, James Wardrop, collected all his publications into two volumes which also included a biography. This work appeared in 1825, just two years after

Baillie's death. The 'Lancet' gave it a warm welcome in a twelve and a half page review and commented that Baillie's work was known for its immense value by the medical world in general. It also stated that the book and its associated Atlas were both in the hands of most practitioners. The text seems to have been much the same from edition to edition and it appears that in some places it was not up-to-date. Mr. Wardrop realised this and added notes which were highly praised, and it was hoped that these might be extended in a later edition.[23]

In his writings, Baillie showed that, while he attached great importance to clinico-pathological correlation, he was also interested in pathogenesis, and emphasised the value of observations rather than hypotheses, which is not unexpected in view of his early training with John Hunter. Between 1797 and 1802 he had published the Atlas supplementary to his book, which consisted of a series of engravings to illustrate the changes observed in Morbid Anatomy.[24] These had been skillfully drawn by a young man, William Clift, who was later to become Museum Conservator at the Royal College of Surgeons in London. it was the first time that drawings had been used to illustrate pathology.

With the rise of the Vienna School of Pathology, Rokitansky published his three-volume 'Handbuch der Pathologischen Anatomie' between the years 1842 and 1846. Based on an enormous amount of autopsy material, it was acclaimed as the best work on Pathology. Much of it was descriptive, but unfortunately Rokitansky also speculated on pathogenesis on the basis of an erroneous theory proposed by Schleiden and Schwann, who had suggested that the body cells developed from a primitive fluid. Rokitansky adopted the presence of such a formative fluid to explain some of the manifestations of pathology and in so doing really revived the old humoral pathology.[25]

In addition to these outstanding works there were other publications which should be briefly mentioned. Extracts of these had sometimes found their way into the 'Lancet', which had just introduced some rather lengthy and not altogether charitable book reviews. Prior to Baillie's work on pathological anatomy the only work on the subject in English was a small book by Samueal Clossy, published in 1763. It was entitled 'Observations on some of the Diseases of the parts of the Human Body', and was based on 53 autopsies performed at Steven's Hospital in Dublin. Its influence was slight as there was only one edition, and it had little chance of survival once Baillie's work had appeared.

Caleb Parry (1755–1822) had published a book entitled 'Elements of Pathology and Therapeutics' in 1815 and a second edition appeared in 1825. Parry was a very celebrated practitioner in Bath, to whom Jenner had dedicated his work 'Inquiry into the causes and effects of

the Variolae Vaccinae' published in 1798. Parry gave the first description of facial hemiatrophy, and of congenital idiopathic dilatation of
the colon.[26] He also wrote an excellent account of eight cases of
exophthalmic goitre, and was the first person to associate angina
pectoris with coronary atherosclerosis ('ossification of the coronary
vessels'). This book was intended to be the forerunner of a series of
volumes, but he died when only a small portion of the second had
been completed. He wrote on haemorrhage, dropsy, and inflammation,
and his description of the latter together with the possible sequelae was
well done. When it comes to causation and pathogenesis his thoughts
show signs of the Vitalistic Theory, still prevalent to some extent at
the time. He thought that inflammation was due to 'increased momentum' of the blood, and that this originated from the heart. When he
tried to distinguish between dropsy with or without inflammation he
fell back on levels of the 'Phlogistic diathesis'. His views on inflammation were not accepted by all, for one contemporary, Dr. Wilson
Philip, stated that 'Inflammation seems to consist in the debility of
the capillaries, followed by an increased action of the larger
arteries'.[27] Parry's writings give a good representation of medical and
pathological knowledge at the time, when descriptive or systematic
pathological anatomy was often relatively accurate. By contrast,
General Pathology and the causation of disease were still being held
back by the Vitalistic Theories.

In 1827 there appeared a translation of the second edition of a
'Manual of Pathology' by L. Martinet. It was something more than
its title implied, as its length had been extended by a number of notes
from the translator, Jones Quain A.B., Demonstrator of Anatomy at
the Medical School in Aldersgate Street. It was a clinical guide with
instructions on clinical examination, as well as providing advice on
autopsy technique and morbid anatomical appearances. The reviewer of
the work thought that it was 'calculated to supply that deficiency of
pathological science, which has long been experienced in this country'.
It was based on the General Anatomy of Bichat, and Jones Quain
lamented the fact that there was no English work on Anatomy, though
he added that he was presently engaged on one which 'will speedily
appear'.[28]

In 1830, an illustrated work with upwards of 250 drawings appeared
under the title of 'A Vade-Mecum of Morbid Anatomy, Medical and
Chirurgical with Pathological Observations and Symptoms'. Unfortunately, the author was not identified. It was essentially a pictorial
guide with descriptions of the plates.[29] The reviewer had little praise
for it, because the subjects for illustration had not been well-chosen
nor were they of high quality. It certainly compared very unfavourably
with Baillie's Atlas of 37 years previously.

In 1829, a Dublin publisher produced a book by Dr. Thomas Mills,
who was a fairly prolific writer. Its title was 'An account of the

morbid Appearances exhibited on Dissection in Disorders of the Trachea, Lungs, and Heart with Pathological Observations; to which a Comparison of the Symptoms with the Morbid Changes has given rise'. The 'Lancet' reviewer gave it detailed attention to the extent of eight and a half pages and criticised it severely because it lacked originality. A further complaint was that while views of other workers were expressed, no acknowledgement was given.[30] Mills probably foresaw this criticism, for in a note he stated that the book was intended 'to give solely the result of my own observation and experience'; he also said that if he quoted many extracts from well-known workers it would confuse his readers. In spite of this title, the pathology is overshadowed by a wealth of detail of clinical symptoms and therapy, and the observations at autopsy were those of others, frequently of a surgeon named McNamara. The book did not have much success, for in addition to its imperfections it had to compete with Laennec's great work on a similar subject, which had just been translated into English by Dr. Forbes. The correlation of symptoms and morbid changes had no special merit, and he revealed himself as a victim of the Vitalistic Theory when he stated that medicines given for a case of phthisis, because of post-mortem findings, 'cannot be useful, and as they lower the tone of the vital powers and impede digestion, it is manifest that they must shorten the life of the patient'.

Later, in the same year, a second edition appeared of a work by Dr. John Abercrombie, the first edition having been published in 1819. Its title was 'Pathological Researches on the Diseases of the Brain and Spinal Chord', and this edition comprised 476 pages.[31] It contained case records with detailed clinical information and in some instances with post-mortem appearances. The discussions on the pathological findings and clinical pictures were of a high standard, and he emphasised the difficulty of such correlation in many spinal diseases. At the time it must have been regarded as one of the leading works on Pathology in a special field.

In 1830 the second volume of a book written by Dr. John Mackintosh[32] was published in Edinburgh. It was essentially a work on Medicine, and the pathology dealt with the pathogenesis of disease rather than with detailed anatomical lesions. The early part dealt with the central nervous system and referred to the conflicting views at the time between Abercrombie, Monro (Alexander tertius) who had written in 1827 'Morbid Anatomy of the Brain', and the author. It seems that there was a surprising amount of interest in the central nervous system and its diseases at the time. One interesting discussion dealt with the nature of hydrocephalus and whether it was due to inflammation, venous obstruction or debility. It was contrasted with inflammation of the brain (called 'phrenitis' in those days) and the symptomatology was compared. It is interesting that Abercrombie in his work refers to slowing of the pulse and its association with drowsiness and coma, yet at the time the connection with cerebral compression does not appear to have been recognised. Dr. Mackintosh's book deals with other aspects of medicine and the causation of disease and was warmly commended for its quality. He made a clear distinction between erysipelas and cellulitis, but surprisingly did not believe that colchicum had any claim to be a specific for gout, though he did admit its occasional value.

One most important work which influenced pathological thought during the first half of the 19th century was written by the French physician, Gabriel Andral (1797–1876). He had studied in Paris under Lermontier, a pupil of Corvisart, and had subsequently aligned himself with the anatomical views of Laennec, rather than with the physiological views of Broussais. Andral then set out to try to unify these two schools of thought and accordingly produced 'A treatise on Pathological Anatomy'.[33] It was in 1829 that Dr. R. Townsend and Dr. W. West translated the work into English and produced the first volume. Andral, like others, wanted to make a classification of lesions, but in defining them there was considerable source of error at a time when identification depended solely on the gross appearances. He was however quick to realise another great difficulty, namely that it was possible to have symptoms without an anatomical lesion and vice versa. Accordingly he attempted to devise a simplified system, and his work was unique in that it was one on General rather than on Special Morbid Anatomy. The only work at the time which resembled it was a series of treatises on pathological anatomy by Johann Friedrick Meckel (1781–1833) of Halle, an eminent Pathologist and Comparative Anatomist. Terms such as inflammation were so ill-defined that Andral dispensed with them and classified conditions according to whether there was too much or too little blood, i.e. hyperaemia or anaemia. At the time there had been much discussion about the nature of miliary tubercles. They were explained on a humoral basis and Andral believed that they were produced by a morbid secretion, which subsequently produced cells and became solid and indurated. This is reminiscent of the later view of Schleiden and Schwann, who stated that cells could arise in a formative fluid, a theory subsequently overthrown by Virchow who proved that cells only arose from other cells, the famous 'Omnis cellula e cellula'. At the time there was remarkable unanimity on the humoral origin of tubercles, which was supported by Andral, Dupuy (a professor of a Veterinary College), Wardrop (an eminent London surgeon), and Meckel referred to above. An interesting new theory, based on experimental work, was now to appear. Cruveilhier in 1827 had injected metallic mercury into the femoral arteries of dogs, and on dissection of the thigh had found a large number of miliary tubercles.[34] On close examination, they were found to consist of 'caseous material' surrounding a minute globule of mercury. Cruveilhier therefore proposed that the lesion was produced by inflammation and further experiments injecting mercury into the trachea gave similar lesions in the lung. During the subsequent years Andral became very interested in blood and its analysis. At the time there was no shortage of blood for the purpose, because therapeutic bleeding was much in vogue. Also, he was fortunate in having as friends the chemist Jean Baptiste Dumas, and another chemist Jules Gavarret who gave him technical assistance. This association is reminiscent of that at Guy's Hospital between Richard Bright and John Bostock. Andral recognised the anaemia caused by lead poisoning and the reduction of fibrin in fevers. These events were important milestones in the history of Pathology for they represent a new development within the subject. Thus, Andral had excited interest in what was later to become Haematology, and in 1845 Virchow and Hughes Bennett added to it with independent descriptions of leukaemia.

Important though these discoveries were, it should be remembered that there had been some interest in the composition of blood many years earlier. In 1772 William Hewson, a pupil of the Hunters, had observed the excessive 'buffy coat' which was associated with rapid red cell sedimentation, and also the shortening of the blood clotting time as animals became exsanguinated.[35] Both of these subjects attracted attention, and in later years there were many reports about the buffy coat in various diseases. In 1834 a book appeared with the title 'An Inquiry into the Nature and Properties of the blood in Health and Disease'.[36] It was the second edition of a work originally written by Dr. Charles T. Thackrah, and published in 1819. This new edition had been a revision of the first by Thos. G. Wright one year after Thackrah's death. The comments of the reviewer were not favourable and it was stated that, probably on account of the author's illness (tuberculosis, from which he died when only 37) and his other duties, he had not had sufficient time to revise the first edition satisfactorily. This may well have been true, for his 'other duties' were probably given priority. Thackrah was a Yorkshireman who was apprenticed to a local practitioner before going to Guy's, where he was a pupil of Sir Astley Cooper. He returned to Leeds, where he took over a prac- tice. He subsequently developed an interest in industrial disease and became one of the main pioneers in its prevention. He published a paper on brass-founders' ague and other dust diseases, and in 1831 produced an enlarged second edition dealing with general aspects of the subject.[37] He must have been very busy, for he also opened a School of Anatomy in Leeds which was so successful that it soon developed into a complete Medical School. His haematological interests were mainly concerned with blood coagulation and his experiments resemble those of Hewson. At that time there was a disagreement amongst workers about the amount of serum in blood at three periods during the slaughter of an animal. This obviously relates to clot retraction and Thackrah seems to have been aware of it for he speaks of a clot which 'does not expel the serum from it'. Two other workers on the subject were Dr. Stevens and Dr. Prater. The latter published a book on the blood at about the same time and the reviewer of Thackrah's work considered Prater's book to be greatly superior.

Some years later, Dr. George E. Day published two articles in the 'Lancet' on 'Report of the Recent Progress of Chemical and Microscopic Physiology and Pathology'.[38] The terminology was very complex and it included a study of the amounts of fibrin and red cells present in 'diseased blood'. The blood was divided into four groups and the nomenclature included such terms as 'hyperinosis', indicating the sinking of red cells prior to coagulation. The second article described in great detail an analysis of blood, urine, and saliva. The application of chemistry to medicine was not new, for Gavarret had assisted Andral in his analysis of blood, and Bostock had given similar help to Bright in his studies of the blood in renal disease. William Prout had given the Goulstonian Lectures on 'The application of chemistry to physiology, pathology and practice' in 1831,[39] and had worked out a method of urine analysis a few years earlier.[40] One obvious application of chemistry to surgery was the analysis of urinary bladder stones, and in 1826 Mr. John Wood, the lecturer in Chemistry at the Windmill Street School, devised a simple series of tests for the purpose.[41] He used these tests to analyse 167 calculi obtained from Mr. Bell of the Windmill St. School, Mr. Cross of the Norfolk and Norwich Hospital, and the surgeons of the Kent and Canterbury Hospital. The interest in chemical analysis was further emphasised when in 1836 G. O. Rees published a book 'On the analysis of the Blood and Urine in Health and Disease.'[42]

With this short consideration of some of the books available at the time, it can be seen that Pathology had already started to branch out from being solely Pathological Anatomy. To appreciate the full development it will be necessary to refer to some other examples from the rest of the medical literature of the period.

In 1815, there appeared a 'Treatise on the Diseases of Arteries and Veins' written by Joseph Hodgson (1788–1869). He was a surgeon for 30 years in Birmingham and this work contained a particularly good description of aneurysms, in which he pointed out the difficulties of diagnosis. Some years later an Edinburgh medical student, James Hope (1801–1841), was to resolve this difficulty. He had gone to Paris to study under Chomal and became devoted to the use of the stethoscope. He wrote a thesis on aneurysm of the aorta, carried out a number of animal experiments, and finally published his 'Diseases of the Heart' in 1831. This was described as being 'a masterly exposition of the principles and practical application of auscultation'. In it he greatly improved the diagnosis of aortic aneurysm by giving a meticulous description of physical signs.[43] Both authors did much to clarify the pathological anatomy of the condition. Meanwhile, with Guy's in its golden era, there were the well-known writings of Addison on pneumonia, Bright on renal disease, and Hodgkin on Morbid Growths. With the Dublin School in full bloom there was the work of Stokes on diseases of the chest, and Graves on fevers. In the latter's clinico-pathological case reports one of exophthalmic goitre impressed Trousseau so much that he referred to the condition as Graves's disease. Other well known names in Dublin included Colles and Corrigan. That there was activity outside of London is indicated by a series of essays on General Pathology published by Mr. J. Bower Harrison, a Manchester surgeon. In one of these he dealt with morbid conditions of the vascular and nervous systems. He believed that most causes of disease operated on the mucous membranes, either directly or indirectly, and this recalls the earlier views of Broussais. Inflammation with its hyperaemia was contrasted with anaemia, as in Andral's writings, and he introduced an unusual term 'adynamia', which meant absence of the vital force necessary to maintain the circulation, and therefore presumably indicated congestion.[44]

There are some subjects which are surprising for this early time. Dr. Blundell published an article on the 'Transfusion of Blood', and this was chiefly devoted to an apparatus to be used for the purpose. It was followed by a leading article based on some recently published work on transfusion and infusion by Dr. Dieffenbach of Berlin.[45] This doctor performed much experimental work, and in 1824 the 'Lancet' quoted an article on transplantation written by him in Grafe and Walther's Journal Chirurgica.[46] The purpose of the experiments was to see whether parts removed from one animal and transferred to another could be made to grow. He was probably stimulated by Hunter's earlier work, for he wrote that it is well-known that the spurs of cocks will readily grow to the living parts of other animals. He described a series of experiments made mostly on birds. He transplanted hair and feathers, for he found that 'other parts separated from the body seldom remained long after transplantation'. With these he had some success and about 3 out of every 12 transplants survived. Of those which were unsuccessful he gives a good description of the inflammation and abscess formation, which led up to the rejection. Some years later, he carried out some studies of corneal transplants. These were published in a quarterly journal which was reviewed in the 'Lancet'.[47] Very disappointingly the article states ' "On Transplantation of the Cornea" being rather curious than useful, we have not room for an analysis of it'. Dieffenbach was ahead of his time and gave his dissertation for Doctorate on 'Regeneration and Transplantation of Tissues.' As Professor of Surgery in Berlin he was best known for the excellence of his plastic surgery of the nose.[48]

At this time, the application of the microscope to pathological problems was to result in enormous progress. The method seems to have been accepted more readily on the Continent than in England, and it became the chief feature of the pathology of the great German schools later in the century. As early as 1827 Dr. Milne Edwards in Paris had published some studies on the 'Intimate Structure of the Organic Tissues of Animals'.[49] For this purpose, he used a microscope which gave a magnification of about 300 diameters. Like other workers of the period he teased out the tissues for examination and described 'globules' of varying size. These were measured with mixed success, though Edwards estimated that the size of the red globules of the blood was 1/150mm., a figure which was not too far out. Surprisingly, he found that the globules of pus and tissues were smaller and about 1/300 mm. By 1839, Schleiden and Schwann had propounded their cell theory, and with further improvements in the microscope progress quickened very considerably. Some idea of this can be gained by reference to the work of Hughes Bennett (see chapter 5). He was Professor of Physiology (or 'Institutes of Medicine' as it was then called) in Edinburgh.[50] The holder of this Chair was also a Physician to the Edinburgh Royal Infirmary, and thus had an opportunity of linking Physiology with Clinical Medicine. Hughes Bennett had been disappointed that Britain was lagging behind the Continent in the use of the microscope. He made his point very strongly in 1845 in an introductory address to a course of lectures on 'Histology and the use of the microscope'.[51] In it, he traced the history of the instrument, emphasising its recent improvements by the reduction of spherical and chromatic abberation. Most important of all he made a special plea for its use in Pathology. Of particular interest were his examples of its usefulness in Forensic Pathology. In one case examination of hair from a murder weapon, which was a hatchet, revealed it to be of animal rather than of human origin. In another case of a lady complaining of haemoptysis, microscopic examination of the sputum revealed that the red blood cells were nucleated and therefore not of human origin. The lady later admitted that she had killed a chicken and added some of its blood to her sputum. Later, in an article in the 'Edinburgh Monthly Journal'[52] he made a similar plea and urged that in arriving at a diagnosis it was essential to use all the means at one's disposal, such as specula, stethoscopes, pleximeters, sounds and the microscope. Although officially a physiologist he was greatly devoted to Pathology and recommended that in all hospitals connected with medical schools, there should be an 'officer well-acquainted with morbid anatomy and the modern means of cultivating it, whose duty it shall be to conduct the post-mortem examinations, keep a minute record of each, teach morbid anatomy to the students, and publish a yearly report', a full time job.

Finally, there are two other text-books which should be mentioned. Firstly there was Carl Rokitansky's treatise on Pathological Anatomy in 1842–46. It embodied a remarkable experience, for he is said to have performed over 30,000 autopsies during his life-time. His descriptive work was excellent and was widely acclaimed, but his views on the nature of disease were severely criticised. He was essentially a descriptive pathologist, and although his school became famous, it was not until Virchow published his famous book on Cellular Pathology that pathological histology and the use of the microscope came into their own. The other work, published in 1829, was the first text-book of Pathology published in the United States. It was written by William Edmonds Horner (1793–1853), a Virginian, who studied medicine in Edinburgh and Philadelphia. He became Professor of Anatomy at the University of Pennsylvania and gained much knowledge of Pathology by performing autopsies for physicians in Philadelphia. It was entitled 'A Treatise on Pathological Anatomy' and, while not a complete guide to the subject, it was useful to practitioners and included many individual reports of post-mortem examinations.[53]

From the examples given, it is clear that at this time there was no shortage of literature on Pathology, and there was also considerable recognition of its importance by many leading physicians and surgeons. It is remarkable that subdivisions of the subject had already appeared, though in their elementary state, and no one could have foreseen the extent of their future development. Bacteriology was the only one missing at the time; this was inevitable as the compound microscope needed further improvement before bacteria could be clearly seen. An additional handicap was the reluctance at that time to believe that diseases could be caused by living agents, and it seemed hard to get away from the theory of miasmas. This is surprising because Schonlein was able to see the relatively large microscopical parasite causing Favus in 1839 (see chapter 17).

REFERENCES

1  'Lancet'. (1823), *1*, 410.
2  Ibid (1823) *1*, 339.
3  Ibid (1825) *8*, 95.
4  Ibid (1835–6) *i*, 550.
5  Ibid (1825) *8*, 349–51.
6  Ibid (1833–34) *i*, 327.
7  'British Medical Journal'. (1927), *i*, 523–4.
8  'Lancet'. (1825–6) *9*, 132–4; 224–8.
9  Ibid (1832–3) *ii*, 172.
10  Winton, W. E., (1975) 'British Medical Journal'. *i*, 505–7.
11  'Lancet'. (1829–30) *ii*, 17–19.
12  'An encyclopaedia of London'. Ed. by W. Kent, J. M. Dent & Sons, London 1937, p. 686.
13  'Lancet'. (1835–6) *i*, 263–4.

14  Ibid (1830–1) *ii*, 125.
15  Ibid (1825–6) *10*, 273.
16  Ibid (1825–6) *9*, 464.
17  Ibid (1823) *1*, 94–8.
18  Ibid (1823) *1*, 383.
19  Ibid (1835–6) *i*, 129–30.
20  Ibid (1826–7) *11*, 258–9.
21  Willis, R. A., 'The Borderland of Embryology and Pathology'. Butterworths, London. 2nd. Ed. 1962. p. 149.
22  Rodin, Alvin E., 'The Influence of Matthew Baillie's Morbid Anatomy'. Charles C. Thomas, Springfield, Illinois 1973. pp. 32–3.
23  'Lancet'. (1825–6) *9*, 184–96.
24  Rodin, Alvin E., 'The Influence of Matthew Baillie's Morbid Anatomy'. Charles C. Thomas, Springfield, Illinois 1973. pp. 32–3.
25  Long, Esmond R., 'Selected readings in Pathology'. Charles C. Thomas, Springfield, Illinois, 2nd edit. 1961. pp. 149–51.
26  Garrison, F. H., 'History of medicine'. W. B. Saunders Company, Philadelphia and London, 4th edit. pp. 360; 373.
27  'Lancet'. (1825) *7*, 138–45.
28  Ibid (1827–8) *i*, 20–2.
29  Ibid (1829–30) *ii*, 463–4.
30  Ibid (1828–9) *ii*, 245–50.
31  Ibid (1829–30) *i*, 222–4.
32  Ibid (1830–1) *i*, 353–8.
33  Ibid (1829–30) *i*, 922–7.
34  Ibid (1826–7) *11*, 243–4.
35  French J. E. & Macfarlane R. G., in 'General Pathology'. Edit. Lord Florey. W. B. Saunders Company Philadelphia and London. 4th Edit. 1970. pp. 264; 320.
36  'Lancet', London. (1834–5) *1*, 522–5.
37  Hunter D., 'Health in Industry'. Penguin Books 1959, pp. 42–6.
38  'Lancet', London. (1845) *1*, 171–7; 202–6.
39  Foster W. D., 'A short history of Clinical Pathology'. E. & S. Livingstone, Edinburgh & London, 1961, p. 45.
40  Partington J. R., 'A short history of Chemistry'. Macmillan & Co. Ltd. London, 1948, p. 213.
41  'Lancet'. (1826–7) *11*, 452–5.
42  Ibid (1835–6) *ii*, 969–71.
43  Mann, Ruth J., Mayo Clin. Proc. (1974), *49*, 889–92.
44  'Lancet'. (1845) *i*, 730–2.
45  Ibid (1828–9) *ii*, 321–6.
46  Ibid (1824) *3*, 280–6.
47  Ibid (1830–1) *ii*, 326–9.
48  Ibid (1830–1) *ii*, 237–8.
49  'Lancet', London. (1827) *12*, 267; 322.
50  Guthrie D., 'A history of medicine'. Thomas Nelson & Sons Ltd, Edinburgh 1945, p. 278.

51 'Lancet'. (1845) *i*, 517–22.
52 Ibid (1846) *ii*, 130.
53 Long, Esmond R., 'Selected readings in Pathology'. Charles C. Thomas, Springfield, Illinois, 2nd edit. 1961, pp. 187–92.

# FOUR
# The Clinician-Pathologists 1820–50

The importance of university recognition in the development of a new subject has already been mentioned. In the case of Pathology this first occurred in 1819 when Johann Martin Lobstein (1777–1835) was appointed to the Chair of Pathological Anatomy at the University of Strasbourg in Alsace. He classified lesions based on their anatomical character rather than on their location, and started an Atlas of Pathological Anatomy which he never finished. In Great Britain the first two Chairs of Pathology were founded in 1831. John Thomson was appointed to Edinburgh and Robert Carswell to University College, London. Carswell's appointment was only part-time and he gave it up after two years because he did not have time to attend to his practice. But although Carswell's sojourn in Pathology was brief, he made some remarkable contributions to the subject in that short time. In addition to being a very good pathologist he was also a very gifted artist and made 2,000 water-colour paintings of lesions, from which he made coloured plates for his series of Fascicules.[1] These were ten in number and dealt with such subjects as Tubercle, Carcinoma, Melanoma, Haemorrhage, Hypertrophy, and Atrophy. Many of the specimens that he drew were obtained from the hospitals in Paris, and it is thought that Magendie, Louis, and others provided him with material. It is generally agreed that his drawings were of the very highest quality. One other important university appointment was that of Cruveilhier to the Chair of Pathological Anatomy in Paris in 1836. This was largely brought about through the influence of the well-known surgeon Dupuytren, who had Cruveilhier as one of his pupils. It was not until 1882 that a full-time Chair was established in Great Britain when D. J. Hamilton was appointed to the University of Aberdeen.

In the interim period between French predominance and the later rise of the German schools under Rokitansky and Virchow, there had been some substantial progress in Great Britain. A number of clinicians appeared whose names have become perpetuated by their association either with diseases or physical signs. Many of these men were responsible for the outstanding achievements of the Dublin School in Ireland, and those of Guy's Hospital. The influence of Laennec was apparent for many of these clinicians were interested in the use of the stethoscope. William Stokes of Dublin published his famous book on diseases of the chest, and Addison of Guy's wrote on pneumonia. Most of these men showed great interest in Pathology, and furthered the progress of the subject by following in Laennec's footsteps and correlating autopsy findings with clinical symptoms and signs. Stoke's enthusiasm for the subject was such that he founded the Pathological Society of Dublin in 1838, the first of its kind. From 1768 until 1815, Guy's was the only school in London which conducted organised teaching of medicine. For the purposes of student instruction Guy's and St. Thomas's had joined forces in 1768 and were known as the United Hospitals of the Borough. Anatomy and Surgery were taught at St. Thomas's and Physiology and Medicine at Guy's. When this arrangement came to an end in 1825, Guy's had a strong staff of physicians which was later to include such well-known names as Addison, Bright, and Hodgkin. Addison was one of the great men of Guy's, an excellent teacher and a commanding figure. Although chiefly remembered for his paper on diseases of the 'Suparenal Capsules', he made his reputation by his observations and writings on pneumonia. Using the diagnostic methods of Laennec and studying the pathology of the condition, he demonstrated that the inflammatory exudate was in the pulmonary alveoli and not in the interstitial tissue, as was believed at the time.[2] Richard Bright's interest in Pathology became obvious in his first major work in 1827, entitled 'Reports on Medical cases' and with a sub-title 'selected with a view of illustrating the symptoms and cure of disease by a reference of morbid anatomy'. Several cases had terminal oedema and his observation of the association of diseased kidneys and albuminuria led him to collect the cases which were the basis of his classic paper in 1836, on what was later to be called Bright's disease. Tests for proteinuria by heat and acetic acid had been known for over a hundred years, and the urine examinations on Bright's cases were carried out by John Bostock, a lecturer in Chemistry. Fortunately Bright's pre-eminence in renal disease was recognised and the Guy's authorities set aside two clinical wards of 42 beds for the study of renal disease, probably the first example of a 'special unit'. With his inspiring personality he was able to influence and encourage two younger physicians, G. H. Barlow and G. O. Rees. On his appointment to the staff Rees was given laboratory space, thus enabling him to make tests on diabetic blood, and on the proportion of urea in 'certain diseased fluids'.[3] Thus, even at this early stage, there were signs of an application of chemical pathology to the study of medicine.

The nearest approach to that of a modern anatomical pathologist was Thomas Hodgkin, but he never occupied a University Chair in the subject. He studied at Guy's Hospital and later in Paris, finally proceeding to Edinburgh where he obtained his MD degree. In 1825 he returned to Guy's where he became curator of the Museum and Demonstrator in Morbid Anatomy. He occupied this post for 12 years and devoted his time to studying various aspects of anatomical pathology. He performed many autopsies and his investigation of the notorious lithotomy case of Bransby Cooper will be recalled (see chapter 2). In 1832, he wrote the paper for which he is best known, namely 'On some morbid appearances of the Absorbent Glands and Spleen'. Some of these resembled the cases later reported in 1859 by Samueal Wilks, who very generously referred to them as Hodgkin's disease in a later paper in 1865. In his early days Hodgkin, no doubt influenced by his studies in Paris, read a paper to the Guy's Physical Society on the 'The application of the stethoscope' in 1822. Once he had turned to Pathology he published a paper 'On the object of post-mortem examination',[4] and this probably reflects the importance placed on autopsies by the clinicians of the time at Guy's Hospital. Had Hodgkin stuck to Pathology, the subject would undoubtedly have benefited for he was a good observer and dissecter. But his whole life changed in 1837 when he made an unsuccessful application for the post of Assistant Physician at Guy's.[5] Bitterly disappointed, he turned to some of his other interests and his Quaker spirit led him to become involved in many philanthropic causes. Finally he died of typhoid fever at Jaffa, while visiting the Holy Land with Sir Moses Montefiore.

One lesser known but important figure was Golding Bird, whose career was cut short by his death from rheumatic heart disease at the age of 40. He was a young chemist of outstanding brilliance, who studied at Guy's and took his MD degree in 1838 at St. Andrew's University. He returned to London, where he was in clinical practice and at the same time carried out chemical research at Guy's. He was well ahead of his time and concentrated on the analysis of stones and urinary deposits, thus affording another example of investigations which were later to develop into Chemical Pathology.[6]

At this time Forensic Medicine appeared and A. S. Taylor was made Professor of Medical Jurisprudence in 1831, a post which he held until 1877. He is best known for his testimony in the trial of Palmer, the notorious strychnine poisoner.[7]

It remains to consider two outstanding figures, even though their influence extended outside the period under discussion. Samueal Wilks (1824–1911) in his long life had served Guy's Hospital well.[8] In his younger days he was greatly interested in morbid anatomy, published his book 'Pathological Anatomy' in 1859, and was even referred to as one of the leading pathologists. His writings covered a number of subjects and he drew attention to the effects of syphilis on internal viscera. He studied cases of Bright's disease and pointed out that one type came on acutely and another insidiously. Most of all, he commands our admiration because he never sought fame for himself and because of his generosity to his predecessors, Addison and Hodgkin, in attaching their names to diseases which they had described. His loyalty and his love for his hospital were characteristic of this great man.

Astley Cooper (1768–1841) belonged to an earlier generation than that of Addison, Bright, and Hodgkin, and was apprenticed to Henry Cline senior at St. Thomas's before studying with John Hunter. He became the leading surgeon of his day in London and was elected President of the Royal College of Surgeons of London for two terms of office. He was devoted to Guy's Hospital and when at the time of his retirement, in 1825, differences arose between the United Hospitals, he played an outstanding part in promoting the independent status of his Medical

School. This separation had adverse effects on St. Thomas's, which only regained its previous prestige many years later. By contrast, it was a moment of triumph for Guy's as students flocked to its medical school, which entered its most prosperous period.[9] His interest in Pathology was considerable, and he was an ardent collector of specimens throughout his life. This led to a private museum which was second only to that of John Hunter. While Astley Cooper's collection of Comparative Anatomy specimens was inferior to John Hunter's, he probably possessed a much more representative collection of surgical pathology. He employed assistants for the dissection of specimens, but he did much of it himself. He felt that if a day passed without his doing some dissection, it had been wasted. Unfortunately few of his specimens remain today, but some may be seen in the museums of Guy's, St. Thomas's, and the Royal College of Surgeons of England. Cooper soon realised that preservation of specimens in alcohol was unsatisfactory because of loss of colour. He therefore made use of artists to paint pictures of pathological lesions in the fresh state. He was also responsible for a wonderful collection of wax models of anatomical and pathological specimens, at present housed in the Gordon Museum at Guy's Hospital. It was at his instigation that a remarkable man, namely Joseph Towne, was given a life appointment as a modeller, which enabled him to carry out this unique work.[10] It is not known whether or not Towne knew about the waxwork museums on the Continent, or whether he had seen the models displayed in England by Madame Tussaud.

At about the same time the Irish School of Medicine blossomed forth when a number of Dublin-born doctors returned to their native city having completed their studies at various centres. Their influence was great and it has been suggested that two of these, namely Graves and Stokes, were mainly responsible for the formation of the British teaching school. Graves was descended from an officer in Cromwell's army, and both he and his brother achieved distinction. He took his medical degree at Trinity College, Dublin and after having studied at various schools on the Continent returned in 1821 to Dublin, where he was appointed Physician to the Meath Hospital.[11] He proceeded to found a new teaching school, in which the students took histories and performed the clinical examination of patients. He criticised the Edinburgh School, because there the teacher performed these duties. In 1843 he published his 'Clinical lectures' which included one case of exophthalmic goitre, and so excellent was this that Armand Trousseau named it Graves's disease. He is chiefly remembered for his interest in fevers, and for his belief in feeding such patients, rather than starving them as was the practice at the time. He was impressive for his kindness and lack of arrogance and was a popular and eloquent lecturer.

William Stokes joined Graves at the Meath Hospital in 1826, and they maintained a lifelong friendship. Stokes was much impressed by Laennec and his methods, and in 1825 published a small treatise on the use of the stethoscope. He was a doctor for the poor and he saw much suffering in the outbreaks of typhus in 1826 and of cholera in 1831. He was much interested in Pathology, and as already mentioned founded the Dublin Society of Pathology in 1838. He is well remembered for his writings, the chief of which were 'Diseases of the Chest' in 1837, 'Diseases of the Heart and Aorta' in 1854, and 'Lectures on Fevers' in 1874.[12] In his work on the heart he gave accounts of Cheyne-Stokes respiration and Stokes-Adams syndrome. Adams had published a paper on some cardiac conditions, which included cases with a pulse rate of 30 per minute, and attributed the fainting attacks to the imperfect supply of blood to the heart. Some years later in 1846, Stokes put together his cases with those of Adams and drew attention to the association of syncopal attacks and a slow pulse. Adams published an interesting case,[13] presumably hypertensive, who had an enlarged heart without any valvular disease. The patient maintained that when he lay down his pulse became very slow. Adams found that it fell suddenly from 90 to 30 per minute when he assumed the horizontal posture.

Another example of a good clinical observation leads us to mention Dominic J. Corrigan. He was a Dublin Physician on the staff at the Jervis Street Hospital, at the time of Graves and Stokes. Although he had only six hospital beds, he made a number of good observations and in 1829 wrote on aneurysm of the aorta and the necessity of the employment of the stethoscope for diagnosis. In 1832 he wrote on 'Permanent Patency of the mouth of the Aorta, or inadequacy of the aortic valves'. One of his patients with this condition told Corrigan that the pulsation of the brachial and palmar arteries could be increased if he raised his arm above his head.[14] This collapsing pulse became known as the 'water-hammer' or Corrigan's pulse. In France, aortic regurgitation was known as 'maladie de Corrigan'.

John Cheyne was a Scotsman, who came to practice in Dublin and is always remembered for Cheyne-Stokes respiration. His interest for pathologists lies in a paper which he published on a case of apoplexy 'in which the fleshy part of the heart was converted into fat'[15] It remains to make brief reference to a Dublin surgeon of the time, Abraham Colles, who had a wide variety of interests though his publications were few. He was the greatest of the Irish surgeons and lived about a generation earlier than Graves and Stokes. He studied in Dublin but obtained his degree in Edinburgh, and subsequently worked for a time in London with Astley Cooper. He was a very good clinical observer and his name is perpetuated for his account of a fracture of the carpal extremity of the radius.[16] It was a classical description for he dealt with the impaction, the characteristic deformity, ease of reduction and difficulty of maintaining it in only 1528 words. He also wrote in 1837 on 'Practical observations on the venereal disease and on the use of mercury', and was, of course, responsible for the well-known Colles' law. He was also interested in subclavian aneurysm and in two cases treated it by ligature of the artery.

In any discussion of the progress made in Clinical Medicine and Pathology, the part played by the Edinburgh School of Medicine should not be forgotton. Many doctors already mentioned studied there and obtained their MD degrees. The activity of the Edinburgh school is illustrated by the fact that between 1781 and 1826 the MD degree was granted to 2,792 students. They came from many places, for 819 were Scottish, 706 English, 843 Irish, 225 from the British Colonies and 193 from various foreign countries.[17]

Apart from the growth of medical literature in the late 18th and early 19th centuries, the number of medical societies which came into existence is also indicative of medical activity. In London two of the earlier ones were the Medical Society of London, and the Physical Society of Guy's Hospital, both of which were founded in 1771. Others soon followed, the movement spreading throughout England, where by 1839 at least 28 had been established.[18] They were essentially clinical societies, and many of the earlier ones had originated from Medical Book Clubs. The 'Lancet' encouraged them to submit reports of their meetings and these were added to the publication of lectures given by eminent medical men. With no full-time pathologists, there was no society entirely devoted to this growing subject until 1838, when as previously mentioned Stokes founded the Dublin Society. In 1839 the Reading Pathological Society made its appearance. London followed suit somewhat tardily and the Pathological Society of London appeared in 1846, under the presidency of Dr. Charles J. B. Williams, the Professor of Medicine at University College. That he had been interested in Pathology for some years is indicated by his publication in 1828 of a book entitled 'A Rational Exposition of the Physical Signs of the Diseases of the Lung and Pleura; illustrating their Pathology and facilitating their Diagnosis'.[19] His choice of subject is not unexpected for he states that his opinions as well as his acquaintance with the physical signs 'are the result of some extent of study and observation, prosecuted chiefly in the Charité in Paris, where Laennec taught and Andral prosecuted his labours'. The book was well-reviewed and it is significant that it achieved success in spite of its competition with Laennec's great work which had just been translated into English by Dr. Forbes. In 1843 Williams produced a large work under the title of 'Principles of Medicine; comprising General Pathology and Therapeutics, and a brief general view of Aetiology, Nosology, Semeiology, Diagnosis and Prognosis'.[20] The pathology is dealt with from a physiological angle and describes diseases of secretion and diseases of the red blood corpuscles amongst others, the basis of classification being conditions with increase, diminution, or alteration of function. The reviewer considered that it was the best text-book on Medicine at that time available for the medical student. But we must return to the foundation of the Pathological Society of London, and some initial events which in retrospect seem very puzzling.

In March 1840[21] the 'Lancet' reported the first meeting of the

Pathological Society of London, held on the 17th and attended by a great number of visitors and Fellows. The President was Dr. Clendinning, a physician to the Marylebone Dispensary. Many well-known men including Bright, Hodgkin, and Erasmus Wilson took part in the discussions. A number of pathological specimens were on view, but such was the interest that some had to be left over for the next meeting, because of the lateness of the hour. It was decided that future meetings would be held on the first and third Tuesdays of April, May, and June. These meetings did take place, the sixth being held on Tuesday the 16th June. When reported in the 'Lancet' it was headed 'Pathological Meeting', and no mention is made of the Pathological Society of London. One of the meetings (24th April), was on a Friday and not on a Tuesday as previously arranged. The report of the meeting on 5th May states that Dr. Clendinning was Vice-President and not President as before. It seems likely that this meeting may have been held in conjunction with the Royal Medico-chirurgical Society, and Clendinning may have been Vice-President of that society. A further two meetings, both held on the 16th June, were reported separately in the 'Lancet' in the issues of the 20th and 27th June. The speakers and the specimens were different, and the predominance of surgeons at one of the meetings suggests that this may have been a pathological meeting of the Royal Medico-chirurgical Society. These details may be of little importance, but what really is significant is the fact that at the 16th June meeting (reported in the 'Lancet' of 20th June), the President announced that the Pathological Society would hold no more meetings.[22] Nothing more seems to have happened until 1846, when the 'Lancet' reported[23] the first meeting, on 20th October, of the Pathological Society of London. This time Dr. C. J. B. Williams, Professor of Medicine at University College, London, was elected President. He gave a presidential address, laying emphasis on the importance of Morbid Anatomy and of autopsies, at which he had assisted in over 2,000 and was still finding new things to learn. He promised that the Society would keep accurate records of the proceedings, and publish selected items annually in the Transactions. He referred to the previous lack of such a society in London, while Paris, Dublin, and even many of the provincial towns of the kingdom had active pathological societies. He opened his address by saying[24] 'In opening the public proceedings of the Pathological Society of London in this first year of its existence ———'. He made no reference to the previous society founded in 1840 and one wonders what thoughts were passing through Dr. Clendinning's mind as he sat in a distinguished audience, which included such well-known men as Bence Jones, Barlow, Hughes Bennett, Golding Bird, Liston, Hilton and others. The meeting concluded after some specimens had been displayed. It was decided to hold future meetings on the first and third Mondays of each month until the end of June. The new society flourished, the meetings were regularly reported in the 'Lancet', and in 1847 the first volume of the Transactions appeared. With its own society Pathology now grew rapidly, stimulated by the development of histopathology in the German schools. The Society's life was a long one and continued until 1907, when with a number of other societies it became incorporated into the Royal Society of Medicine. It was succeeded by the Pathological Society of Great Britain and Ireland in 1906 (see chapter 6).

The 1840 meetings of the Pathological Society of London are of some interest in regard to priority because it has always been said that the distinction of the first pathological society in England belonged to the Reading Pathological Society, which was founded in 1841.

The problem of the growing number of societies caused some concern at the time. While announcing the 'christening' of the Pathological Society of London and wishing it success, the 'Lancet' devoted a leading article to societies. It criticised some for the length of their names, but felt that the number of societies joined will in the end be a matter of financial economy. In retrospect it is easy to see how pathology was developing even at this relatively early stage. At the time this was not possible, for no one could have foreseen the enormous developments of the future. Also, its close association with the clinical subjects and the fact that the leading pathologists were often practising surgeons or physicians hindered the recognition of Pathology as an independent subject. At the beginning of this period it was purely Anatomical Pathology, but at the end the branches Haematology and Chemical Pathology had made their appearances.

One problem was clearly stated in a letter to the 'Lancet' in 1847, namely, 'What is Physiology and what is Pathology?'[25] It was the perennial problem of what was normal and what was abnormal. This lack of a clear distinction must have existed for some time, for in 1829 a review of Andral's work on Pathological Anatomy appeared. The concluding sentence reads as follows; 'M. Andral had struck out on a new path and the work, with all its imperfections, entitles him to a place amongst the first Physiologists of the age'.[26]

The Pathological Society of London seems to have resembled a London Club, for of its 81 original members only five had an address outside London. It had 10 Honorary Members, the list of which contains such well-known names as William Alison (Edinburgh), Gabriel Andral (Paris), Sir Robert Carswell (Brussells), J. C. Cruveilhier (Paris), J. Henle (Zurich), Carl Rokitansky (Vienna), and William Stokes (Dublin).[27] Virchow, then a young man, was elected an Honorary Member some few years later. The first President was a London Physician and the Professor of Medicine at University College and it is noteworthy that out of a list of the 30 Presidents of the Society only one – the last but one, Burdon Sanderson – was a Pathologist. The Society was an active and flourishing one and by 1897 had 655 members. Its ten Honorary Members then included Sir William Jenner (London), R. Koch (Berlin), E. Metchnikoff (Paris), E. Rindfleisch (Bonn), Sir John Simon

(London), R. Virchow (Berlin), W. H. Welch (Baltimore), and E. Ziegler (Freiburg).[28] A glance at the membership list at this time shows the names of mostly English clinicians from all parts of the country to say nothing of a number of foreign members. The Society had by now very much changed from the London club that had started half-a-century before.

The early meetings showed a strong bias towards Pathological Anatomy in the number of specimens displayed. In the year 1853 there were 121 specimens on exhibit which had been examined histologically. In one case of 'hypertrophy of the stomach,' Beale had examined it chemico-microscopically by adding strong nitric acid, acetic acid, and potash as well as submitting the tissue to boiling water. Several specimens of teratoma of the testis (called enchondroma) were also on view.[29] In 1854 a case of 'bronchitis' was found to have fruiting bodies and was presumably aspergillosis.[30] In 1865 there was some attention given to occupational pulmonary disease and material was shown from a man who had worked for 38 years in the Cornish tin and copper mines.[31] In the subsequent years the Transactions changed their character and the articles published became scientific papers. In 1897 Kanthack submitted a paper on the newly-discovered fixation method of formalin for preserving museum specimens[32]. Three years later there was a discussion on blood in disease by a very distinguished group including Sidney Martin, C. S. Sherrington, A. Wright, J. Lorrain Smith, and William Hunter.[33] At about this time it was noted in the Transactions that 'the Members of Council forming each Section (A. Pathological Anatomy and Histology; B, Bacteriology; C, Experimental Pathology; D, Chemical Pathology) constitute committees of reference in the subjects enumerated, with power to add to their numbers in particular cases.'

The Pathological Society of London existed for approximately sixty years, a vital period in the consolidation of Pathology. Its drive came from the high percentage of Clinicians. There were very few pathologists at the close of the century and it would to be a few more years before Universities recognised the subject as an independent subject. By then the Pathologists would have a Society of their own, namely the Pathological Society of Great Britain and Ireland, which was founded in 1907 (see Chapter 6).

REFERENCES

1 'Lancet'. (1833–4) i, 326–31.
2 'Great men of Guy's'. edited W. B. Ober, Scarecrow Reprint Corporation, Metuchen, New Jersey 1973. Intro. pp. x–xii.
3 Ibid Intro. pp. x–xiv; xviii–xix.
4 Ibid Intro. pp. xvii–xviii.
5 Ibid Intro. pp. xix–xx.
6 Ibid Intro. pp. xx–xxi.

7 Hodgkin T., 'London med. Gazette'. (1828) *2* 423–31.
8 Major, R. H., 'Classic descriptions of disease'. Charles C. Thomas, Springfield, Illinois, 3rd edit. 1948, pp. 467–9.
9 Brock, R. C. E. & S. Livingstone Ltd. Edinburgh & London 1952, pp. 131–9.
10 Ibid pp. 121–30.
11 'Medical Classics'. The Williams and Wilkins Company, Baltimore, *5*, no. 1, 22.
12 Ibid (1939) *3*, No. 7, 711–46.
13 Ibid (1939) *3*, No. 6, 648–9.
14 Ibid (1936) *1*, No. 6, 707.
15 Ibid (1939) *3*, No. 7, 705–9.
16 Ibid (1940) *4*, No. 10, 1043–72.
17 'Lancet'. (1827) *12*, 335.
18 McMenemey, W. H., 'The life and times of Thomas Hastings'. E. & S. Livingstone Ltd., Edinburgh & London 1959. pp. 42–3.
19 'Lancet'. (1827–8) ii, 501–2.
20 Ibid (1843–44) ii, 580–2.
21 Ibid (1839–40) ii, 25–7.
22 Ibid (1839–40) ii, 462; 479.
23 Ibid (1846) ii, 462–3.
24 Ibid (1846) ii, 481–3.
25 Ibid (1847) i, 319.
26 Ibid (1829–30) i, 926.
27 Trans. Path. Soc. London. (1855) *6*, iii–vii.
28 Ibid (1897) *8*, viii–xxvii.
29 Ibid (1853) *4*, 180–6.
30 Ibid (1854) *5*, 38–41.
31 Ibid (1865) *16*, 57–8.
32 Ibid (1897) *48*, 282–337.
33 Ibid (1900) *51*, 285–337.

# FIVE

# Microscopy, Museums and the Birth of Public Health 1840–55

The progress of Pathology in the early part of the 19th century under the influence of the Paris School has been described. These advances were mainly in Anatomical Pathology and were to extend into Pathological Histology during the remainder of the century. The microscope had undergone several technical improvements and the cellular theory of Schleiden and Schwann had been propounded in 1839. As a result the German School now came to lead the way, firstly under the influence of Rokitansky in Vienna and later under Virchow at Berlin and Wurzburg. With the publication of Virchow's famous work on cellular pathology in 1858 pathological histology became studied even more widely until it became overshadowed by the discovery of pathogenic bacteria during the last two decades of the century.

Some idea of the early development of Pathological Anatomy can be gained by the mention of a few books on the subject. In 1794, Matthew Baillie published 'The Morbid Anatomy of some of the most important parts of the human body' and those that followed included Conradi's 'Handbuch der pathologischen Anatomie' in 1796; Otto in 1814 and Voigtel in 1824 also produced similar handbooks. More important still were a number of beautifully illustrated atlases, the first one in 1799 by Matthew Baillie being a supplement to his earlier work. This was followed in 1829 by Cruveilhier's 'Anatomie Pathologigne du Corps Humain,' in 1833 by Hope's 'Atlas of Morbid Anatomy,' and in 1838 by Carswell's 'Illustrations of the elementary forms of disease', many of which were drawn by the hand of this talented author. Other works of the time noted for their illustrations were Bright's 'Reports on medical cases' (1827–31) and Hodgson's 'Treatise on the diseases of arteries and veins' (1815). The enthusiasm for the subject resulted in the establishment of a number of anatomical and pathological museums in many European centres. Most of these earlier workers were anatomists and their collections consisted largely of malformations, monstrosities, and curiosities. All this changed when physicians realised the value of correlating symptoms and signs in life with anatomical lesions of autopsy and expanded museum collections with such specimens. In the early years of the 19th century, France led the field with such outstanding names as Andral, Bayle, Corvisant, Cruveilhier, and Laennec. But there had also been similar developments in Austria and these are important because they lead up to the growth of the German school later in the century.

Although it has been stated that the use of the microscope was less well-recognised in England than the Continent, it would be a mistake to conclude that it did not have its devotees. Already attention has been drawn to the work of Hughes Bennett in Edinburgh and his enthusiastic advocacy of its use (see Chapter 3) and London also had at least one centre of activity. This was at the Royal College of Surgeons where the council foresaw its importance and resolved to appoint a Professor of Histology in 1841.[1] The idea stemmed from work related to specimens in the Hunterian Museum. When the College first received these specimens, the first task was the compilation of a catalogue. This duty was entrusted to a young man named William Clift who had worked as Hunter's Assistant during the last two years of Hunter's life. A talented artist, he is remembered for his illustrations in Matthew Baillie's atlas. It has been said that without Clift there would have been no Hunterian Museum today,[2] and fifty years of his life were devoted to its care. He had been appointed Conservator of the museum, the specimens of which included a pathological section illustrating the General Principles of Pathology, and these Clift dealt with personally for they had not been formally arranged in any set plan. Before long he was in need of assistance for the museum had grown tremendously, partly from gifts and partly from the acquisition of specimens obtained at sales of various smaller or private collections. In 1827 a young man who had studied in Edinburgh and at St. Bartholomew's Hospital, London had been recommended for the post of Assistant Conservator by the surgeon John Abernethy. This man, Richard Owen, was appointed and proved himself to possess outstanding ability; he was an authority on Comparative Anatomy, and eventually succeeded Clift on the latter's retirement in 1842. Owen must have had some interest in microscopy, for with others he had been instrumental in the founding of the Microscopical Society of London (later the Royal Microscopical Society) in 1839. Amongst the founders was John T. Quekett who in the same year was appointed to a studentship in Human and Comparative Anatomy at the Royal College of Surgeons, where he was to work in the museums until his death in 1861. In 1843 he was appointed Assistant Conservator and as well as assisting Owen in his researches, he was engaged in routine museum duties. But Quekett's real interest was microscopy for at the age of sixteen he had given a course of lectures on the microscope and demonstrated an instrument which he had built himself. In his early years at the College he made a collection of over 2,000 microscope slides illustrating human and comparative Anatomy. These were purchased by the College in 1846 to supplement the small number already in their possession, many of which had been acquired by John Hunter at the sale of William Hewson's museum.[3] It is likely that Quekett was the foremost English microscopist of his day, and in 1857 he gave a course of twelve Museum lectures on histology at the College. He suffered very bad health for many years and died at the age of 46. His chief published works were 'Lectures on Histology' and a 'Practical treatise on the use of the microscope'.[4] A tribute was paid to him when in 1865 the Quekett Microscopical Club was founded, which still remains very active at the present time.

It therefore appears that there was much enthusiasm in England for Microscopy, though it might be wondered why there were two societies in London. The Microscopical Society was the learned society which catered for experienced and professional microscopists. The Quekett Club, the 'Father' of which was Mordecai Cubitt Cooke, a well-known Mycologist of the time, was chiefly for those who used microscopy as a hobby and for young microscopists who needed experience; it had grown from Cooke's Society of Amateur Botanists.[5] Finally Jabez Hogg's work on Microscopy confirms the interest in the subject at the time. It was published in 1854 and by 1861 the fifth edition consisting of 615 pages had appeared. The first three editions each of five thousand copies had been completely sold.

Meanwhile in Great Britain there was much interest in Anatomical Pathology, though the persons concerned were mostly physicians, surgeons and anatomists. There were few appointments in Pathology and those that did exist were usually part-time. For instance, when in 1831 King's College, London established a Chair of Morbid Anatomy, it was combined with the Chairs of Anatomy and Physiology and the first holder was Herbert Mayo, who was a surgeon at the Middlesex Hospital. However, any society which devoted itself to Pathology was likely to be a great stimulus to its eventual emergence as an independent subject. Yet we find that when the Pathological Society of London was founded there were 130 members; the vast majority were clinicians and all but four of them were from London. There was only one pathologist, namely W. H. Walshe, who was Professor of Pathology at University College, London and, of course, he was part-time. During the life of the Society, which extended until 1907 there were 30 Presidents. The first of these was C. J. B. Williams, Professor of Medicine at University College, London and the second was Charles Aston Key, an eminent Guy's Hospital surgeon. In the whole life of the Society there was only one President who was a pathologist, namely Sir John Burdon Sanderson (Regius Professor of Medicine at Oxford) and he was the last President but one.[6] The contribution to Pathology of this society, however, cannot be overestimated and its Transactions are a mine of information on Morbid Anatomy. Thus a strong clinical influence existed in the subject throughout the 19th and even into the early years of the 20th century.[7]

By this time Pathology had developed into something much more extensive than Pathological Anatomy as a result of a number of discoveries made during the second half of the 19th century. These transformed the face of medicine as a whole, and influenced the development of Pathology though often in an indirect way.

The end of the 18th and the beginning of the 19th centuries were characterised in England by a considerable population increase and a rapid growth of the towns. Epidemics were by no means infrequent and included smallpox, typhus and typhoid fever. In 1772 according to the Bills of Mortality there were 3,392 deaths from smallpox.[8] Thereafter there seems to have been a decline in the mortality of these diseases, although there were no specific measures (except some vaccination) directed against them. It has been suggested that improvements in farming had made food more plentiful, but this would probably have been offset by a deterioration in living conditions in towns. The migration to the towns during the Industrial Revolution led not only to overcrowding but to a change in the style of living, which was to prove detrimental to health. Little was known of either the identity or the cause of these epidemic diseases, but their association with unpleasant odours gave rise to the popular view that they were caused by 'miasmas' or vapours in the air. It had been noted that typhus was associated with poverty and famine, and was almost confined to the poorer classes. However, although the ill-effects of bad living conditions may not have been generally recognised in the late 18th century, physicians such as Lettsom in London, Clerk in Newcastle and Currie in Liverpool knew only too well of the appalling conditions in the slums and had begun to write about them.[9] In Lancashire, where the overcrowding was at its worst, John Ferriar, a physician to the Manchester Royal Infirmary, directed his attention to the improvement of living conditions in the lodgings occupied by cotton operatives.[10] The last straw may well have been the horrifying scenes of Asiatic cholera which appeared for the first time in England in 1831. Dr. Kay-Shuttleworth, the medical officer to the Ancoats and Ardwick Dispensary in Manchester,[11] by his reports of the epidemic did much to make people realise that attention to the general health of the public was an urgent necessity. Thus it came about that the philanthropy of the 18th century, which was responsible for the extensive building of hospitals, now gave way to a new wave of humanism in the early 19th century when several persons showed concern for the conditions under which their less fortunate brethren were living.

The social reformers were a strange mixture, some being deeply religious and others secular. Jeremy Bentham was a politician and thinker, who had little idea of the practical world. He propounded his theory of Utilitarianism (or Benthamism as it was sometimes called) which is usually summed up as 'the greatest good for the greatest number'. His chief importance here was the tremendous influence that he had on two men, Edwin Chadwick and Southwood Smith. When the public health problems of poverty, bad sanitation and overcrowding came to be tackled in earnest the outstanding figures were Chadwick, Southwood Smith, and Anthony Ashley Cooper, the Seventh Earl of Shaftesbury. It seems strange that a group dealing with medical problems should have only one member who was medically qualified. Yet this is less surprising when it is appreciated that the early changes brought about were legislative and administrative. Chadwick was a lawyer though he never practised, and after a short period as a journalist he became a civil servant. A man of tremendous drive and great administrative ability, he first achieved prominence as a member of the Poor Law Commission, which in 1834 instituted drastic changes through the Poor Law Amendment Act. Outdoor relief was abolished and paupers were forced to obtain relief by living in workhouses or infirmaries. This Act was exceedingly unpopular and Chadwick, who was considered the chief architect, attained an unpopularity which was to stick to him for the rest of his life. Without medical advice Chadwick would have been helpless and it was here that Southwood Smith proved to be his salvation. He not only gave information of the deplorable medical conditions, but more importantly indicated those which were most likely to be amenable to public health measures. In earlier years Smith had been the medical officer of the London Fever Hospital and in 1830 had published his 'Treatise on Fevers'. This was followed by his 'Philosophy of Health' in 1835, which established him as the leading public health authority of the time. Two other doctors, Neil Arnott and James Philip Kay (later Sir James Shuttleworth-Kay) were also interested in these problems and in 1839 published with Southwood Smith two reports, one on the causes of fevers and the other on the deplorable housing conditions of the working classes. Shaftesbury, who literally devoted his life to the poor, was chiefly concerned with alleviating the inhuman working conditions for women and children in factories, with the abolition of the use of children ('climbing boys') for sweeping chimneys, and with improvements in the treatment of lunatics in asylums.

For a period of about 15 years these men campaigned for improvements in Public Health, and the details of their efforts have been excellently described in the Fitzpatrick Lectures for 1946 and 1947 by Sir Arthur Salusbury MacNalty.[12] Several reports on both the living and working conditions of the poor in the rapidly developing towns created quite a shock in Parliament. It was pointed out that the annual death rate from typhus fever was double the losses on the Allied armies at the battle of Waterloo (about 30,000). A Royal Commission was appointed in 1843 which led to the Public Health Act of 1848, one of the main provisions of which was the constitution of a Central Board of Health. In many ways this was an unfortunate venture, though it would be wrong to call it a failure. The Board consisted of three members, Lord Morpeth, the Earl of Shaftesbury and Chadwick. The presence of Chadwick was one source of its immediate unpopularity. The Royal College of Physicians resented health proposals which came from a non-medical body, though this was rectified in 1850 by the appointment of Southwood Smith. When this was approved under the Medical Interments Act it prompted Mr. Rumsey to say that 'the whimsical experiment had been actually tried of appointing three non-medical authorities, i.e. two Lords and a Barrister, to preserve the health of the living and then after a year or so of doubtful success, calling in a physician to bury the dead'.[13] The aims of the Board were reasonable enough. They included the provision of a safe water supply, the promotion of cleanliness and the eradication of vermin, the proper disposal of sewage, the proper maintenance of cemeteries, and the provision of sufficient air and light by reducing overcrowding. Conflict over the water supplies soon followed. The Board had laid down certain conditions and the fulfilment of these would involve the water companies (many of whom were private) in additional and, as they thought, unnecessary expense. The difficulties are obvious when it is remembered that there was at the time no knowledge of the aetiology of the diseases which were being attacked. To Chadwick, disease was synonymous with 'dirt and smell' and one member of Parliament had remarked that 'England wanted to be clean, but not to be cleansed by Mr. Chadwick'.[14] The Board had been decidedly unlucky for after Chadwick had threatened cholera to those who did not keep clean, an explosive outbreak of cholera with 54,000 deaths occurred in the first year of the Board's existence. A fresh outbreak occurred in 1853 and people began to doubt the validity of the Board's proposals for reducing disease. In 1854 the Board was disbanded in all but name and Chadwick retired from public life. Probably the Croydon typhoid outbreak had been the last straw. Chadwick had installed a new drainage system in the town and given it a certain amount of publicity. The reaction of individuals can be imagined when the installation was followed by the worst outbreak of fever in the town's history. The Board of Health was completely disbanded in 1858 and the medical duties and public health functions then became transferred to the Privy Council. Southwood Smith continued his work but died in 1860.

The public health reforms mentioned had done much to focus attention on infective diseases, though it would be another generation before their causes were understood. There are however two aspects of progress which must be mentioned. The importance of statistics had been realised and, largely because of Chadwick, William Farr (1807–83) had been appointed Compiler of Statistics to the General Register Office in 1839. He had studied in Paris with Andral and Louis, who probably interested him in the subject. He was the first to study the pattern of epidemics and to show that these could be represented mathematically.[15]

Another advance related to the mode and spread of infection came from an unexpected quarter. The story is now well-known of how John Snow, the first English anaesthetist, had in his spare time traced a cholera epidemic in 1853 to water from the Broad Street Pump. This demonstration of transmission of infection by water was not immediately accepted by all, but John Simon, who was to be the foremost public health authority for the next 30 years, accepted it straightaway. Similar information on the spread of disease came when William Budd, a Bristol practitioner, showed that typhoid could be spread by water and in 1858 Michael Taylor of Penrith traced an epidemic of typhoid to infected milk.[16]

Such was the new thinking in England when it was realised that the medical care of the community was of even greater importance than that of the individual patient. As a result hygiene and sanitation became greatly improved. But at this time a similar and worse state of affairs existed in the Crimea, where the outbreak of war in 1854 had been accompanied by epidemics of cholera and typhus. There was no proper medical care and reports of the atrociously bad hygienic conditions soon reached home. Public health measures were urgently needed, and in 1855 Shaftesbury was responsible for the sending of a Sanitary Commission to the theatre of war. These events abroad are dealt with in chapter 14.

REFERENCES

1 Hogg, Jabez, 'The Microscope'. Routledge, Warne & Routledge, 1861. 5th Ed. Preface ix.
2 Dobson, Jessie, Chapter in 'History of the Royal College of Surgeons' by Zachary Cope. Anthony Blond, London, 1959, pp. 282.
3 Ibid p. 286.
4 'Illustrated London News' (1861) J. T. Quekett, Obituary notice *2*, 227.
5 English, Mary P., 'Microscopy'. (1978) *33*, 329–338.
6 Dible, J. H., J. Path. Bact. (1957) *73*, 3–4.
7 Rolleston, Sir Humphrey, Ann. med. History (1939) *1*, (3rd series) 236.
8 Gale, A. H., 'Epidemic diseases'. Penguin Books 1959. p. 132.
9 Ibid p. 133.
10 Singer C., & Underwood, E. A., 'A short history of medicine'. Oxford, Clarendon Press 1962. 2nd ed. p. 189.
11 Ibid pp. 210–11.
12 MacNalty, Sir Arthur Salusbury, Fitzpatrick Lectures 1946 & 1947. Royal Institute of Public Health & Hygiene, London. pp. 9–15.
13 Ibid p. 21.
14 Singer, C. & Underwood, E. A., 'A short history of medicine'. Oxford, Clarendon Press 1962. p. 219.
15 Idem p. 732.
16 MacNalty, Sir Arthur Salusbury, Fitzpatrick Lectures 1946 & 1947. Royal Institute of Public Health & Hygiene, London. p. 25.

# SIX
# Advances of Pathology, 1830–1900

The first full-time European pathologists made their appearance in the early years of the 19th century and it is important to see how this came about. In past years it had been the custom of the universities to teach the clinical subjects, namely Medicine and Surgery, in two halves, the Theory and the Practice of the subject. The Professor of Anatomy often played a large part in the teaching of Surgery, but in the case of Medicine there were two Professors, one for the Practice and one for the Theory or 'Institutes of Medicine'. The latter part of the subject also included the principles of Physiology, Pathology, and Materia Medica, and as these subjects advanced they attained independent status. In the case of Pathology there might be two types of teacher, the Pathological Anatomist who was trained in Anatomy and the General Pathologist who took over the teaching of the principles of the subject from the Professor of the Institutes. A few details may clarify the situation.

When the first Chair of Pathology was founded in Strasbourgh in 1819, and Lobstein appointed, it was largely due to the influence of the great Comparative Anatomist, Georges Cuvier; when in 1836 Cruveilhier became the first occupant of a similar Chair in Paris it was due to the famous French surgeon, Dupuytren. It is easy to understand why the two Chairs were designated for 'Pathological Anatomy'. In Vienna a similar Chair was established in 1845 and Rokitansky became the first holder, though the process was rather protracted. In 1812 a museum had been founded and put in charge of a Prosector, whose duties included the performance of autopsies. In 1819 the holder, Dr. Biermayer, gave some lectures on 'Pathological Anatomy with dissection of subjects.' He became Adjunct Professor in 1823 and was succeeded in this post by Rokitansky in 1834.[1] A similar process was responsible for the development of the subject in the German universities. The hospital prosector, in addition to making dissections and giving lectures, started to make museum collections which became invaluable for teaching pathological anatomy.

In the meanwhile, the first two part-time Chairs of Pathology had been founded in Great Britain. One was occupied by Robert Carswell (1793–1857) at the University of London and the other at the University of Edinburgh by John Thomson (1765–1846). One surprising feature of these appointments was that whilst the London Chair was one of 'Morbid Anatomy', that in Edinburgh was of 'General Pathology', and this, as will be seen, was related to some unusual happenings. Prior to this time the Edinburgh medical student received tuition in Pathology as part of two other subjects. Some practical aspects were introduced into the Clinical Surgery lectures given by the Professor, James Russell (1755–1836). The principles of the subject formed part of the Institutes of

59

Medicine Course which included Pathology, Physiology and Therapeutics.[2] The holder of this Chair was William Pulteney Alison (1790–
1859), who was well-versed in his subjects, having published his 'Outlines
of Physiology' in 1831 and his 'Outlines of Pathology and the practice
of Medicine' in 1844. In these surroundings, the new Professor of
General Pathology must have been regarded as an interloper, for his
course would have been very similar to that given as part of 'the
Institutes'. In the event General Pathology became a subject on its own.
But apart from this, it was the method of appointment that caused
resentment. It had been made by the Crown without University consultation and the antagonism aroused amongst the local authorities and other
teachers was considerable.[3] It is interesting to note that there was a
parallel event in 1830 when Louis Philippe created a similar Chair of
General Pathology in Paris, apparently also without consulting the
University, and Broussais was the first occupant.[4]

John Thomson, the new professor in Edinburgh, gave the first course
of lectures on General Pathology in 1831 and it was continued by his
successors throughout the remainder of the century. It would be
interesting to know the content of such a course in those early days, as
from the literature it appears that several 18th century views were still
prevalent. For example, William P. Alison, the Professor of the
Institutes in Edinburgh from 1821 until 1842, had written of his belief
in the 'vital attraction and repulsion' which he thought were
characteristics of life as exhibited by the tissues.[5] A much fuller idea of
such a viewpoint is given by James Bower Harrison MRCS London, who
published sixteen lectures on General Pathology in the 1844, 1845, and
1846 issues of the 'Lancet'. Some ideas of the beliefs of the time can be
obtained by reference to these lectures.

At this time in England it was customary for the teaching of Pathology
to be given by a member who held a junior staff position such as Assistant Physician. This may have been so in the case of Harrison who is
described as 'late Surgeon to the Ardwick and Ancoats Dispensary and
formerly one of the Resident Medical Officers of the Manchester Royal
Infirmary'. He seems to have been well acquainted with the work of the
leading medical men of the day, such as Andral, Bright, Christison, John
Hunter, Latham, and Muller. He emphasised the value of clinical
experiences as compared with book knowledge and he illustrated his
lectures with a few clinical cases. He dealt at some length with constitu-
tional peculiarities, some hereditary, in predisposing to disease.[6] His
main aim seemed to be to divide disease into 'elemental conditions' but
admitted that he found difficulty with the effects of one system on
another due to the lack of knowledge of the functions of the various
parts of the body.[7] Perhaps because of his extensive clinical experience
he realised, in this study of disease, the importance of distinguishing
what is only a symptom, and whether a particular manifestation is
primary or secondary.[8] He was less advanced when he revealed himself

as a vitalist who followed Hunter in his belief in the vitality of the blood.[9] It may be recalled that Hunter believed that food became converted into chyle, a process of 'animalisation', and was then changed into blood by 'vivivication' in the lungs.[10] Harrison discussed diseases caused by 'vitiated states of the blood, produced by a faulty process of vivivication'. He believed that these changes in the lungs had a chemical basis for he referred to them as 'vito-chemical', not surprising in view of the strong influence of Liebig, the German chemist, at the time. But he admitted that 'when we approach discussions which concern vitality it is no reflection to acknowledge ignorance, and we may be pardoned some conjecture'.[11]

At home in the clinical field, he gave a good description of local and general vascular congestion, especially that associated with diseases of the mitral and aortic valves. But in these lectures there is no mention of thrombosis and this is unexpected in view of the beliefs of Cruveilhier who considered phlebitis to be the basis of all Pathology. The discussion of inflammation is hard to follow and this process was regarded as an error of the nervous as well as the vascular system. He believed that there was a derangement of the blood vessels which might affect the nutrition of the body. Surprisingly he illustrated this process with an interesting clinical case which is very clearly one of myositis ossificians progressiva.[12]

Another case quoted under conditions of 'vitiated states of the blood' revealed at autopsy multiple nodules in the skin and throughout the rest of the body. Harrison was familiar with this tendence to widespread growth of carcinoma for he had seen another case very similar to the above. He quoted Muller[13] who had found, by microscopy, in such cases that such deposits were made up of minute cells possessing an inherent vitality which he thought was responsible for their widespread propagation. At this time there seems to have been no idea of spread through the vascular system.

Amongst other pathological features was the coexistence of several morbid conditions which Harrison called 'cumulative disease'.[14] These conditions would 'have induced or succeeded each other during the course of life.' Many examples occurred in the elderly and the majority had chronic bronchitis, though age was not the only factor. Other instances were 'failing of the constitution' connected with Bright's disease of the kidneys.[15]

These fragmentary references give some indication of one aspect of the teaching of General Pathology. It was not advanced and the author's approach, theoretical and speculative, was based on Natural Philosophy rather than on the Natural Sciences.

This General Pathology was very different from that which was taught at the German Schools during the next 15 years (see chapter 7). At that time the cell theory of Virchow had become established and the 'blastema' theory of Schleiden and Schwann discredited. Virchow linked

Pathology to Clinical Medicine and at the same time clarified much of General Pathology by his work on inflammation, thrombosis, embolism and tumours. Rokitansky's famous work had been written in two parts, one on General and one on Systematic Pathology. This pattern came to be followed by future text-book authors in Germany, as well as by teachers of Pathology in medical schools. New staining methods and techniques of tissue preparation did much to advance Pathology in Germany.

In Great Britain there was no such striking progress though there were a number of outstanding clinicians such as Astley Cooper, Addision, Bright, Hodgkin, Stokes, Wilks, and others who made substantial contributions to Pathological Anatomy. When further advances were made in England they were related to the natural history of infectious disease. For these we are indebted to Sir John Simon, a leader in the field of Public Health, and his assistants (see chapter 13). By the application of the rules of simple hygiene, there was considerable reduction in the incidence of infectious diseases, even forty years before the causes of these had been discovered. Simon, who started his medical career as a surgeon, held a lectureship in Pathology for most of his life and stimulated interest in the natural history of infectious diseases amongst his assistants. He became well-known in Europe and was described by Virchow as an excellent pathologist. He gave a series of twelve lectures on General Pathology at St. Thomas's Hospital. Fortunately these were published in the 'Lancet'[16] and a brief comparison of their content with that of the lectures given by James B. Harrison provides a striking contrast in their content of General Pathology. This is all the more surprising when it is noted that the two sets of lectures were published within a period of five years.

In his opening lecture Simon made a plea for Pathology to be recognised as a science.[17] He realised that progress in Pathology could only be made by accurate observations, hence the value of the experimental method. But such phenomena as witnessed were only of value when compared with similar states in health. As a result this had led to some confusion in the use of the terms Physiology and Pathology. Some workers used Physiology in a wide sense to include both states of health and disease, and therefore Pathology. Others confined Physiology to health and Pathology to disease.

The physiology of blood was described as being responsible for providing material for new growth of tissue while washing away those elements which are worn out and no longer of use.[18] Red cells were in one of three stages, namely:

(1) developing or not yet 'ripe'
(2) fully developed or normal
(3) 'worn out'

This was a theoretical concept for there was no known method of isolating the cells of these groups. But included in abnormal red cell development was chlorosis which it was noted could be cured by administration of iron. Blood seems to have been given a kind of primacy in the body over other tissues. It was pointed out that in prussic acid poisoning the poison reached the blood before the tissues. It was even suggested that blood, receiving nutritive elements first, was able to grow first, and that other organs then grew only at the expense of it. It was noted that interference with the normal excretions of carbon dioxide caused rapid death in warm-blooded animals, though less rapidly in cold-blooded. The arterial blood in such cases was less easily distinguished from venous blood which was very dark and failed to coagulate normally.

Simon believed in the importance of blood in facilitating the spread throughout the body of the infectious diseases in which he, as a Medical Officer of Health, was especially interested. His fourth lecture dealt with the quantitative aspects of the irregular distribution of blood. For this purpose he described two states, passive congestion, and active hyperaemia.[19] He dealt with the former which was much simpler and described some of the complications such as increased exudation and haemorrhage which may follow venous obstruction. With active hyperaemia things were much more complex and the condition became confused with inflammation and with hypertrophy. In acute inflammation there was excess of blood but in order to produce tissue in excess as in hypertrophy the presence of a special substance, 'developable blastema,' was postulated. It emphasised that passive congestion was not associated with hypertrophy.

The idea of the prime importance of the blood in health and disease fitted in well with the prevalent theory of Humoral Pathology. It was believed that the earliest changes appeared in the blood where the 'morbid poison' causing the disease accumulated and gave rise to its symptoms. It seemed likely that drugs which were administered also found their way first into the blood.[20] A cure of the disease was effected by excretion of the noxious substance, or 'peccant humor', and confirmation of this seemed very clear in the case of gout in which relief of severe acute pain occurred following the removal of 'lithic acid' from the blood. At this time there were a number of drugs in current usage which promoted excretions.[21] In some conditions like chronic Bright's disease, when renal excretion was impaired it was thought that the accompanying vomiting and diarrhoea were compensatory by providing alternative routes of excretion.

One surprising application of Humoral Pathology was given in the case of Cancer.[22] The classification of tumours given included other conditions such as cysts and elephantiasis, the famous case of the Chinaman Hoo Loo at Guy's Hospital (see chapter 2) being quoted of the latter.[23,24] It is really a classification of 'lumps'. When he came to cancer, which was divided into scirrhus, colloid, and encephaloid, a very clear account was given of how malignant emboli spread along blood and lymphatic channels to give rise to metastases. But there is one major error in his concept of cancer which seems to have arisen from his observation of ulcerating or fungating encephaloid cancers. Observing the discharge from such a lesion he came to regard cancer as a purposeful process beneficial to the patient and 'substantially a new excretory organ.' If this were so it would preclude the use of surgical treatment of the disease. As he wrote 'to speak of curing a cancer by operation is an absurdity'.[25]

Drugs which promoted the evacuation of excretions naturally found their way into Humoral Pathology. It was pointed out that medicines often contained twenty ingredients and that their action was often quite unknown. At the time Materia Medica was in an empirical state and Simon recognised that no progress could be made until it became based on a true scientific pharmacolgy.[26] This did not occur till 1885 when Lauder Brunton (1844–1916) published his well-known text-book, 'Pharmacology, Therapeutics, and Materia Medica'.[27] It was the first comprehensive treatise on Pharmacology.

Simon's concluding lecture was on a subject which must have been dear to his heart, namely morbid poisons.[28] These substances were thought to be the specific poisons which brought about the phenomena of infectious diseases. They possessed two striking differences when compared with ordinary poisons, i.e. drugs. Firstly the full effects of morbid poison could be produced by the smallest dose whereas the effects of drugs increased proportionally to the dosage. Secondly, as the condition developed ordinary poisons decreased while morbid poisons underwent a striking increase. This latter point was exemplified in the case of smallpox when the material from any one pustule was capable of producing the disease. This 'multiplication of the morbid poison' led Simon to comment on the view of Dr. Holland and Professor Henle that the essence of the morbid poison might be a living thing, a 'contagium animatum' or the 'contagium vivum' of Frascatorius. Holland's essay, 'The Hypothesis of Insect Life as a Cause of Disease', led Simon to consider insect as synonymous with animalcule, and he dealt with both under 'the parasitic theory of fever'. But he was never able to bring himself to accept this theory. Based on the parasites known at the time, Simon believed parasitic effects to be only local. Also he was not able to detect parasites in certain lesions though he was unlucky in his choice, namely smallpox pustules, scarlet fever kidney, and syphilitic periostitis. He believed that changes were produced in the blood and that the agent was a chemical one, possibly of the nature of a catalyst. For the future he looked for the discovery of a chemical which would neutralise the morbid poison of infective diseases just as smallpox had been neutralised by Jenner's vaccination.

The lectures given in 1850 by John Simon are remarkable for the time and show the progress that was being made now that Basic Sciences were being applied to Pathology.

Back in Edinburgh, John Thomson's course of General Pathology was being given by his successors. In 1869 Professor W. R. Sanders, realising the importance of Pathology as a branch of Clinical Medicine, added a course in Systematic Pathology and established laboratories for practical instruction. This pattern of instruction proved to be very successful and subsequently became adopted in most of the Medical Schools of the British Isles. It was still in Lorrain Smith's mind when in 1904 on his appointment to the Chair of Pathology in Manchester he expressed his intention of providing students with a course in General Pathology as well as one in Morbid Anatomy.[29]

The remaining years of the century were to witness tremendous advances on the continent, chiefly in Germany. Virchow was succeeded by such worthy men as Rindfleisch, Weigert, Ehlich, and many others. University Institutes of Pathology sprang up at Wurzburg and Berlin under the influence of Virchow and also at Strasbourg under von Recklinghausen. Julius Cohnheim (1839–1884) carried out his classical experimental work on inflammation first at Breslau and later at Leipzig. Brief reference should be made to the versatile Edwin Klebs (1834–1913) whose name is thought of in connection with diptheria, it being sometimes forgotten that he produced experimental endocardits, and also introduced the technique of paraffin wax embedding to histology in 1869.[30] He held five Chairs of Pathology at such diverse locations as Bern, Wurzburg, Prague, Zürich, and Chicago. Lastly he even had the temerity to oppose the views of his master, the great Virchow. The theory of Humoral Pathology supported by Cohnheim's experimental work on inflammation was now opposed by that of Cellular Pathology, chiefly supported by Elie Metchnikoff (1845–1916), a Russian who was working with Pasteur in Paris. The century concluded with the discovery of many pathogenic bacteria which gave a new lease of life to the study of infectious disease and Public Health.

In Great Britain progress was less spectacular though there were a number of interesting developments. The Pathological Society of London, founded in 1847, spanned half the century and was run chiefly by clinicians with an interest in Pathological Anatomy. They held regular meetings at which cases might be shown, though it was more customary to show Pathological specimens, and it will be remembered that in 1907 the Society became the Section of Pathology of the newly-formed Royal Society of Medicine. These clinico-pathological meetings must have done much to stimulate interest in Pathology as must similar activities of the British Medical Association (BMA). This society was founded in 1832 by Charles Hastings (1794–1866) in Worcester. It was essentially a provincial medical society but in 1862 it was decided to issue a weekly journal (the British Medical Journal or BMJ) which over the years has gone from strength to strength. One of its earlier activities was the Annual Meeting which was held in one of the provincial towns of the British Isles, and at the meeting of 1867 the programme included an item called 'Annual Museum'. This became a regular feature and grew to such an extent that it was divided into sections. For instance, in the Annual meeting at Glasgow in 1888 it included sections dealing with:

A.  Food and drugs
B.  Pathology including Casts, Medals, Diagrams, Microscopical preparations and Microorganisms
C.  Anatomy – dissections, etc.
D.  Physiology – apparatus, microscopes, etc.
E.  Instruments and books
F.  Sanitation – Domestic Sanitary Appliances, Personal Hygiene, Ambulances and Carriages[31]

In 1891 at the Bournemouth meeting there was a division devoted to Pathology, and also a series of wax models illustrating skin diseases.[32] In 1895 the meeting was arranged for London and from all accounts this surpassed any of its predecessors. By this time the titles of the exhibits had become changed. For instance, the term 'Annual Museum' referred to the commercial exhibit of food, drugs and surgical instruments which was surprisingly large for the time. In 1895 there was also a separate division called 'Pathological or Clinico-pathological Museum'. As such, it included (1) morbid anatomy specimens, many of which were on loan from other museums in London; (2) bacteriological exhibits; and (3) patients who were shown each day.[33]

It would therefore seem that with a number of sources of museum specimens and such a fine museum collection as that possessed by the Royal College of Surgeons of England, pathological specimens did much to stimulate interest in the subject.

A chance reference to the subject of museums should be mentioned. In 1889 the British Association for the Advancement of Science was held in Newcastle-on-Tyne for the third time, the previous meetings being in 1838 and 1863. The President on this occasion was the Director of the British Museum of Natural History, Professor W. H. Flower, and he gave his inaugural address on the subject of Museums[34].

He pointed out that nearly all the collections used to teach Anatomy or Pathology were the private property of the professors. For museums as a whole, he felt that they were little understood though they were beginning to attract attention. He was encouraged by the formation in that year of an association of Curators and others interested in Museums. In 1906 Maude E. S. Abott (1869–1940) of McGill University, Montreal founded the International Association of Medical Museums. In 1908 at the Royal College of Surgeons of England, demonstrations were given by Sir Arthur Keith and Professor Shattock explaining certain sections of the Museum.[35]

Throughout the century it is interesting to find that the post of Museum Curator was frequently held by clinicians at an early stage of their career. A list of these includes such distinguished names as S. Delépine (later Professor of Pathology in Manchester), L. S. Beale (later

Professor of Pathology, King's College London), A. A. Kanthack (Director of Pathology, St. Bartholomew's Hospital, London), and John Goodsir (later Professor of Anatomy in Edinburgh).

By the end of the century Pathology had become recognised as an independent subject which had also proved its value in the practical application of Bacteriology to Clinical Medicine. This was seen in the career of Sheridan Delépine, the first full-time Professor of Pathology in Manchester and who in a few years (1901) became the first Professor of Bacteriology. In 1896 the Annual BMA meeting was held in Carlisle and Delépine, as President of the Section of Pathology, addressed his audience on 'The Place of Pathology in Medical Education'.[36] It was an appropriate subject as the General Medical Council had recently been considering educational reform. This seemed to apply especially to Pathology in view of the relatively recent recognition of the subject by some universities.[37] The activity in these circles can be imagined when it is pointed out that the seven Chairs existing in 1896 had risen to eleven by 1906 (see Chapter 11).

This great advance in Pathology was really part of the development of the Basic Sciences. It is of some interest to study the dates of foundation of the scientific societies connected with these disciplines. One of the earliest was the Pharmaceutical Society, founded in 1837, presumably at this date because of the long-associated study of Botany and Materia Medica as part of medical education. The Society of its basic science subject, Pharmacology, was delayed till near the end of the century probably because it was long treated as an offshoot of Physiology. Physiology in Great Britain had a long and difficult path because of the opposition of the anti-vivisectionists (see chapter 12) and had no Society till 1876. Even more surprising is Anatomy whose Society was not established until 1886. Sir George Humphry was instrumental in its foundation and was its first President. With Sir William Turner he had founded the 'Journal of Anatomy' twenty years earlier. This delay might be related to the relatively small number of Human Anatomists, because this subject was often taught by surgeons. The pure anatomists often devoted themselves to the comparative aspects of the subject, and to Embryology. The first societies of Pathology in the United Kingdom were local, namely the Dublin Society (founded by William Stokes in 1838) and the Reading Society in 1841. As previously mentioned, the Pathological Society of London was founded in 1846, and flourished throughout the remainder of the century. Its early foundation can be related to the dominance of Pathology by clinicians of the time. As a result the membership was largely composed of clinicians with special interest in Pathological Anatomy. It is significant that as late as 1881, at the International Congress of Medicine held in London, the representative for Pathology was Sir Samueal Wilks; he is remembered and respected for his knowledge of Pathology, but he was essentially a physician.

It will be recalled that in 1907 the Royal Society of Medicine was founded and the Pathological Society of London became incorporated in it as its Section of Pathology.

Pathology was now recognised as an independent discipline, its numbers increasing, the scope of the subject widening, and university recognition advancing. But yet there were some things lacking. The Pathologists had no society of their own and as Greenfield[38] had said in 1884, they badly needed a journal.

In 1906 when there were thirteen Chairs of Pathology the Pathological Society of Great Britain and Ireland was founded. It was to prove a vital step which greatly furthered the scientific growth of the subject. An excellent history of the first fifty years of the Society had been published by the late Professor J. H. Dible and punctuated with delightfully humorous touches so characteristic of the author.[39] For the present purpose only special relevant points will be mentioned and for these the author is indebted to Professor Dible.

In June 1906 a letter had been circulated inviting those 'actually engaged in Pathological teaching or research' to join the proposed society and it was signed by fifty-four pathologists including all the holders of the thirteen university Chairs of Pathology. The inaugural meeting was held in July 1906 in Manchester and the second meeting at the Lister Institute in London in January 1907.

With the diverse developments in Pathology many pathologists felt the need of a Society, especially as the Societies of Anatomy and Physiology were proving so successful. One feature of the new society and one which has persisted over the years was the strong influence of Scotland and the North, and the relatively minor role played by London and the South. In the original letter circulated less than one-third of the signatories were from London. This is probably related to the development of Pathology in the universities. Of the whole-time Chairs of Pathology, Cambridge and the Scottish schools led the way; a few years later there were the English provincial and the Irish medical schools; it was not until 1912 that a London school appointed a full-time professor in the subject. The London schools regarded Pathology as a subject ancillary to Medicine and Surgery, while those of Scotland, Ireland, and the English provinces established it as a basic science discipline in its own right.

The society was run by a Committee and had for its Officers two Secretaries and a Treasurer. There was no permanent President nor Chairman, and at the meetings the Chair was taken by the head of the laboratory in which the meeting was held. The present author once spent an entire afternoon trying to convince some American visitors that there was a reputable society of Pathology which had neither a President nor a Chairman!

One of the earliest needs of the Society was for a Journal. As far back as 1884 Greenfield pointed out the great need for a journal of pathology as there existed none at that time in the English language.[38] In 1892

Dr. Sims Woodhead (Director of the Conjoint Research Laboratories in London) in association with an Edinburgh publisher, Young J. Pentland, had produced a 'Journal of Pathology and Bacteriology'. This was still in existence in 1907 when the matter arose and when Sims Woodhead had become Professor of Pathology in Cambridge University. It was an unusual thing for a private individual to produce such a journal. The explanation lies probably in his home circumstances for Sims Woodhead was brought up in Huddersfield where his father was editor of the local newspaper. The Committee approached Sims Woodhead and over the next few years arranged to purchase the Journal, the deal being completed in 1914.

Although most of the Society members were pathologists who were medically qualified, this was not a prerequisite. Amongst the original members was a well-known veterinarian, J. McFadyean, and in later years an outstanding technician called Richard Muir was admitted to the Society. From the earliest years encouragement was given to technicians and this resulted in the formation of the Laboratory Assistants Association in 1912. The membership of the Society numbered 264 in 1908, and it grew steadily to 317 in 1914. By 1938 it was 641 and after World War II it rose rapidly reaching 1230 in 1956. This phenomenal rise was partly due to the influx of a number of Dutch pathologists, which followed the very successful and desirable institution of joint Anglo-Dutch meetings in 1950 and 1956. In 1924 a proposal to limit the size of the Society to 400 was defeated. In 1950 it was decided to set a limit of 800, but this does not appear to have been followed, possibly because it conflicted with the advent of the Anglo-Dutch association.

The growth of membership also had repercussions relating to the presentation of scientific communications. When the Society was founded the papers were presented in the order in which they had been submitted. Normally 15 minutes were allocated for a paper but the timing was not always strict. The programme consisted of a list of papers without any specific times, and it became impossible to tell when exactly a paper would be presented. There was no grouping of papers related to similar topics and it was customary to listen to all papers whether related to one's particular interest or not. Many members enjoyed this for it helped them maintain interest in the developments in Pathology as a whole. But with a sharp increase in the number of papers submitted it was suggested that meetings be divided into two sections, namely Pathology and Bacteriology. In 1923 this proposal was defeated unanimously and it was not until 1948 that it was approved. This tended to split the Society, but it was inevitable, and had the advantage that papers on allied topics could be grouped together.

The service which the Society did for Pathology cannot be overestimated, and in many ways it developed into the ideal scientific society. Many pathologists, particularly the younger members, enjoyed the hours spent in the pleasant and friendly atmosphere of the meetings.

Scientific projects were sponsored as for example the establishment of the National Collection of Type Cultures in 1919. But from the beginning and throughout its existence the Society insisted on its limitation to scientific matters and would have nothing whatever to do with anything which smacked of Medical Politics. The main clash over such an issue came in 1927 when a breakaway group formed the future Association of Clinical Pathologists (see chapter 19).

There is one point on which this admirable Society had received criticism which does not appear to be unjustified. It was founded mostly by Morbid Anatomists, though at the time of foundation there was a number of Bacteriologists, and their subject was recognised. But when in later years numerous other sub-divisions were making their appearance the Society was strangely reluctant to recognise them. Had this been done, new subjects such as Haematology and Immunology could have had their own sections in the parent Society, thus preserving the unity of the subject. But this was not to be and so the Society became criticised for being 'A Society of Morbid Anatomy'.

In the teaching of Pathology the Universities were coming to play an ever increasing part. This was partly due to the realisation that there were many disorders which could not be explained in terms of structure only. From the time of Harvey function had been considered, but only by a few individuals whose thoughts were decidedly in advance of those of the time. The outlook began to change with John Hunter, who was trained primarily as an anatomist and surgeon, but also realised the importance of the function of organs.

It was at this time that Medicine changed direction and the force impelling it came from newer knowledge of the Basic Sciences. So far there had been only a limited application of these subjects, though Physics and Chemistry had been the basis of the Old Iatromechanical and Iatrochemical schools of thought. Botany, as the basis of Materia Medica and Pharmacy, was an essential subject and maintained its importance until well into the 19th century. Anatomy, as already indicated, was closely attached to Surgery, and both subjects were often taught by the same person. During the century under consideration these basic subjects continued to progress, but the pathological scene was dominated by the development of new subjects such as Microscopical Anatomy, Physiology and General Pathology. This led to a new type of Medicine, often called 'Laboratory Medicine', in which experimental methods formed an important part. Experiments with drugs eventually led to Pharmacology, which for a long time remained an offshoot of Physiology before becoming a discipline in its own right. It follows that Research and the training of individuals to carry it out became urgent necessities. As a result, the Medical Course of the future came to consist of two parts. The clinical subjects dealing with the care of the sick were taught in hospitals, but the Basic Sciences required a different atmosphere and facilities, and the ideal place was in the University. In practice, this would entail recognition of a subject by the University to the extent of setting up a department and the appointment of relevant staff. Advances resulting from research would be transmitted to the clinical workers for practical application in the hospital. Obviously, such aims would be best achieved if the hospital and the university were closely adjacent, and under ideal conditions each would benefit the other. Such a system was later seen at its best in 19th century Germany where, in many places, the two were side by side, and the hospital was staffed by the university. This concept of the University Hospital was mainly responsible for the rapid advances in clinical medicine in that country.[40]

It is now appropriate to consider the constitution of a university medical faculty when originally founded, and the early steps in its development. This presents some difficulty because there were many variations from a set pattern not only between the British universities themselves but also between them and the Continental Schools. The two groups influenced one another because in the 18th and 19th centuries it was customary for prosperous young men to do the 'grand tour' of Europe to complete their education. Such men as Richard Bright spent about two years abroad, and were much influenced by their contacts with some of the leading professors of the Continental Universities. Also, there were universities such as Edinburgh and Leyden in which there was a free interchange of students. We even find that in 1692 Dr. Archibald Pitcairne (1652–1713) of Edinburgh became Professor of Physic in Leyden, where Boerhaave and the future English physician, Richard Mead, were amongst his pupils. Students might commence their studies at a 'home' university, proceed to take courses abroad and finally take their degree at any of the universities attended. Such a procedure was not difficult because Latin was the recognised university language. Pitcairne graduated MA in Edinburgh, then studied mathematics there and also in Paris, where he became interested in Medicine and finally graduated MD at the University of Rheims.[41].

In Europe, the influence of the University of Leyden in the teaching of Medicine was particularly great, especially in the early days of the 18th century when the famous physician, Hermann Boerhaave (1668–1738) was in his prime (see chapter 7).

Some general details of the structure of the early Medical Faculties will now be given. It should be realised that when a university recognised a subject by the appointment of a professor, the main concern seems to have been to test the proficiency of the students. It was often many years before lecturing was considered to be one of the professor's duties. Even when this was so, he might only be expected to lecture at the request of a set number of students. Although there was variation from place to place, the general pattern was similar. The subjects first recognised were Anatomy, Botany, Chemistry, Theory and Practice of Medicine, Natural Philosophy, and Surgery. Not infrequently a Chair would include more than one subject. The professor of Anatomy was often also the professor of Surgery, and in Edinburgh the three Alexander Monros successively held such a joint appointment for 126 years, from 1720 till 1846 (see chapter 9). Sometimes the combination of subjects was unusual as in the case of Alexander Donaldson, who for 38 years held the Chairs of Medicine and Oriental languages in Aberdeen.[42] In 1850, at St. Andrew's University, Dr. William MacDonald was appointed Professor of Civil History on condition that he also taught Natural History, and some of his successors continued to do so.[43] Again, William Cullen (1710–1790) showed remarkable versatility in holding the Chair of Medicine, and at the same time giving lectures on Chemistry, Materia Medica, and Botany.[44] Botany, because of its association with plant remedies, was greatly emphasised, and Yale University will be taken as an example. Here, a College was first founded at Saybrook in 1700 and moved in 1718 to Newhaven. In 1810 a Medical Institution was added and the following professors appointed to teach the whole medical course, namely (1) Professor of Materia Medica and Botany, (2) an adjunct professor in the same subjects, (3) Professor of the Theory and Practice of Physic, Surgery and Obstetrics, (4) Professor of Anatomy and Physiology. Today two out of four professors would seem a decidedly generous allocation for Botany, but it indicates the importance of the subject at the time.[45]

The development of a full medical Course took many years to evolve for it required not only a University Faculty, but also a General Hospital where clinical teaching could be carried out. In general, these two arms of medical education seem to have developed in an unrelated way. In the case of the Scottish Schools the provision of a university course in medicine was complete by the early years of the 18th century, presumably as part of the general university development of the period. Large general hospitals tended to be built (except in the case of Edinburgh, which was already in existence) towards the end of the century – a tendency seen throughout England as part of the 18th century Age of Philanthropy.

REFERENCES

1 Billroth. T., 'The Medical Sciences of the German Universities'. Macmillan Co. 1924, pp. 37–8.
2 Comrie. J. D., 'History of Scottish Medicine' Vol II 1932, p. 607. Wellcome Historical Medical Museum. Balliere, Tindall & Cox.
3 Duvall. E. & Currie A., 'Edinburgh Dept. of Pathology, the first hundred years 1831–1931' Edinburgh University Press 1931, p.1.
4 Greenfield, W. S., 'British Medical Journal'. 1881, ii, p. 695.
5 Comrie, J. D., 'History of Scottish Medicine' Vol II 1932, p. 11. Wellcome Historical Medical Museum. Bailliere, Tindall & Cox.
6 'Lancet'. (1844) ii, pp. 37; 100.

7   Ibid (1844) i, p. 633.
8   Ibid (1844) i, p. 623.
9   Ibid (1844) ii, p. 363.
10  Palmer, J. F., 'The Works of John Hunter, FRS'. Vol. I. Longman, Rees, Orme, Brown, Green & Longman. 1835, pp. 230–1.
11  'Lancet' (1844) ii, p. 364.
12  Ibid (1845) i, p. 781.
13  Harrison, J. B., 'Lancet'. (1844) ii, p. 365.
14  'Lancet'. (1845) ii, p. 559.
15  Ibid (1846) i, pp. 521–3.
16  Ibid (1850) i, p. 683.
17  Ibid (1850) i, p. 684.
18  Harrison, J. B., 'Lancet'. (1850) i, p. 709.
19  'Lancet'. (1850) i, pp. 769–70.
20  Ibid (1850) ii, p. 194.
21  Ibid (1850) ii, pp. 193–200.
22  Ibid (1850) ii, p. 107.
23  'Lancet'. (1830–1) ii, pp. 86–8.
24  Ibid (1850) ii, p. 69.
25  Ibid (1850) ii, p. 109.
26  Ibid (1850) ii, p. 193.
27  Dict. Nat. Biography. 1927. pp. 75–6.
28  'Lancet'. (1850) ii, pp. 227–234.
29  Loraine Smith, J., 'British Medical Journal'. (1904) ii, p. 884.
30  Long, E. R., 'History of Pathology'. Williams & Williams Co., 1928, p. 213.
31  'British Medical Journal'. (1888) ii, p. 99.
32  Ibid (1801) ii, p. 272.
33  'Lancet'. (1895) ii, p. 311.
34  'British Medical Journal'. (1889) ii, pp. 615–6.
35  Ibid (1908) ii, p. 1130.
36  'Lancet'. (1896) ii, pp. 349–51.
37  'British Medical Journal'. (1896) i, pp. 1370; 1397.
38  Ibid (1884) ii, p. 259.
39  Dible, J. H., 'J. Path. Bact.' (1957) *73*. pp. 1–35.
40  Patey, D. H., 'The University Hospital'. 'Lancet'. (1957) i. pp. 420–2.
41  Underwood, E. A., 'Boerhaave's Men'. Edinburgh University Press, 1977, pp. 90–1.
42  Ibid p. 87.
43  'History of Scottish Universities'. Vol. 2. p. 580.
44  Guthrie, D., 'History of Medicine'. Thomas Nelson & Sons Ltd, 1945, pp. 222–3.

# SEVEN
# The continental background 1700–1870

We must now consider the spectacular development of the Continental Universities in the 18th and 19th centuries, which had a considerable effect in Britain. To understand how this came about it will be necessary for us to retrace our steps.

In the northern part of the old kingdom of Lotharingia, the Counts of Flanders had built up a province in the 10th and 11th centuries, which comprised the Holland and Belgium of today. It became an active trading area and seems to have been well in advance of the rest of Europe. Towns had sprung up and, by the beginning of the 14th century, included Bruges which was a flourishing port with a population of 35,000. There were others even larger, as for example Ghent and Ypres which had 60,000 and 30,000 inhabitants respectively. In 1648, when the Thirty Years War ended, the northern part of the province (Holland) was given her independence. The southern part (Belgium) was put under the Spaniards and became the 'Spanish Netherlands' until 1713, when they were transferred to the Austrian Habsburgs to become the 'Austrian Netherlands'. It was not until 1830 that Belgium was given independence. The new Dutch Republic flourished and had been granted control of the mouth of the river Scheldt. This had the effect of strangling the large port of Antwerp and resulted in its replacement by Rotterdam. It was just about this time that the Dutch Medical Schools entered their most fruitful period.

The main Dutch Universities with their dates of foundation were Leyden (1575), Groningen (1614), Amsterdam (1634), and Utrecht (1634). Such institutions were mostly city formations and located at centres which had enjoyed prosperous trade for some time.[1]

The influence of the University of Leyden on the teaching of Medicine was very great, especially in Britain. It began with Francesco Sylvius (1614–1672), the iatrochemical physician who first introduced clinical training in his medical course. By the early days of the 18th century it had attained great prominence, largely due to the famous physician, Hermann Boerhaave (1668–1738). As previously indicated, there was a close association between Edinburgh and Leyden. Boerhaave had studied Natural Philosophy and Divinity at Leyden before turning to Medicine and taking his MD degree at the University of Harderwyck in Holland in 1693. In 1701 he became a Reader in Medicine at the University of Leyden. He believed in the study of Medicine at the bedside and was consequently a great admirer of the English physician, Thomas Sydenham. The most outstanding features of his career were the number of students that he attracted to Leyden for study, and the influence that they subsequently exerted on other universities. Many students of Boerhaave's graduated at Leyden or Rheims, but there were many others who followed a course at Leyden and then took their degrees at Utrecht, Cambridge, Edinburgh, St. Andrew's, Dublin and Harderwyck.[2] When the medical faculty at Edinburgh was founded in 1726, all of the nine medical men associated with it had been pupils of Boerhaave, and five of these became the first professors, namely, Alexander Monro (primus), John Rutherford, Andrew St. Clair, Andrew Plummer, and John Innes. In 1736 the University of Göttingen was founded by Albrecht Von Haller, another pupil of Boerhaave's. Finally in 1745 two other pupils, Gerard Van Swieten and Anton de Haen, founded what is now known as the 'Old Vienna School'[3] and more of this will be mentioned later.[4]

Academic developments were influenced by Maria Theresa who, aided by the Pragmatic Sanction, had become Empress of Austria in 1740. She inherited problems which kept her at war for much of her reign, and also some enemies of which Frederick the Great was the most formidable. Her empire was heterogenous, but she did much to unite her several peoples and has been described as the first modern monarch of Austria. She had genuine concern for the welfare of her people, tried to alleviate suffering of the poor, and instituted reforms in taxation, finance, and legislation. By the time of the conclusion of the Seven Years War in 1763, her son Joseph, then 22 years of age, had shown some interest in the governing of the empire. As a result she decided to make him a co-regent in 1765 when her consort Francis of Lorraine died, and they reigned together until her death in 1780. They were not always of one mind, and there were important differences. Maria Theresa remained a devout Catholic till the end of her days, while Joseph strongly believed in religious freedom even though he received his earlier education from the Jesuits. He is believed to have influenced the Pope to abolish that Order – and this did nothing to narrow the gap between mother and son. Joseph was far ahead of his time and had admired the views of the 'philosophes' of the Enlightenment. With the death of his mother he pressed on hurriedly with a series of reforms. Believing that speed could only be achieved if carried out by one person, the remainder of his reign became that of an 'enlightened despot'. He was largely responsible for making education a secular matter and taking it out of the hands of the Church. In his later years his health deteriorated and in 1790 he died a disappointed man who felt that he had accomplished nothing.[5] He was twice married and in each instance smallpox proved fatal to his wife within a short time of the marriage. In later years Maria Theresa nearly died from the same disease, and these tragedies must have stimulated the physicians to consider inoculation which was being practised at the time. We know that in 1798 Jenner described vaccination with cowpox, and that it was tried on Joseph's three children by a public health officer, Pasqual Joseph Ferro (1753–1809), in 1799 in Vienna. It was the first time that vaccination had been carried out in a Continental city.[6]

But Maria Theresa, although much more conservative than her son, realised the need for improved education at both school and university level, and was agreeable to its being taken out of the hands of the clergy. Thus, in an attempt to advance medical education, she invited Gerhard Von Swieten (1710–1772), one of Boerhaave's best pupils at Leyden, to come to Vienna in 1745 as her personal physician. It does her credit that such a constructive step was taken while she was in the midst of the War of the Austrian Succession, but its importance was paramount as it led to the formation of what we now call the 'Old Vienna School'.

To understand the influence that Von Swieten exerted in Vienna, a few words must be said about the medical faculty at the time. It was really the relic of a mediaeval guild for it consisted not only of the academic teachers, but also all the medical practitioners of the city. This gave rise to two difficulties in that the university teachers could easily be outvoted on any matter, and the head of the faculty need not necessarily be a member of the academic staff. In fact, this latter position was occupied by the 'first physician' to the reigning monarch, and was sometimes referred to as the 'Protomedicus'. Holding this position he had a combination of offices, viz.:

(1) Head of the Faculty of the University
(2) Director of University studies
(3) Head of the public health of the Empire[7]

Thus, in his new position von Swieten did not lack authority. In 1749 he laid before the Empress his plan for a sweeping reorganisation of medical education.[8] With his Leyden background he naturally instituted clinical teaching and in 1754 opened a clinic at the city hospital or 'Burgespital' as it was called. It was a modest beginning for like Boerhaave's clinic in Leyden it consisted of twelve beds, six for men and six for women. To organise this aspect of the teaching von Swieten suggested that another of Boerhaave's pupils, Andon de Haen (1704–1776), be invited to join the staff. He himself presided over the clinic, conducted bedside tutorial sessions and also carried out the first routine autopsies before students. He encouraged careful observation and gave only the simplest treatment. The fame of the Vienna Clinic soon became known, and began to attract many foreign students. By 1772, when von Swieten died of senile gangrene the Vienna School was developing rapidly. His successor Anton Steorck (1731–1803) was noted as an administrator rather than a teacher, though he is remembered for his experiments on drugs and for being a great champion of emetics. By contrast de Haen's successor in 1776 was Maximilian Stoll (1742–1787), an able clinician and a brilliant teacher, and it was during his term of office that the Old Vienna School reached its zenith.[9] He had advanced views and favoured smallpox inoculation which had been strongly opposed by de Haen.[10] It is sad to relate that Stoll's life was cut short in 1787, when he died of cerebral haemorrhage.[11] However, he did live to see one of the greatest landmarks in Viennese medicine. The Emperor Joseph II, always interested in matters medical, gave help and encouragement to the establishment of a large general hospital, the Allgemeines Krankenhaus, which was opened in 1784. It included the 'Narrenturm' or tower for mental patients and also the Clinic which was now moved from the Burgespital. Progress did not stop here, for in the following year the Emperor opened the magnificent 'Academia medico-chirurgica Josephina' or the 'Josephinum'. This was provided for the training of competent military doctors and was given the rank of a university. In addition to the usual lecture rooms and library, there was a museum containing a fine collection of anatomical wax models which had been made in Florence.[12] Teaching had advanced considerably, a full medical course was available, and students were encouraged to visit France and England.

Administrative changes were in evidence, for in 1790 the Emperor Leopold II abolished the faculty directorates, and logically decided that the management and supervision of medical education should be the function solely of academic teachers.[13] Thus, what might be called the 'directoral despotism' of von Swieten's day came to an end. However, it did not last long for the successor of Stoeck, namely Joseph Andreas von Stifft (1760–1836), put the clock back by reviving the position of Protomedicus in 1803. It enabled him to extend his authority and ushered in a less happy period in Viennese medical history. Stifft was a hard-working and energetic man who had been a pupil of Stoll and one who followed his beliefs with avidity. He resented the current views of the time associated with Joseph II's reforms and therefore set forth on a 'restorative programme' which would recall the days of von Swieten. Having revived the office of Protomedicus, he felt that he had sufficient power to proceed with his aims. His first act was to revise the curriculum which he wished to make more difficult, and to reorganise it so that it closely resembled that originated by von Swieten. He took over public health responsibilities but soon found that in order to achieve his ambitions there were certain figures whom he did not like and of whom he must rid himself.

This brings us to one of the most outstanding characters of the Vienna School, Johann Peter Frank (1745–1821). Stoll had been succeeded by Jacob von Rheinlein, whose lack of competence was shown by the rapid decline in the attendance of students at the Clinic, and in 1795 he was relieved of his duties.[14] In that year he was followed by Johann Peter Frank, a native of the Bavarian Palatinate who had studied at Heidelberg and Strasbourg prior to becoming professor at Gottingen. At Heidelberg he had first become interested in public hygiene and had written a work of six volumes, the first of which appeared in 1789. It covered such subjects as water supply, sewerage, school hygiene, and his idea for a scientific 'medical police'. He came to Vienna to be Director of the Josephinum, but on arrival was made Director of the Allgemeines Krankenhaus and the Medical Clinic. He was an immediate success. He was an excellent teacher and the prestige of the Clinic was soon restored. He made many improvements in the hygiene of the city, and by the beginning of the 19th century the terms 'forensic medicine' and 'medical police' had been combined into 'State Medicine'. It is ironical that he was never allowed to teach this subject in Vienna. Frank's lectures in Vienna were soon to have some serious repercussions. John Brown (1735–1788), the wine-loving Scotsman, had recently propounded his new theory of disease, which stated that disease was not due to a change in body fluids (the humoral theory), but was related to a force in the body known as 'excitability'. Disease could be due either to too much or too little stimulation of the excitability and could therefore be treated by the appropriate drug. The theory became known as Brunonianism and it was badly received by the Viennese who were highly suspicious of hypotheses. Many must have been shocked when Frank, as the new Director, showed himself to be in sympathy. In spite of this the theory claimed a number of supporters, including a group of doctors at the Josephinum who at the time had founded a Society of Physicians. Under their leadership, the support for Brunonianism was increasing. Amongst its greatest opponents was Stifft, who regarded it as 'medical Jacobinism' and went out of his way to discredit it. This brought him into collision with Frank, and he even tried to prove that there had been higher mortality figures in the Allgemeines Krankenhaus since Frank took over. Relations between Frank and Stifft had never been cordial, but they steadily grew worse and in 1804 Frank, very disillusioned, decided to leave Vienna. Brunonianism did not last long in Europe, but it did leave its mark in Vienna. Frank seems to have thought less and less of it as the years went by.

At about the same time certain differences arose between Stifft and a capable young surgeon, Johann Nepomuk Rust (1775–1840), who as a result left Vienna. There were others of whom two must be mentioned.

Franz Joseph Gall (1757–1828), a friend of Frank, suffered persecution at the hands of Stifft. A native of Swabia, he had been educated at Rastatt and Strasbourg prior to graduating in Vienna. He introduced a new science of the skull which he called 'organology' and which was later referred to by his pupil Spurzheim as 'phrenology'. In a period when physical examination was in vogue palpation of the skull did not seem unreasonable. He was encouraged by Frank and given facilities by him to examine mental patients in the Narrenturm of the Allgemeines Krankenhaus. Although regarded by many as a charlatan, he had carried out some good neurological studies on the cranial nerve nuclei, and thus was responsible for some of the earliest studies of 'localisation' within the brain. At last weary of Vienna, he went to Paris in 1805 with his pupil Spurzheim. There he was well received and was very successful. He stayed there for the rest of his life and died a very rich man.

Brief mention should also be made of Franz A. Mesmer, a graduate of Vienna who soon became widely known for his theory of 'animal magnetism'. This caused suspicion and he too was soon regarded as a charlatan. In 1778 Maria Theresa appointed a Commission to investigate his claims. These were discredited and he was given 24 hours to leave the city.[15] Like Gall he went to Paris where he was well received.

But the Old Vienna School had also produced some outstanding figures, the chief of whom were Georg Prochanska (Anatomist and Physiologist), Georg Joseph Beer (Ophthalmologist), Lucas Johann Boer (Obstetrician), Vincent von Kern (Surgeon), and Valentin von Hilderbrand (Physician).

It is sometimes said that the New Vienna School began with the foundation of the Allgemeines Krankenhaus in 1784. By that time the Faculty of the Old School had become famous in Europe. There followed a period of decline before the New School came to fruition. In the intervening years the School at Paris came to lead European Medicine and maintained this position till mid-19th Century. Strangely enough, an Austrian was to make a significant contribution to this advance. An innkeeper's son, Leopold Auenbrugger (1722–1809), graduated in Vienna, where he became a practising physician and was on the staff of the Spanish Hospital. In 1761 he published a 95 page article on percussion. The uncharitable de Haen sneered at the idea, and although it was noted by a few individuals it was not generally thought to be important. Stoll introduced the method into his clinic but failed to realise its value. Finally Corvisant, Napoleon's physician, ran across the article accidentally about 1788. Having used the technique for 20 years he published his findings, together with Auenbrugger's original paper. Now, with Laennec's stethoscope it became an important contribution to Clinical Medicine in Paris. Some years were to elapse before the New Vienna School reached its peak with names such as Rokitansky and Skoda in the 1840's and by this time French medicine was on the wane.

Since the days of Boerhaave there had been many changes. One striking feature of the 18th century was the rapid population growth accompanied by the increased number and size of the towns. It was also a period when large hospitals were built and we read of the great overcrowding of such institutions in Paris. Here, compared with the days of Boerhaave, medicine came to be practised on a much larger scale. The famous French physician Bouillard could claim to have seen 25,000 cases in five years.[16] Attempts were being made to correlate not only symptoms but also the new physical signs with autopsy findings. This was particularly so in the new Allgemeines Krankenhaus in Vienna where about 14,000 patients were being treated per year.[17] With the Paris Schools and the New Vienna School adopting similar methods it is interesting to consider why the latter advanced and the former declined. As will be seen it lay in the difference of the practise of Pathological Anatomy. In Paris this was carried out by the clinicians themselves or by their assistants. In Vienna it had become a separate discipline and obviously assistants appointed solely for this special work could handle much more material more effectively. There was also more centralisation in the large Allgemeines Krankenhaus which provided autopsies in plenty.[18]

From the time of von Swieten and de Haen, it was customary for physicians to be their own prosectors for autopsy material. When Frank came to Vienna in 1795 and saw the wealth of pathological material he immediately appointed a prosector to deal with it. Alois Rudolph Vetter became the first full-time voluntary prosector and he was also given charge of the Museum. For the promotion of Pathology he was an ideal choice. He had studied medicine at Innsbruck and Vienna and after graduation had given some instruction in autopsy technique.[19] His basic training had been good and in 1788 he published a Manual of Anatomy; this was followed by a similar work on Physiology in 1794. He enjoyed his association with Frank, performed several autopsies within the next seven years and increased the number of museum specimens from 4 to 400. With such training it is not surprising that he became interested in two cases of gastric fistula which had been described by Jacob Anton Helm (1761–1831).[20,21] Of these cases one was traumatic and had healed satisfactorily; the other was spontaneous and the patient died some five years later. During this time Helm made observations and carried out experiments on both himself and his patient. Vetter continued his work and in 1803 published his 'Aphorisms on Pathological Anatomy'. He never received the appreciation that he deserved, though Hyrtl, a most outstanding anatomist of the time, said he was 'the first thinker in Pathological Anatomy'.[22] But Vetter was not happy for he felt that he was not receiving the cooperation from his colleagues that he needed. Worse still, he was beset by bureaucratic irritation and envy from other staff members. He left Vienna in 1803 to be Professor of Anatomy and Physiology at the University of Cracow. There his health broke down and he died in 1806 at the early age of 41 of pulmonary tuberculosis.

With Frank gone and Stifft in control as Protomedicus, the post of Prosector lapsed. In 1806 Valentin von Hildebrand (1763–1818) was appointed Professor of Internal Medicine and Director of the Clinic. He had been a pupil of Stoll and a fellow student with Stifft. He proved to be the most outstanding of Frank's successors and soon revived the Annual Reports of the Clinic which had not been issued since the death of Stoll. As one of Stoll's students he realised the value of Pathological Anatomy. It was therefore to his credit that in 1811 he persuaded Stifft (possibly with support from Türkheim)[23] to create a Prosectorship which would be salaried. In 1812 Lorenz Biermayer was appointed and worked to such good purpose that he produced a Museum Catalogue in 1816. This earned him a reappointment for 4 years, responsibility for forensic autopsies in 1818, and a promotion to Assistant Professor of Pathology in 1821. For four years all went well and he was given an assistant, Johann Wagner (1800–1832). Then Biermayer became discouraged as had Vetter, and commenced to neglect his duties. He became an alcoholic and was dismissed in 1829. It was now left to Wagner, aided by a young unpaid student apprentice who had joined him in November 1827, to continue the work of the department. Wagner died after 3 years at the age of 32, and was succeeded by his student-assistant, Carl Rokitansky (1804–1878), who became Assistant Professor in 1832 and Professor in 1834. In his short life Wagner had shown himself to be a very skillful dissector, and with him Rokitansky learned the autopsy technique which was to prove so useful to him in his subsequent career. He had studied at the universities of Prague and Vienna, and had been greatly influenced by the work of Martin Lobstein (Strasbourg), Gabriel Andral (Paris), and Johann Frederick Meckel the Younger (Halle), a Comparative Anatomist and Pathologist.

The teaching of Pathological Anatomy was first instituted in 1819 when Biermayer gave lectures on the subject at the General Hospital.[24] This led to the appointment of a Professor of Pathological Anatomy and the way it occurred is described because a similar pattern was followed later in other universities. In 1812, a new pathological museum had been founded and a permanent Prosector appointed.[25] One of the duties of the latter was to provide demonstrations of Pathological Anatomy in the Clinic. Rokitansky became Assistant Prosector to Johann Wagner in 1830 and Prosector in 1834. At that time the post became upgraded to Assistant Professor and eleven years later Rokitansky became Full Professor of General Pathology. As such, Rokitansky taught General and Special Pathology but the real strength of his department lay in Pathological Anatomy and the enormous numbers of autopsies which it handled. His contribution to this subject cannot be overestimated and his 'Manual of Pathological Anatomy' became the classical text of the day. The first volume of this work, which was published last (1846) and dealt with General Pathology, contained one very unfortunate error. In his attempt to reconcile humoral pathology with the recent cellular theories, he had expressed his belief in the 'blastema' theory of Schleiden and Schwann, which Virchow denounced in his two articles in the 'Berline Medizinische Zeitung' in December of the same year. There is one other criticism which has been levelled at Rokitansky and is related to the fact that his knowledge was based on about 30,000 autopsies. Because he saw mostly the end stage of disease his attitude towards Pathology was pessimistic and he often failed to appreciate the earlier stages in the disease process.

We must now return to the Annual Reports issued from the Clinic in Vienna. As already mentioned these had ceased with the death of Stoll and been later resumed by Hildebrand. They now included details of the patients in the 24 beds of Hildebrand's Clinic. Rokitansky, when appointed, found a vast amount of autopsy material at his disposal and was soon including articles on various aspects of Pathology in these Annual Reports. He had performed thousands of autopsies and his approach to the subject was strictly anatomical. He classified the lesions in this vast amount of material and by 1840 an Institute of Pathology had grown up. Wunderlich (1815–1877), the Tübingen physician, had been much impressed at the School of Paris in 1837 but at least as much by the School of Vienna which he visited two years later. As a result he published a book intended to be a students' guide for further studies at these places. William Wilde (1815–1876), the famous Irish Ophthalmologist and Aural Surgeon, visited Vienna and spoke of the School of Pathological Anatomy and the Museum as being the best in Europe.[26] This was certainly true, for during the 1840s students from many European countries were flocking to the University. The New Vienna Medical School had surpassed the fame of its predecessor.

Rokitansky's contribution to the School had been considerable, but there had been others, including a physician who worked in close association with him. Joseph Skoda (1805–1881), like Rokitansky, came from Bohemia, had studied in Vienna, and had become very interested in the use of physical signs as introduced by the Paris physicians. Not content with their empirical approach he investigated the exact method of production. He eventually became Professor of Clinical Medicine in 1846, seven years after the publication of his monograph on 'Percussion and Auscultation'.[27] He was always more interested in diagnosis then in treatment and this was doubtless the reason for the accusation of his being a 'therapeutic nihilist'. At this time in Vienna, a number of physicians had become sceptical of the value of drugs given therapeutically, hence the term. It seems that this was more correctly applicable to Skoda's assistants, one of the best of whom, Joseph Dietl (1804–1878), had been particularly outspoken.[28] In spite of this it was unfortunate that many of the attacks on nihilism were levelled at Skoda. But apart from this he was a good diagnostician and teacher and did much to attract students to the Vienna School.

In 1811 a student of Frank's attained prominence when given public health duties as well as being made Vice-Director of Medical Studies at the Faculty.[29] His name was Ludwig von Türkheim (1777–1846) and he was destined to play a prominent part in the further evolution of the School. Stifft had died in 1836 and been succeeded as Protomedicus by his brother-in-law, Johann Nepomuk Raimann (1780–1847), who appears to have done little. With his new appointments Türkheim had the opportunity to show his remarkable organisational ability and this earned him, according to Skoda, the title of 'the second von Swieten'. He systematically replanned the medical curriculum, but he never saw it put into force for he died in 1846, two years before the reforms which followed the revolution of 1848. At that time Türkheim's draft plan of 1845 was submitted by Ernst Baron von Feuchtersleben (1806–1849) with only minor alterations. These proposed reforms carried with them the slogan 'Freedom of Teaching and Freedom of Learning'. This is only one aspect of Türkheim's achievements for he also did much to develop the Clinic at the General Hospital. By forming the Vienna Society of Physicians in 1837 he promoted unity amongst staff members. In 1840 he established, for Skoda, a department for chest diseases occurring in the poor. In 1842 he enabled Ferdinand Von Hebra (1816–1880), one of the foremost teachers, to conduct clinical courses on skin diseases. In 1844 Rokitansky was made a Full Professor and Pathological Anatomy was given the status of a regular chair. He played a part in establishing Heller's Chemical Pathology laboratory, and in 1846 founded a neurological department for Ludwig Turck (1810–1868). These are just a few examples of the way in which the Clinic developed. Many departments made use of the pathological material classified by Rokitansky.[30] At the same time academic staff had been expanding, and it was all of these special clinics which by 1874 made Vienna the leading centre in Europe for postgraduate study.[31]

The progress of Pathology and Rokitansky must now be studied further. By now his department had become the leading one in Europe for Pathology, and in the years 1842–1846, his famous three-volume work was published. It was a classic and two of the volumes were devoted to pathological anatomy based on an enormous experience of autopsy material. He had really transplanted the French version of clinico-pathological study into Vienna. But although the use of the microscope was being advocated by people like Hughes Bennett in Edinburgh, Rokitansky appears to have used it little, though we do know that on a visit to Paris in 1842 he returned with a Brunner microscope. He realised that all pathology could not be explained on an anatomical basis. There were many cases in which the paucity of anatomical findings simply could not account for the severity of the clinical symptoms – and these were sometimes known as 'dynamic diseases'. As a supporter of humoral pathology he proposed his theory of 'crases'. The blood was everywhere in the body so the changes must be present there. There might be alterations in the fibrin or albumin content. He therefore believed that the solution to the problem would be a chemical one, and it was for this reason that the chemical laboratory was set up. In it John Florian Heller carried out tests not only on blood, but on other body secretions such as urine, sweat, sputa, and faeces. He also suggested that the 'crasis' might become localised and thus involve a single organ. It was all highly speculative.

Volumes II and III of Rokitansky's great work appeared first. They dealt with pathological anatomy and were acclaimed by all, including the young German pathologist, Rudolf Virchow. Volume I appeared last and contained the theory of 'crases'. At the time when Rokitansky was preparing his book, the cellular theory of Schleiden and Schwann was announced in 1839. In describing cells which Schleiden had observed in plant and Schwann in animal tissues, they also proposed their 'blastemia' theory. According to this, cells could be formed in a primitive, protein-rich fluid and of course this started afresh the arguments of the previous century on spontaneous generation. This was unfortunate as Rokitansky, encouraged by his enthusiastic assistant, Joseph Engel (1816–1899), introduced the idea of a 'blastema' which was responsible for producing changes which would account for the large number of 'crases' which had been described.[32] If this were so, then further elucidation of 'crases' would be achieved by chemical examination of the blood and other body secretions – and this was the work that Heller set out to do in his new laboratory of chemical pathology.

Such a speculative theory was bound to cause controversy but it also excited severe criticism from the young 26-year-old pathologist in Berlin, Rudolf Virchow 1821–1903). He pointed out that Rokitansky had tried to explain matters of anatomy by matters of chemistry. The destruction of the theory was so complete that in subsequent editions of the book, Rokitansky did not reprint the disputed passages. From now onwards the work of Virchow would grow ever more prominent and German Medicine would take over the lead in Europe.

At the beginning of the 19th century, German Medicine, still struggling with the problems of 'nature philosophy', lagged far behind France. With the rise of the New Vienna School, it became customary for young medical men to complete their education by visiting Paris and Vienna, and this included a number from Germany. The second half of the century saw the rise of a number of centres in Germany, many stemming from the work of Virchow and his pupils and their extensive use of the light microscope. There were also advances in knowledge of the Basic Sciences, especially Pathology and Physiology.

These advances were closely linked with a remarkably rapid development of the university centres. Before dealing with the German scientists of the period, it will be necessary to examine the factors which contributed to this surprising university advance, and the essentially German institution, the University Hospital.

Some of the German Universities were of relatively ancient foundation, as for instance, Heidelberg in 1386 and Leipzig in 1409. A medical faculty was formed in Heidelberg in 1387 and in Leipzig in 1415. A greater number had a Medical Faculty at the time of their foundation, as for example, Greifswald (1456), Freiburg (1457), Basel (1460), Tübingen (1477), Marburg (1529), Jena (1558), Wurzburg (1582), Gratz (1585), and Giessen (1607).[33] These early universities were originally private institutions, but were very much under the influence of the Church. In fact, until 1482 all medical teachers had to be members of the clergy. Gradually many universities lost their independence and after the 17th century many had become state institutions, but in spite of this development they had several favourable features. They were relatively well supported, the teachers had academic freedom, and the students were given a free choice in selecting their courses and instructors. It was characteristic of the German student that his medical training might be obtained in half a dozen schools. In general each university had four Faculties, namely Theology, Law, Medicine, and Philosophy. In this way the German Universities developed, but medical thought tended to lag behind the leader of Europe, namely France. Elsewhere it has been explained that French Medicine progressed rapidly by means of an empirical approach, whilst the Germans stagnated by attempting to establish a universal and systematic solution to medical problems which was confused by metaphysical theories and Vitalism. It was not until the 19th century that Germany was to make some spectacular advances, which were related to European political events, and these must be briefly outlined.

It has often been said that the history of Germany is the history of Prussia which, by 1786 when Frederick the Great died, had become a considerable power in Continental Europe. The two factors which brought this about were a succession of strong rulers and the development of a very efficient military machine. But two weak rulers followed Frederick the Great, namely Kings William II and III, and with a growing complacency in the Army Prussia entered into a period of decline. Frederick William III was only 27 when he became King in 1797 and there were high hopes for the success of his reign. He had many admirable personal qualities but when it came to making political decisions he proved to be sadly lacking. He could not make up his mind and his policy of neutrality in regard to Coalitions in the Napoleonic Wars was the result of vacillation which was to cost Prussia dear. When he finally did decide to join the Russians against the French Emperor, the Prussian forces sustained a most humiliating defeat at the Battle of Jena in 1806. The harshness of the terms of the Peace Treaty of Tilsit which followed included a loss of about half the territory and population of Prussia, in addition to a heavy indemnity (120 million francs) to pay for the French occupation, and led to a phase of pessimism not altogether surprising. Much of the unity which had been gained in the past was now lost, and the policy of Napoleon was calculated to make it worse. He had encouraged the kingdoms of the south, namely Bavaria, Baden, and Wurttemberg, with their Catholic population, and deliberately thwarted the unity of Protestant Prussia in the north. As a result the former showed no reluctance to be under the aegis of the French. By his action he was aiming at making Prussia a Hohenzollern kingdom of the north, which would effectively neutralise the Austrian Habsburg kingdom in the south and so discourage unity amongst the Germans as a whole. Apart from geographical considerations there was little unity of thought amongst the Germans. Those who favoured the views of the Enlightment naturally turned to France as the leader of that movement, whilst the romantics looked towards Habsburg Vienna. Also it was obvious that many Germans were little concerned with what might happen to their fellow countrymen in Prussia. It was a time of considerable confusion amongst German-speaking peoples and the future held out many possibilities.[34]

If lack of unity had been at the root of German troubles it could not be overcome until national consciousness resulted from a national movement. Soon this appeared in Prussia, mostly brought about by anti-French feeling as a result of the severe terms of the Treaty of Tilsit.

Thus, by 1813 the struggle against the French started with the War of Liberation. It is often referred to as the Prussian Reform movement and its thought was made up of several ingredients, including: (1) ideas from the Enlightenment; (2) the idealistic philosophy of Kant and his successors; (3) theories and practices of the French Revolution; and (4) anti-French feeling which stimulated German patriotism. These developments owe much to one of the greatest of German philosophers, Johann Gottlieb Fichte (1762–1814). He emphasised the importance of education but, as will be seen later, Wilhelm von Humboldt was the one most responsible for the new educational developments of this Reform era. Fichte had been Professor of Philosophy at Jena but came to Berlin in 1799, and gave regular courses of public lectures for several years. In his earlier years he felt that his views were in line with the new France but by 1806, disillusioned by the French conquest, he became a German patriot. His lectures in Berlin aroused national consciousness in Prussia, and led to an enthusiasm which replaced the existing pessimistic mood. It is significant that he addressed his lectures, not to the Prussian people, but to the German nation.[35] Patriotic feelings was also stimulated in the literature of the time, especially by the greatest dramatist amongst the Romantics, Heinrich von Kleist, who since 1807 had lived in Dresden, a centre of anti-French sentiment. Historians of law, such as Savigny and Eichhorn, also lent their support. Friedrich Ludwig Jahn, a lesser political figure, organised corps of national volunteers who later fought in the wars of Liberation. After the Treaty of Vienna (1815), when Metternich was striving to suppress nationalism and to restore the *status quo*, Jahn kept Nationalism alive in German by his activity in the nationalist student associations, the 'Burschenschaften.'[36]

When the era of Reform came about there were three outstanding figures, Stein, Hardenburg, and Wilhelm von Humboldt. Heinrich Friedrich Karl Baron von Stein (1757–1831) was probably the greatest of the three. He studied law and political science, attending in part at the University of Göttingen, where he learned English history and became interested in English political institutions. He did not practice law, but entered the Civil Service and eventually, in 1807, became first minister to King Frederick William III. His task of instituting reforms must have been the most difficult that he had ever faced, for at the time the social and economic structure was entirely feudal. The most immediate problem he faced was that of finance, as money had to be raised to pay the large indemnity levied by the French under the terms of the Treaty of Tilsit. In a short space of time he instituted a number of social, economic and administrative reforms and emancipated the peasants. He made municipal reforms and relieved the towns from control by feudal lords and by the central government. But with his work half done he was dismissed by Napoleon in 1808 and the remainder was left to be completed by his successor. Stein was a German patriot and had much in common with Fichte, though surprisingly he was quite prepared for a foreign power, especially if it was Great Britain, to assume the role of guardian of German integrity.

Stein was succeeded by Carl August von Hardenburg (1750–1822), who was a Hanoverian, and an aristocrat of the *ancien regime*. In spite of this he was able to absorb ideas from the French Revolution and was in fact more radical than his predecessor. His foreign policy was related solely to Prussian considerations. He owed much of his success to his quality of diplomacy, conspicuously absent in Stein, and in this way was able to guide the King to his way of thinking.

By its complacency the Army had declined and had suffered a resounding defeat in 1806 at the Battle of Jena. Now it was due for reform and this was brought about by two distinguished soldiers. Gerhard von Scharnhorst (1755–1813) was born in Hanover and served in the army of the Electorate in the campaigns of 1793–4, but in 1801 transferred to the Prussian forces. He wrote on military topics and became a Professor in the Military Academy in Berlin. He fought at Jena, and after the Peace became the head of the military administration in Stein's 'Ministry'. August Neithardt von Gneisenau (1760–1831), like Scharnhorst, had fought at Jena. Born in Saxony he had entered the service of the emperor, though later he was among the German mercenaries hired by England for service against the American colonies. He had a distinguished career and took part in the defeat of Napoleon at the battle of Leipzig, finally attaining the rank of Field Marshal. He was a member of Scharnhorst's Commission for the reorganisation of the Prussian Army, and these two soldiers did much to prepare it for the part that it would play in the wars of Liberation.

In 1809 the matter of education was placed in the hands of Karl Wilhelm Baron von Humboldt (1767–1835), a Prussian and the brother of Alexander, a famous traveller. He was a scholar of great distinction and a friend of many literary men and intellectuals, including Schiller. Appointed Head of the Department of Cultural Affairs he, like Stein, held office for only a year, though in this short time he achieved a great deal. His thoughts were based on ideas of the Enlightenment and Kantian idealism. Like Stein, he was anxious to emancipate the peasant class, and he also aimed at increasing the number of educated citizens who might be able to take part in local government affairs. He reformed education at all levels, elementary, secondary, and university. He was most concerned with the highest form of secondary education which was given in the Gymnasium. This type of school was staffed with university-trained teachers, and those who wanted to attend university had to pass a 10-year course at the Gymnasium commencing at the age of 10.[37] University education was at a low ebb and by the Treaty of Tilsit, Prussia had lost its best university at Halle. Of the remainder Königsberg was too remote, and Frankfurt-on-the-Oder was inadequately endowed. Von Humboldt therefore founded the University of Berlin in 1809 and it is for this that he is chiefly remembered,[38] though Fichte, Schleiermacher, and Stein had all contributed ideas. This university was planned to be different and would pursue pure knowledge, recognise the unity of knowledge, and have freedom to teach and pursue research and to ensure interchange between teachers and research workers. To the traditional faculties of Theology, Law, and Medicine were added subjects such as History, Linguistics, Natural Sciences and Philosophy with equal status. A promising start was made by the recruitment of such distinguished men to the staff as Fichte, Schleiermacher, Niebuhr, and Savigny. In 1817 Hegel (1770–1831), the eminent philosopher, was invited to Berlin where his presence attracted large numbers of students.

The most important features of the new university were its insistence on the unity of knowledge and the pursuit of it for its own sake. It was not a new idea for it had been encouraged in the later 18th century at universities such as Göttingen where both Humboldt and Stein had studied. An exchange of information between members of the academic staff was encouraged. This was particularly important in the Faculty of Medicine, where basic science was liable to be divorced from clinical teaching. Now at Berlin, the university remedied this defect by locating the University Hospital in close proximity to the University, setting a pattern for German medicine for the next 100 years.

The pattern of development of German Medicine was in general based on that in Vienna. But there were many differences in the atmosphere of Austria and Germany. In the latter, following the Wars of Liberation and the defeat of Napoleon, a spirit of optimism had suddenly appeared. The approach to learning had become more practical compared with that of the last century and was now 'natural scientific' rather than 'natural philosophical'. The new Berlin University, founded in 1809 largely through the activities of Alexander von Humboldt, provided an example which would later be followed in many other German towns. Many of these were either State institutions or at least in receipt of state support, and as such faced a dual challenge. As a school, they needed to provide doctors, teachers, and lawyers for the community; as universities, they should advance knowledge of their subject. To provide for the latter, students had to realise the importance of research and to be familiar with its methods. It became established that a Professor should not only teach research but was also required to be engaged in active research himself. The triumph of German medical education lay in the University Hospital where both types of instruction could go on side by side.

It was a period of very rapid growth of the Natural Science subjects and their value as a preliminary to Medicine was becoming realised. In past times any such teaching had been purely theoretical, but the day had arrived for practical instruction. For this to occur, independent laboratories became necessary and the dates on which they were first founded in Germany are of some interest: in 1814, Anatomy at Breslau; in 1824, Physiology at Breslau; in 1825, Chemistry at Giessen; in 1849, Pharmacology at Dorpat; in 1856, Pathology at Berlin.[39]

In the earliest days of the University Medical Faculty, it was customary to appoint two Professors of Medicine, one to teach the Principles of the subject and the other the Practice of it. In some centres the former became known as 'The Institutes' and included Anatomy, Physiology, General Pathology and General Therapeutics. The date for the foundation of the Physiological Institute is probably incorrect. Purkinje went to Breslau in 1823 as Professor and set up a small laboratory in his house. It was not until 1842 that the Prussian Government erected an Institute.[40] As knowledge accumulated it became necessary to divide off some of them. In some instances Physiology joined with Anatomy as one subject, and similarly Pathology with Therapeutics; in others, Physiology was linked to General Pathology and some lectures on the History of Medicine added; in yet others, a separate Chair of Physiology was founded. This last change occurred much later and it is interesting to note that the great Johannes Muller (1801–1858), usually referred to as a physiologist, occupied a Chair in Berlin which up to 1850 had included Anatomy, Physiology, Pathology, and Embryology.[41]

During the formative years, the new German University schools had trained many scientific workers with a real enthusiasm for research. Now was the time for them to apply the latest basic scientific techniques to the problems of Medicine. By employing the methods of Physics, Chemistry, and Microscopy, rapid advances in Physiology and Pathology resulted and these furthered the progress of Clinical Medicine later in the century. Mention of a few of the outstanding workers will illustrate the way in which all this occurred.

It will be suitable to commence with Johannes Muller, a Rhinelander of humble origin. He became the greatest teacher of the 19th century and was the originator of the meteoric rise of German Medicine. As a pupil of the well-known physiologist Rudolphi, he succeeded his master as Professor at the University of Berlin. Knowledgeable in all branches of science, he directed his students into many fertile fields of research to which as we shall see, they made substantial contributions. In spite of this, he made no major discovery himself, though his name has been perpetuated in embryological circles because of the Mullerian duct. He was farsighted enough to realise that Anatomy had made its contribution to Medicine, and that the future lay elsewhere. As a result he became one of the first to advocate the use of the microscope in Pathology. This was in 1830 and by 1833 his studies enabled him to produce his 'Manual of Human Physiology'. Stimulated by his pupil Schwann's work on the cellular structure of tissues, he embarked in 1836 on a study of the histological appearances of tumours. This resulted in his volume, 'On the finer structure and form of Morbid Tumours' in 1838, but the whole work which he had planned was never completed. A voluminous writer, he published papers on an amazing variety of subjects in addition to founding Muller's Archives, a series of annual reports on all branches of anatomical and physiological science. As a leader of the Natural Sciences in Germany and one with very advanced ideas, surprisingly he remained a confirmed 'vitalist' throughout his life.

Amongst his most outstanding students were Theodor Schwann (1810–1882), Jacob Henle (1809–1855), Hermann Helmholtz (1821–1894), and greatest of all, Rudolf Virchow (1821-1902). Schwann had discovered pepsin in the gastric juice and yeast as the active agent in fermentation. But following his master, his real interest was in microscopy and in 1839 he became well known for his cell theory which he proposed with his botanist friend Matthias Jacob Schleiden (1804–1881). This was a great step forward and it maintained that all tissues, both animal and vegetable, were composed of cells. It was unfortunate that they went further with the ill-fated 'blastema theory' which Virchow demolished some years later. Henle too was a devotee of Schwann's microscopy. He worked with Muller in Bonn and Berlin before becoming Professor of Anatomy at Zuerich, Heidelberg, and finally Göttingen. He was the first to describe the structure of epithelium (1837) and subsequently wrote a standard text on Histology. In advance of his time, he suggested that a living agent might be the cause of 'fevers' at a time when the theory of 'miasma and contagion' was generally accepted.

There were two other men notable at this early stage for their microscopical observations. Robert Remak (1815–1865) from Posen was the favourite pupil of Schönlein at the Charité Hospital in Berlin. In his studies of the structure of the central nervous system he had in 1838 first described the presence of non-medullated nerve fibres. In 1845 an interest in embryology led to his discovery of the primary germ layers (ectoderm, endoderm, and mesoderm). Seven years later, he recognised that the enlargement of tissues was produced by cellular proliferation and not from the 'blastema' of Schleiden and Schwann.[42] The other worker was Johannes Evangelista Purkinje (1787–1869), and in studying his life one is struck not only by the number of scientific observations that he made but by their early date. A Czech from Bohemia, he studied Philosophy and Physics prior to developing an interest in Physiology when he became an assistant in the department of Anatomy at the University of Prägue. Rudolphi in Berlin, knowing of his ability, was influential in his appointment in 1823 to the Chair of Physiology in Breslau and in 1827 he married Rudolphi's daughter, Julia. His early work was on the sense organs, chiefly on subjective visual phenomena and on vertigo. He believed in accurate observation in his pursuit of physiology and he carried out many experiments on himself and animals, some of which included the toxic effects of drugs such as digitalis and belladonna. One surprising product of his early work was the classification of fingerprint patterns. In 1832 he obtained an achromatic microscope and from that moment histology became his main interest. Using living tissue, he and Gabriel Valentin (1810–1883) described ciliary motion in higher animals. In his new institute he and his pupils investigated the structure of skin, bone, cartilage, and gastric glands. In the central nervous system he showed that nerve fibres were not hollow tubes, and his name is still attached to the large flask-like cells of the cerebellum as well as to some specialised cells in cardiac muscle. In 1850 he returned to Prage to be Professor of Physiology, but spent most of his later years promoting scientific education amongst his fellow countrymen.

Surveying this remarkable field of work by Purkinje, one wonders how it could have been achieved with methods of tissue preparation which were decidedly primitive at the time, namely 1832–1850. We know that by adding acetic acid the cell nuclei were better visualised and it is said that his assistant Oschatz designed a microtome for cutting sections. But it was many years before W. His (senior) (1831–1904) brought his instrument into general use and it was not perfected until 1875. It is said that Purkinje also used methods of hardening, fixation, and staining as well as the use of Canada balsam for embedding.[43] This may be so but it is generally stated that hardening agents and stains were not in general use until 1847. It was then that Joseph von Gerlach senior (1820–1896) injected capillaries with carmine, which he also used as a nuclear stain in 1855. Most important of all, it is said that Virchow used this stain for practically all his work. The technique of staining is of importance for it developed dramatically in the next 30 years and this period coincided with the ascendancy of German pathology. The basic event occurred in 1856 when Perkin, the young English chemist, accidentally made the first aniline dye when attempting to synthesise quinine. The aniline dye industry flourished rapidly in Germany and a young pathologist found that some of the dyes were suitable for histological staining. This was Carl Weigert (1845–1904) who, first taught by Virchow in Berlin and then by Cohnheim in Leipzig, made a classical study of tissue degenerations. He extended the use of these dyes and was the first to stain bacteria with them. His basic work was taken up by his famous cousin, Paul Ehrlich (1854–1915), under whom it reached full fruition. It is significant that a number of methods devised at the time are still in use today.

It will now be necessary to trace the career of Rudolf Virchow (1821–1902) who was destined to become the 'Father of Pathology'. Due to his great contribution, German Pathology became foremost in Europe.

Virchow became a medical student at the University of Berlin, and we last met him as a pupil of Johannes Muller in company with Du Bois Reymond, Brucke, and Helmholtz. He graduated in 1843 and subsequently worked at the Charité where he studied Chemistry with Linde and assisted the prosector Robert Froriep (1804–1861), whom he succeeded in 1846. Virchow was not long attracting attention for in 1845 he performed an autopsy which led to his description of leukaemia. Froriep had advised him to investigate Cruveilhier's theory that phlebitis was the basis of most of pathology and his classical study of thrombosis and embolism followed. It has sometimes been erroneously stated that Virchow's contribution was confined to pathological anatomy. Great advances had been made in this subject by the classical studies of Rokitansky, but relatively little using microscopical techniques. The other aspect of Pathology, i.e., the general principles or 'General Pathology', had made little progress and workers such as Virchow faced many puzzling problems. He soon realised that abnormal function was an important factor in explaining disease and to detect this more than the technique of one discipline would be needed. In 1845 he had been invited to give an oration and chose for his title, 'On the Need and Correctness of a Medicine based on a Mechanistic Approach'. In it he suggests that future research should be based on

(1) clinical observation (including physical and chemical examination)
(2) animal experiment
(3) necropsy (including microscopy)

He now believed that spontaneous generation was disproved and that life was essentially cellular activity.[44]

In previous years of the century, the theory of humoral pathology had prevailed and Rokitansky had attempted to link it with pathological anatomy by adopting Schleiden and Schwann's 'blastema theory'. In December, 1846 the Berliner Medizinische Zeitung published two articles by Virchow demolishing Rokitansky's idea in rather summary fashion. At the time Virchow was only 26, and in the next year he and Benno Reinhardt founded a journal called 'The Archives of Pathology and Physiology for Clinical Medicine'. Reinhardt died young and the journal was renamed 'Virchow's Archives', a name which it still bears today.

In 1847 his researches were interrupted when he was asked by the government to head an investigation of a typhus epidemic in Upper Silesia. He stayed there till 1848 but on his return played an active part in the great German medical reform movement. He had soon realised that the problem of the typhus epidemic was a social rather than a medical one and he wrote a report highly critical of the government for allowing such appalling living conditions. It was reminiscent of the findings in England of John Simon for whom Virchow had a great respect. These events resulted in his being temporarily suspended, but when reinstated he decided in 1849 to accept an invitation to the Chair of Pathological Anatomy at the University of Wurzburg, the first of its kind in Germany. In the seven years that he stayed there he carried out a great deal of work. He maintained his interest in public health and spent much time developing his cellular theory. More surprisingly, he commenced a new interest, namely anthropology, and he examined the skulls from a number of cretins. In 1856, probably because of the influence of Johannes Muller, he was invited to fill the new Chair of Pathological Anatomy at Berlin. A new Institute was built for him at the Charité and he stayed there for the rest of his life.[45]

If Virchow was at this time remarkable for his early erudition, this was soon to be matched by a corresponding versatility. He entered politics, pursued his research in pathology and anthropology, and became recognised as the leading pathologist of the day. This is no place to attempt to follow these many activities for this had been admirably done by Ackerknecht, who describes him in his book[44] as 'Doctor, Statesman, and Anthropologist'. For the present purpose we are concerned with his activities in Pathology. These were considerable for in the early years after his return to Berlin he published a small book on Trichinosis, a three-volume work on Tumours, and in 1858, his famous work on Cellular Pathology. His real contribution was the foundation of a school of Pathology which turned out important figures like Cohnheim, Klebs, Langhans, Rindfleisch, and von Recklinghausen. Mention of Cohnheim reminds one of Virchow's work on inflammation and his disagreement with his former pupil. The facts are of some interest. Augustus Waller (1816–1870), better known for his work on nerve degeneration, had in 1846 described diapedesis of white cells which he saw passing through the walls of some blood vessels.[46] Apparently Dutrochet (1776–1847) in 1824[47] and Barry (1802–1855) in 1841 had made similar observations[48]. This work was unknown to Cohnheim who between the years 1867 and 1873 made his classical description of diapedesis as seen in the cornea and mesentery of frogs. He went on to say that pus cells in inflammation were merely escaped leukocytes. It was here that Virchow made one of his rare mistakes for he stated with some determination that pus cells were derived from the proliferation of fixed connective tissue cells.

By the early 1860's German Pathology was in the forefront and Virchow was recognised as the leading pathologist in Europe. He became universally acclaimed in international circles, he was in constant demand at meetings, especially in England, and honours were conferred on him in a regular sequence. Not only had he put Pathology 'on the map', but he had changed it radically from what it was in the early days of Rokitansky. At that time Pathological Anatomy was confined to the description of anatomical dissections and therefore clear-cut. General Pathology, embodying the principles of the subject, was less defined, less understood, and thus more problematical. Virchow, realising that abnormal function was the basis of disease, studied the latter from all view points, clinical, experimental, anatomical, and histological. In doing this, he created a new and wider Pathological Physiology based on Pathological Anatomy. With the rapid growth of this new subject, the scope of 'General Pathology' became curtailed.

His cellular research was carried out with cells whose properties varied considerably from the normal as, for instance, tumour cells with enhanced proliferation. In the past it had become customary to draw a sharp line of demarcation between 'normal' and 'abnormal'. But Virchow soon observed that in some instances the cellular differences were quite slight and that it was by no means always easy to say where 'normal' ended and where 'abnormal' began. This was to prove a great problem throughout the century and caused some to ask, 'What is physiology and what is pathology?' The nomenclature of the time did not simplify matters. Some called Physiology a study of bodily function, thus including Pathology with it; others described Physiology as a study of normal and Pathology a study of abnormal function.

The outstanding feature of German pathology during the remainder of the century was the growth of Pathological Institutes and the large number of eminent pathologists which issued from them. These graduates, trained in research methods, were now ready to take over new schools. Foreign students flocked to Germany and German text-books such as those by Rindfleisch and Ziegler became widely used. It was significant that an English translation by F. Chance of Virchow's famous work on Cellular Pathology appeared only two years after it was published in Germany.

REFERENCES

1 Ornstein, M., 'Role of Scientific Societies in the 17th Century'. University of Chicago Press, 1975, pp. 250–1.
2 Underwood, E. A., 'Boerhaave's Men'. Edinburgh University Press, 1977, p. 34.
3 Underwood, E. A., 'Boerhaave after 300 years'.
4 'British Medical Journal' (1868) ii. p. 824.
5 Durabt, W. and A., 'Rousseau and Revolution'. Simon & Schuster, New York 1967, pp. 342–364.
6 Lesky, E., 'The Vienna Medical School of the 19th century'. Johns Hopkins University Press, Baltimore 1976, p. 13.
7 Ibid pp. 1–2.
8 Korns, H. M., Ann. Med. Hist. 1937. 9, p. 351.
9 Baas, J. H., 'History of Medicine'. J. H. Vail & Co, New York 1889, pp. 619–23.
10 Neuberger, M., 'British Medicine and the Vienna School'. Heinemann Medical Books, 1943, p. 11.
11 Korns., H. M., Ann. Med. Hist. 1937. 9, p. 359.
12 Neuberger, M., 'British Medicine and the Vienna School'. Heinemann Medical Books Ltd, 1943, p. 18.
13 Losky, E., 'The Vienna Medical School of the 19th Century'. Johns Hopkins University Press, Baltimore 1976, p. 18.
14 Korns, H. M., Ann. Med. Hist. 1937, 9, p. 466.
15 Baas, J. H., 'A History of Medicine'. J. H. Vail & Co. New York 1889, pp. 629–30.
16 Ackerknecht., 'A short History of Medicine'. Ronald Press Co, New York 1955, p. 134.
17 Schryock, R. H., 'The Development of Modern Medicine'. University of Wisconsin Press 1936, p. 188.
18 Sigerist, H. E., 'The Great Doctors'. Doubleday Anchor Books, Doubleday & Co 1933, p. 277.
19 Ann. Hist. of Med. 1937. 9, 467.

20 Kisch, B. J., 'Hist. Med & Allied Services'. (1954) 9, pp. 311–328.

21 Ibid (1967) 22, pp. 54–81.

22 Ann. Hist. of Med. 1937, 9, 467.

23 Lesky, E., 'The Vienna Medical School of the 19th Century'. Johns Hopkins University Press, Baltimore 1976. pp. 121–2.

24 Billroth, T., 'Medical Sciences in the German Universities'. MacMillan Co. 1924, pp. 37–8.

25 Menne, F. R., Ann. Hist. Med. 1925. 7, 380.

26 Neuberger, M., 'British Medicine and the Vienna School'. Heinemann Medical Books 1943, p. 42.

27 Sigerist, H. E., 'The Great Doctors'. Doubleday Anchor Books 1933, pp. 281–6.

28 Lesky, E., 'The Vienna Medical School of the 19th Century'. Johns Hopkins University Press, Baltimore 1975, pp. 121–2.

29 Ibid p. 19.

30 Ibid pp. 88–9.

31 Neuberger, M., 'British Medicine and the Vienna School'. Heinemann Medical Books 1943, p. 108.

32 Lesky, E., 'The Vienna Medical School of the 19th Century'. Johns Hopkins University Press, Baltimore 1976, pp. 110–11.

33 Commission on Medical Education. 'Medical Education and Related Problems'. April 1980. p. 59.

34 Feuchtwanger, E. F., 'Prussia, Myth and Reality'. Henry Regnery Company, Chicago 1970, pp. 99–102.

35 Marriott, J. A. R. & Robertson, C. G., 'The Evolution of Prussia'. Clarendon Press, Oxford 1963, p. 231.

36 Feuchtwanger, E. F., 'Prussia, Myth and Reality'. Henry Regnery Company, Chicago 1970, pp. 102–8.

37 Ibid pp. 123–4.

38 Marriott, J. A. R. & Robertson, C. G., 'The Evolution of Prussia'. Clarendon Press. Oxford Rev. Ed. 1946, pp. 228–38.

39 Flexner, A., 'Medical Education in Europe'. 576 Fifth Avenue, New York 1912, p. 3.

40 Garrison, F. H., 'Introduction to the History of Medicine'. W. B. Saunders Co, Philadelphia. p. 460.

41 Flexner, A., 'Medical Education in Europe'. 576 Fifth Avenue, New York 1912, p. 8.

42 Ibid pp. 453, 459.

43 Kruta, V., Dict. Scientific Biography. 1975, Vol. xi, p. 216.

44 Ackerknecht, E. H., 'Rudolf Virchow'. University of Wisconsin Press 1953, p. 9.

45 Ibid pp. 22–3.

46 'British Medical Journal'. (1987) i, 1548.

47 Castiglioni, A., 'History of Medicine'. Alfred A. Knopf. 2nd Ed 1947, p. 697.

48 Ackerknecht, E. H., 'Rudolf Virchow'. University of Wisconsin Press 1955, p. 65.

# EIGHT
# Developments at Oxford and Cambridge 1830–1920

British, and especially English Universities, were less advanced than those on the Continent, hence the importance of the latter in British medical education.

Oxford and Cambridge, the oldest Universities in England and founded in the 13th century, retained their mediaeval character for over 400 years. When Victoria came to the throne in 1837 it was said that Cambridge was being governed by the Elizabethan statutes of 1570 and Oxford by the Laudian statutes of 1636.[1] As such they were dominated by the Church and their main aim was to produce members of the clergy. They were thus in no state to meet the educational demands of the sciences in the 19th century.

In their early days the functions of a university, namely to house students and to provide education, were controlled by the Colleges, and as a result the university consisted of a collection of private schools. These bodies were dominated by the heads of the Colleges who tended to operate under their own set of rules. Because of the high cost, students were usually sons of the rich, and were further limited by the religious tests to members of the Anglican church. There was no control over the quality of the student because there were no entrance examinations and a number of them were more concerned with living in the town for a period and did not trouble to obtain a degree. Tuition was poor and often bore little relationship to the curriculum for the degree. Lecturing was not considered to be part of a professor's duties until the early 1800s. A student anxious to obtain good teaching might be able to go to a local 'coach' whose services were very expensive.

The changes required in education were great, related as they were to new social needs in a changing social structure. The universities were slow to react to these new demands though in the early decades of the 19th century there were some encouraging signs. In 1802, Oxford introduced an Honours Examination and some of the Colleges, notably Christchurch, became well known for the scholarship of many of their students. Lecturing by professors was introduced, and at Oxford Edward Nares was only appointed on condition that he gave an annual course of lectures on History.[2] At Cambridge the Regius Professor of Physic from 1817 till 1851, John Haviland, gave lectures on General and Special Pathology.[3] But on the whole progress was very slow. The educational needs were no longer for theologians, as in the past, but for a wide variety of middle-class students who would fill the growing need for lawyers, doctors, schoolmasters, civil servants, politicians, and colonial administrators. The real question was whether the universities would

96

implement such necessary reforms of their own accord or whether only because of outside pressure.

In 1837, Lord Radnor, a politician with strong Liberal views and a special interest in university reform, demanded the setting-up of a Royal Commission of inquiry into the universities. In the controversy which followed the Whig government fell and the matter was delayed. In 1845 a Liberal pressure group raised it again and in 1850 Lord John Russell, the Whig Prime Minister, informed the House that the government proposed to conduct an inquiry into the state of the universities. When the commission commenced its work it was confronted with frank obstruction on the part of the universities. However, they pursued their inquiry with commendable determination and issued a report with widespread recommendations. Many of these were accepted and incorporated in the University Reform Bills which were passed in 1854 in the case of Cambridge and in 1856 in the case of Oxford.

Many improvements followed the implementation of the Bills, but there were some Liberals who felt that the recommendations had not gone far enough. The universities had been requested to provide additional professorships, lecture rooms, laboratories and libraries, though there had been no action to provide the necessary finance. Also there was still the burning question of the religious tests and it was not until 1871 that a Bill was passed allowing the universities to admit non-Anglicans.

It now remained to provide students suitably prepared for entry into the universities and this meant a fundamental change in the educational system. The demands came from the expanding affluent middle-class, and the development of a large number of 'Public Schools' provided students suitably prepared for the higher education which was now becoming available.

With reform still in the air, yet another Royal Commission was appointed in 1872. Its terms of reference were to inquire into the revenues and properties of the two universities. Further changes were made in the statutes and the universities given until 1878 to implement them. New chairs and readerships were established and the richer colleges called upon to contribute towards their upkeep. By 1880 the modernisation of the older universities was well under way. New standards of scholarship had been reached and natural science and its constituent subjects had found its place. Such progress could not have occurred without a small group of far-sighted men, and it is now our purpose to consider some of them.

## Oxford

At Oxford, at the beginning of the 19th century, there was on average one medical graduate per year, but in the next 30 years there was a revival. The leading men at that time were the Regius Professor of

Medicine, John Kidd (1775–1851) and Dr. Daubeny, a physician to the Radcliffe Infirmary and Professor of a number of subjects such as Botany, Agriculture, and Chemistry. Associated with these two men was James Adey Ogle (1792–1857), who had been appointed clinical professor of medicine in 1830. As such he gave lectures on the Theory and Practice of Medicine at the Radcliffe Infirmary, and at the same time, although there was no regular course in Surgery, there was some informal teaching on the wards of this institution. In addition the Radcliffe and Bodleian libraries were available for study. It was this small group which had recently obtained the institution of a public examination for the degree of MB. In 1841 Ogle issued a pamphlet of suggestions for remodelling the Examinations Statutes which is noteworthy for containing the first suggestion of a Natural Sciences School at Oxford. In 1851 it was embodied in a statute proposed by H. W. Acland.[4] In the same year John Kidd resigned the Regius Professorship of Medicine, following some unkind criticism of his lectures by Victor Carus, a visitor from Leipzig[5] (of whom more later on) and was succeeded by Ogle who held it until his death in 1857.

Throughout the second half of the 19th century, progress at Oxford was dominated by two outstanding men, namely Henry Acland (1815–1900) and John Burdon Sanderson (1828–1905).

Henry Wentworth Acland came from a wealthy family and attended Oxford University. His early studies there had been interrupted by a two-year breakdown in health which he treated by going for a cruise on a man-of-war. During this time he visited many places in the Mediterranean and showed his interest and ability by making an accurate plan of the site of Priam's palace. Returning to Oxford he obtained a Bachelor's Degree, and on the advice of Sir Benjamin Brodie, a friend of his father's, went to St. George's Hospital to study Medicine. One unusual feature in his education at this time was a private course on the use of the microscope, given to him by John Quekett, the leading microscopist of the day. It is likely that this was the start of Acland's interest in museums for at the time Richard Owen was Conservator of the Museum of the Royal College of Surgeons and Quekett was his assistant. He must also have been a mature student for he became concerned for the welfare of his fellow students, exposed as they were to the dangers and temptations of 'the big city'. He therefore wrote a pamphlet advocating the provision of residential colleges, and it is noteworthy that a few years later such an establishment was instituted at St. Bartholomew's Hospital, the first Warden being James Paget, a friend of Acland. Licensed to practice Medicine, he proceeded to Edinburgh where he worked for and resided with the Professor of Medicine, W. P. Alison, for two years. In 1845 he was appointed to the Lee Readership in Anatomy at Christ Church College, Oxford, a town in which he was destined to spend the rest of his life. His experience at Edinburgh was valuable, as Alison's interest in matters of public health influenced him later in showing concern for the sanitary conditions in Oxford. Also, when cholera came in 1854, he did much to secure a safe water supply and to improve drainage.

When Acland first came to Oxford his main aim was to introduce the Natural Sciences into university teaching with the aid of a museum. As Lee's Reader he was responsible for some anatomical specimens housed in Christ Church College and the use of them for his lectures in Anatomy, given to a small number of students. The new establishment which he planned resembled the ancient Museum at Alexandria – a seat of learning for teaching and research in the Natural Sciences, and one where a school of anatomy would be the basis for a physician's education. He envisaged a new building and this was designed by his lifelong friend, John Ruskin. It was an ambitious undertaking for the sum of money available was £30,000. In 1847 he was appointed Physician to the Radcliffe Infirmary, a post which he held for 40 years. On becoming Lee's Reader, his first action had been to collect a large number of physiological specimens to add to those already in Christ Church College. It seems likely that he obtained much help from the hard-working Lionel S. Beale, who came to him from King's College, London in 1847 and stayed with him for about two years. It is stated that when Beale returned to London, Victor Carus of Leipzig took his place.[6] It is not known how long or in what capacity he stayed with Acland but some details of his visit are of interest. Victor Carus, born in 1789, had graduated in Leipzig and become Physician-in-ordinary to the King of Saxony in 1827. In 1844 the King made a visit to England and Carus accompanied him.[7] With the rapid progress of Medicine in Germany at the time he set about making a comparison with the state of medicine in England. Amongst many leading figures he met the Queen's Physician, Sir James Clark, Sir William Lawrence and Michael Faraday, the famous physicist. He visited the London Hospitals, Bart's, Guy's, and St. George's and many special hospitals. He was especially interested in museums for he had himself written a treatise on Comparative Anatomy and Physiology. At the museum of the Royal College of Surgeons he met Sir Richard Owen for whom he developed a great regard. Other museums included the Ashmolean at Oxford, the Anatomical in Edinburgh, and a considerable collection at St. George's and Guy's. Obviously we were fast approaching the time when a teaching museum was a prerequisite of every large teaching hospital. He completed his survey with a visit to some factories in the Midlands and the North to observe the conditions of work of the employees. His criticism of John Kidd's lectures, referred to earlier, was a sad ending to his visit.

To return to Acland's activities, the first examination in Natural Sciences was held in 1853.[8] There had been a good deal of opposition to the new museum but it was at last begun in 1855 and opened in 1860. Its history was told in 1879 in a volume written by Henry Acland and John Ruskin.[9] The new university museum building now contained the original anatomical specimens from Christ Church College and the physiological ones which Acland had collected. It was further augmented by a private collection of van der Kolk which had been purchased. The Radcliffe Camera Library was also incorporated. The new building contained lecture rooms whilst the Galleries were used to display the teaching specimens. The Lee Reader moved there from Christ Church. By this time Acland was well-established for he had become Radcliffe Librarian in 1851 and Regius Professor of Medicine in 1857. He had also made a large number of friends by his unique ability in handling all grades of person. A number of changes were now made involving a rearrangement of the University Chairs.[10] Merton College in 1860 endowed the Linacre Chair of Anatomy and Physiology and George Rolleston was the first holder until he died in 1881.[11] During that period he made no great original contribution, but established himself as a fine teacher of his disciplines. In 1865 Professor Clifton was made head of the Physics Laboratory, and in 1866 the Waynflete Chair of Chemistry was endowed by Magdalen College, the first holder being Dr. Odling in 1872. These appointments were important for they indicated the part that the Colleges with their adequate resources were going to play in helping the University to finance its future expansion.

The introduction of the Natural Sciences into the University curriculum in 1851 and the opening of his museum in 1860 must have been viewed by Acland with some satisfaction. But there was still much to be done and in the succeeding years he was to become very influential and therefore well able to help bring this about. When the General Medical Council was formed in 1858 Acland was the representative of Oxford University,[12] and between 1874 and 1887 he was President of the Council. As such he had great influence on the structure of the medical curriculum and needless to say he favoured a more extensive scientific training. As a member of the Hebdomadal Council of the University he had a say in local educational matters. But all was not well as the number of Oxford medical students was small. The Natural Sciences curriculum, though improved, was not providing the medical student with the help that he needed for his future professional career. It was considered by most that the subjects ancillary to medicine, even including pathology, were best studied at the University. Some clinical instruction was being given at the Radcliffe Infirmary, founded in 1770. These were confined to the rudiments of clinical observation and had originated many years ago from an endowment to the hospital from the third Earl of Lichfield.[13] The majority believed that the main clinical studies were better carried out at one of the large London teaching hospitals for the resources of the Radcliffe Infirmary were too slender to give adequate clinical instruction. Yet there were some who differed and in 1878 an unsuccessful attempt was made to create a full medical school within the university. Already, the contributions of Acland had been enormous but he now took one further great step when in 1882 he persuaded John Burdon Sanderson to come to Oxford.

When George Rolleston died in 1881 there were further changes in the teaching staff when the Linacre Chair was divided, Burdon Sanderson becoming Waynflete Professor of Physiology and Arthur Thomson, Professor of Human Anatomy. Henry Nottidge Moseley (1844–1891), who had been a naturalist on the 'Challenger' expedition, became Professor of Biology, but died when only 47. He will be remembered as the father of H. G. J. Moseley (1887–1915), so tragically killed at Gallipoli in World War I. Moseley was succeeded by Professor Ray Lankester, and Dr. Tylor was made keeper of the Oxford Museum.

Burdon Sanderson (1828–1905) had had an unusual career. Educated privately, he had studied Medicine at Edinburgh and obtained his MD degree in 1851. There were many fine teachers there at the time, such as Goodsir, Syme, and Alison, but he was most influenced by Hughes Bennett, Professor of the Institutes of Medicine and a great advocate of the use of the microscope. Sanderson worked as his Demonstrator, and after a short period of study in Chemistry with Wurzt in Paris, he returned to London where he became Lecturer in Botany and subsequently Medical Jurisprudence at St. Mary's Hospital.[11] In 1856 he was Medical Officer of Health for Paddington under Sir John Simon and by this time was becoming interested in Pathology as well as in Public Health. He held some clinical posts for a short period and even went into general practice. But he was attracted by physiology between 1866 and 1870 when Lecturer in that subject at the Middlesex Hospital and he had his own research laboratory in Howland Street. His early research in experimental physiology dealt with resuscitation in cases of drowning. From 1871–1878 he was Physician Superintendent at the Brown Institute (see chapter 16) and his researches on pyaemia will be dealt with in chapter 18. He was now able to pursue his real interest, for in 1870 he had become Professor of Practical Physiology and Histology and, in 1874, Professor of Human Physiology at University College, London. The latter was an important appointment for at that time the Regulations of the University of London and the Royal College of Surgeons had been changed and now laid down that the study of practical physiology was mandatory for all medical students. As a result Sanderson had no difficulty in obtaining adequate laboratory accommodation for his classes.[15] When apparently settled in London, he was in 1882 persuaded by Henry Acland to come to Oxford to become Waynflete Professor of Physiology, an office which he held until 1895. At University College he had not proved to be a striking lecturer for the average student because his main aim had been to stimulate interest in the practical aspect of his subject. In this he was brilliantly successful and aided by his encouragement many turned to research. In this respect his department of physiology was probably the leading one of the day.

When Sanderson reached Oxford his reception was not a warm one. He had been appointed in the face of much local opposition and he became the target of the antivivisectionists, chiefly because of 'The

Handbook of the Physiological Laboratory', which he had published in collaboration with Michael Foster, Emmanuel Klein, and Lauder Brunton (1872). He found a department at Oxford with no practical facilities and one can imagine his dismay when there was local opposition to the erection of a new building which he had been promised and in which he could provide practical instruction. These difficulties were gradually overcome, thanks largely to the support and encouragement of Acland, who was still Regius Professor of Medicine and continued as such until 1894. Throughout these frustrating days he had the support of two colleagues who had accompanied him from University College to Oxford, namely Francis Gotch as Demonstrator of Physiology and F. A. Dixey as Lecturer in Histology. In future years he had valuable help from J. S. Haldane, and from M. S. Pembrey who subsequently became Professor of Physiology at Guy's Hospital and co-author with James Ritchie (see below) of a text book entitled 'General Pathology'. In 1894, Sir Henry Acland resigned from the Regius Chair of Medicine and in the following year Burdon Sanderson took his place. A new Professor of Physiology had to be found and in spite of strong competition from J. S. Haldane (1860–1936) and C. S. Sherrington (1858–1952), Francis Gotch (1953–1913) was appointed and held the post for the remainder of his life.

At the end of the century Oxford had a modern Natural Sciences programme and flourishing departments of Anatomy under Arthur Thomson and Physiology under Francis Gotch. But the question of Pathology was as yet unsettled and the clinical facilities at the Radcliffe Infirmary were insufficient for teaching medicine. In the case of Pathology the first step was taken when Sanderson, always an enthusiast for the subject, used his influence to introduce Pathology, Public Health, and Forensic Medicine as separate subjects in the Final Examination. But there was as yet no department of Pathology and no tuition in the subject.

In 1892 a young Edinburgh graduate, James Ritchie (1864–1923), came to Oxford to work with a surgeon, Mr. Horatio P. Symonds (1851–1923). It seems that this arrangement had been made through Professor Chiene in Edinburgh, for whom Ritchie had worked as House Surgeon. Symonds was a member of a remarkable family in which he was the seventh in line in uninterrupted descent to practice surgery, the last three being in Oxford.[16] In his new post Ritchie found that he had ample leisure time and was able to embark on some pathological and bacteriological studies. The clinical staff of the Radcliffe Infirmary found that some of his work was most useful to them.[17] The delay in establishing a department of pathology resulted from the prevalent view that Oxford was not a suitable place for studying it. But when Burdon Sanderson became Regius Professor of Medicine all this became alerted. In 1896 regular classes were instituted by Ritchie for a few students who were doing an extra year of Anatomy with Thomson, and Burdon Sanderson gave a few lectures on General Pathology. There is also mention of assistance from 'Edwin' and this probably refers to Arthur Edwin

Boycott, who was an Honours Student in the Natural Sciences between 1894 and 1898.[18] In 1897 Ritchie was appointed Lecturer in Pathology, an excellent choice for he was a first-class teacher. The course progressed and over the next few years attracted many outstanding students such as Boycott, Dean, Sholtos Douglas, and Turnbull, all of whom subsequently reached the top rank in pathology. In 1901 Ritchie was promoted Reader in Pathology, and it should not be forgotten that in 1897 he had published a standard work, namely a 'System of Bacteriology' in collaboration with Robert Muir. With the rapid advances in both Pathology and Bacteriology many thought that the time was ripe for the establishment of a Chair in these subjects. In 1904, when Sir John Burdon Sanderson retired from the Regius Chair of Medicine, there was a movement to add its emoluments (about £400 a year) to the Readership in Pathology and make it a Professorship, but it was defeated.[19] It was decided to retain the Regius Professorship, William Osler being the new incumbent, and Ritchie remained a Reader. In 1905 Ritchie was given the title of Professor, but as the years passed by he became disappointed and in 1907 he accepted an invitation to return to Edinburgh as Director of the Laboratory of the Royal College of Physicians. He held this post until 1913 when he became the first holder of the University Chair of Bacteriology, founded under the unusual bequest of a man named Robert Irvine. Christmas Island in the Indian Ocean has as its sole industry the export of phosphates and a share of the company owning the island was left to the University, and the monies were to accumulate until they were sufficient to found a Chair of Bacteriology. This was made possible in 1913 following an unusually favourable trading year[20] and Ritchie retained his Chair for the rest of his life. He could claim to have been the founder of Pathology in Oxford and it was ironical that in the year in which he left, the University at last established a Chair of Pathology.

If the disappointment at Ritchie's departure from Oxford had been great, it was probably equalled by the surprise at the appointment of a foreigner, Georges Dreyer (1873–1934), of Danish extraction, as the first holder of the Chair. Yet this need not have been so for in recent years there had been frequent interchange of students and scientific workers between Copenhagen and Oxford.

Copenhagen had become known in medical circles for a report made by Peter Ludwig Panum (1820–1885) on a severe outbreak of measles in the Faroe Islands in which 6,000 out of a 9,000 population became affected.[21] This was in 1846, and Panum, who had been born on the island of Bornholm, had graduated in Medicine in the previous year at the University of Copenhagen. He then travelled in Europe and after postgraduate studies with Virchow, von Kolliker, Wurtz and Claude Bernard, he became Professor of Physiology, Medical Chemistry, and General Pathology in the University of Kiel, where he built up a suitable department. This university within Schleswig-Holstein became lost to

Denmark in the Danish-German war and Panum moved to Copenhagen where he became Professor of Physiology from 1864 until 1885. He was interested in experimental work and had published some valuable studies on the effects of artificial embolism.

Amongst his pupils was Carl Julius Salomonsen (1847–1924), whose father was a friend of Panum.[22] Having graduated in Medicine, he embarked on some studies of pyaemia at the instigation of his master and wrote his MD thesis in 1877 on 'Decomposition of the blood.' A period of foreign travel followed and he visited many centres, being particularly impressed by Cohnheim and his studies at Breslau. Returning to Copenhagen, he set up a small laboratory. In 1883 he became Lecturer in Bacteriology and in 1885 published his text-book on bacteriological technique. He was a great enthusiast and a magnificent teacher and students flocked to him. In 1893 his Lectureship was advanced to a Chair in General Pathology, and his department grew in size. Although his main interest was in Bacteriology, he extended his teaching by introducing experimental pathological courses largely based on Cohnheim's example. The department expanded so much that in 1902 a separate Serum Institute became necessary and he was its Director until 1909. Amongst his assistants he worked with Madsen on immunity and with Dreyer on the effects of radium on amoebae and trypanosomes. But the department had become famed for Bacteriology and it is said that this University was the first to create an individual chair in the subject.[23] Some of the visiting scientists came from Oxford, such as Sholtos Douglas and Turnbull. It was in this way that Dreyer got interested in Oxford and came to spend a period of study with Burdon Sanderson. Further visits followed and he collected a number of friends who not only liked him but greatly admired his work. Thus, when the Chair of Pathology was created they suggested that he should apply.

Georges Dreyer had been a brilliant student and graduated from the University of Copenhagen. With this early promise he became an assistant to Salomonsen. He was essentially an experimental pathologist and had his heart in Bacteriology. Like a number of others at the time, he believed that Morbid Anatomy was defunct because it had all been worked out by Virchow and given the coup de grace by the growing subject of Bacteriology. When Turnbull went to Copenhagen, he first had a course in Experimental Pathology and then one in Serology by Dreyer. By this time he too may have felt that there was little future in Morbid Anatomy. But Ritchie, who had been Turnbull's advisor, insisted that he should end his study by working with Schmorl in Leipzig. Inspired by Schmorl, Turnbull returned to London and was a Morbid Anatomist for the rest of his life.

When Dreyer took over in Oxford he had only two part-time assistants and his first duty was to convince the University that he must have some full-time staff. He was to be served for the rest of his life by the loyal Ainley Walker. He worked hard and with great enthusiasm following up previous studies on agglutination and blood volume. By the beginning of the first World War he had established his position. He volunteered for World War I and his services were recognised when he was awarded a CBE. Just after the end of the war he had an unfortunate experience with his research. He was preparing a 'diaphyte' vaccine which it was hoped would prevent tuberculosis. He was forced to make a premature publication which led to a controlled trial by the Medical Research Council to confirm or refute the validity of the claim. The vaccine was shown to be of no value and obviously this was a severe blow, for it has been suggested that from that time his research was on the wane.

At this stage Dreyer turned his attention to improving the teaching of Pathology. The Natural Sciences were now established, for the Department of Anatomy was an excellent one and the Physiology Department second to none. Also the Honour School of Physiology was flourishing and Dreyer felt that a similar School for Pathology was needed. But the University would not agree, possibly because the two subjects were too close to one another.[24] In 1922 the Sir William Dunn Trustees made available a sum of money to build a new Department of Pathology. Dreyer worked extremely hard on this project and after the laying of the Foundation Stone in 1924 the building was opened in 1927. Now it seemed that all was set for a new phase of progress. But unfortunately this never happened and the number of visiting students which was envisaged never materialised.

Georges Dreyer had done many good things and his setting up (with the aid of the Medical Research Council) of the 'Standards Laboratory' is something that no Pathologist in the country is likely to forget. When Dreyer died, Oxford had come a long way, but there was much yet to be done. The next professor, Howard (later Lord) Florey was to transform the Department of Pathology and to make it one of the foremost in the world. The story of this development is admirably told by Gwyn Macfarlane in his recent book 'Howard Florey – the making of a great scientist'.

## Cambridge

There was some resemblance in the overall development of medical education in the two universities in the latter half of the 19th century. This is not surprising for the recommendations of the Royal Commissions had been applied to both. But if the seed was similar, the soil was different and Cambridge was more receptive to scientific changes. Throughout the 18th century the influence of Sir Isaac Newton's great work was still being felt and Cambridge, now renowned for Mathematics and its allied subjects, had left Oxford far behind. Signs of scientific activity were manifest when in 1819 the Cambridge Philosophical Society was founded. It promoted discussions on Natural Science subjects and encouraged publication; it also maintained the only zoological museum in the University. In 1837 a group of naturalists gave rise to the Ray Society. University teaching at the turn of the century was unsatisfactory. It was still in the hands of the colleges and therefore not co-ordinated. Many professors were honorary, and medical students as few as about five every year.[25] Having obtained their BA degree, these students went to London where they attended one of the large general hospitals, and possibly one or more of the private schools of the time for clinical instruction.

The Cambridge medical undergraduates were required to attend lectures on Botany, Chemistry, and Anatomy, and there is some information about one of the early teachers, namely Busick (later Sir Busick) Harwood (1745–1814). His career was a remarkable one.[26] Having served as an apprentice to an apothecary, he qualified as a surgeon, spent some years in practice in India, and returned to England where he taught Botany at the London Hospital. He next went to Christ's College, Cambridge, where in 1785 he graduated MB with a thesis on blood transfusion, based on a number of experiments in which exsanguinated dogs were revived by infusion of sheep's blood. In the same year he was appointed Professor of Anatomy and subsequently in 1800 the first Downing Professor of Medicine. He held both of these posts until his death in 1814. During these years he gave a series of lectures which were later published in six volumes. His lectures were very popular, possibly because they were enlivened by demonstrations of his transfusion experiments. Although his main subject was Anatomy, he drifted into others such as Comparative Anatomy, Pathology, and Physiology. One other of his activities was the collection of anatomical specimens, which he used for his lectures, and which became the nucleus of a University Museum at a later date.

So far the teaching of medical undergraduates had been haphazard, but a great change occurred when John Haviland (1785–1851) succeeded Harwood as Professor of Anatomy in 1814. He held this Chair for only three years, having resigned from it in 1817 when he became Regius Professor of Medicine (1817–1851). Even in this short time he had brought some organisation into the teaching of Anatomy. As a Cambridge undergraduate, Haviland obtained his BA degree in 1807. With medical teaching in Cambridge at a low ebb, he wisely decided to go for his clinical training to Edinburgh where he spent two sessions and to St. Bartholomew's, London where he stayed three years. Returning to Cambridge, he obtained the ML (the University License to Practice) and was elected Professor of Anatomy and Regius Professor of Medicine.[27] As such he gave regular courses first in Anatomy and later in Pathology and Medicine, but his great contribution was in the organisation of the medical curriculum and he was one of the pioneers of Cambridge medical education. His influence was great and he was anxious to make Cambridge a complete medical school, and in 1841 a great step forward was taken by the introduction of clinical lectures in Medicine and Surgery.

Some clinical teaching in hospitals did occur in the 18th century. John Bellers (1654–1725), the Quaker philanthropist, had expressed concern about the teaching of Medicine following a visit to the Continent, and suggested in 1714 that each of the Universities should have a hospital. Five years later, John Addenbrooke, a Cambridge physician, left a sum of money to build a small hospital, though this did not materialise until 1766. Some months later, the Governors of Addenbrooke's Hospital (as it had been named) 'ordered that in any doubtful case the Physicians and Surgeons shall have power to open the body of any person dying in the Infirmary without asking any person leave'.[28] From the time of the opening of the hospital, physicians and surgeons were permitted to have pupils apprenticed to them and in 1824 a similar privilege was extended to the House Apothecary. These pupils were probably taught from autopsy material. But it is important to realise that these pupils rarely if ever became medical undergraduates. It all changed in 1841 when, almost certainly at the instigation of Haviland, medical students were for the first time granted permission to attend the hospital at certain hours for clinical instruction.[29]

In the meanwhile there was progress in the teaching of Anatomy. Harwood had given lectures and illustrated them with his collection of specimens. The value of a museum was realised and he commenced to compile a catalogue. But it remained unfinished at the time of his death and was not completed till 1820 by William Clark (1788–1869), who had become Professor of Anatomy in 1817. Clark occupied the Chair for many years and built up a good teaching department and an excellent museum. Like other anatomists of the time, he encountered many difficulties. Bodies were in short supply and when dissections were performed they had to be done in the Anatomical Theatre. Consequently tuition was still mainly by lecture and a course of fifty were given. It was also the age of 'body snatching' of which the public was well aware. Thus the crux of these difficulties was reached in 1833 when a body was taken from the hospital to the Anatomy department. A riot followed in which a crowd tore up the pavement, smashed the College windows and broke into the Museum where they damaged many specimens.[30] It should be added that the Museum had expanded considerably over the years for Clark had added his specimens of Comparative Anatomy and in 1836 had purchased a collection made by Macartney, a well-known Dublin anatomist. But the specimens were badly housed and there was great overcrowding. There were also collections of Geology and Mineralogy which were scattered about in odd places. In 1837 there had been a proposal to rebuild the Library and to add to it some lecture rooms and museums. Delay followed because of lack of money and when it was started three years later only part of the scheme was eventually completed. Indeed, it was almost thirty years (1865) before the New

Museum was opened. As an example of the financial stringency of the time, it might be mentioned that the Museum of Comparative Anatomy could not have been built had not the Professor loaned the money to the University at a nominal interest rate.[31]

By 1839 the influence of John Haviland on the curriculum and the examination system had already been felt. In the same year he resigned his post as physician to Addenbrooke's Hospital but retained his Regius Professorship. There were now some far-reaching developments. As physician to Addenbrooke's Hospital in succession to Haviland, George Paget (1809–1892), a brother of Sir James Paget, was elected without opposition. He was to remain in this office for the next 45 years. In 1842 there were further changes in the clinical staff, when three surgeons were appointed. Among them was George Murray Humphry (1820–1896), chosen in the face of considerable local opposition and at the early age of 22. Some few months later, medical students were permitted to attend the hospital at certain hours. This was not only the commencement of clinical instruction, but also of a long period of co-operation between Paget and Humphry. These two outstanding men with the later assistance of Sir Michael Foster (1836–1907) were to be the architects of the modern Cambridge medical school.

The curriculum was still not satisfactory for Natural Science subjects were not yet included. This was surprising for there was much interest in science and the time was ripe for a change. The Prince Consort, well in touch with developments in his native Germany, was so impressed by Liebig's chemical research work in Giessen that he lent his support to the establishment of the Royal College of Chemistry in London in 1845. Six years later the Prince launched the Great Exhibition in London which stimulated interest in scientific matters to say nothing of bringing together scientists from many different countries. Visitors to the Continent at the time had been greatly impressed particularly by what they saw in Germany. There was great enthusiasm for extending scientific knowledge and promoting original research.[32] It was also felt that England was lagging behind in technical education; there were fears that repercussions would be soon felt in industry, and for this the older universities were blamed.

In the introduction of science into the curriculum a number of men such as Paget and Humphry played a part, but mention should also be made of one remarkable figure.

William Whewell (1794–1866) was born in Lancaster and, showing early promise, had been sent to Cambridge where he became second Wrangler. His subsequent studies were exceedingly diverse and he held the posts of Tutor at Trinity College, and later the Professorships of Mineralogy and Moral Philosophy. By 1841 he was recognised as an authority on the Sciences, and regarded as greatly superior to any of the heads of the Colleges. In this year he was appointed Master of Trinity College, and in the year 1842–3 Vice-Chancellor of the University.[33] In

1847 when the Chancellor died, Whewell was instrumental in securing the appointment of the Prince Consort. It was a wise move for the Prince had very progressive ideas and was very sympathetic towards promoting science. As a result, in 1848 a Natural Sciences Tripos was established which included Comparative Anatomy, Human Anatomy, Physiology, Chemistry, Botany, and Geology. In 1853 St. John's College became the first to appoint a Lecturer in Natural Science and he was provided with a small chemical laboratory. The establishment of the Natural Sciences Tripos in 1848 was a great step forward and the first examination was held in 1851. But there was still something lacking for the examination did not carry with it degree status. Happily this was rectified in 1860, and in 1871 and 1876 regulations were changed in order to make the study of Natural Sciences more suitable for medical students. The new Tripos examination had increased the teaching load and William Clark, the Professor of Anatomy,looked around for assistance. He found George Humphry willing to help and in 1857 arranged for him to give lectures and demonstrations on Human Anatomy. This worked well and was continued until 1866 when Clark retired. The Chair was now divided, George Humphry becoming Professor of Human Anatomy and Alfred Newton (1829–1907), Professor of Zoology and Comparative Anatomy. In this same year that outstanding scholar, William Whewell, died and it is ironical to read that Humphry said his brain weighed only 49 ounces.[34]

The 1852 Royal Commission was given the task of enquiring into the state, discipline, studies, and revenues of the Colleges and the Universities. This certainly confirmed that the Colleges were rich and the Universities poor, but the matter was not dealt with for some years. One of the most important recommendations, which ensured the future progress of education, was the constitution of a Board of Medical Studies.

By 1865 there had been a substantial improvement in accommodation of the Medical School. The New Museum was at last opened and the new building housed the collections of Anatomy, Comparative Anatomy, and Botany. The old building was now converted into a dissecting room and a chemical laboratory. A laboratory of Experimental Physics was built and the first Cavendish Professor, Clerk-Maxwell, appointed. Most important of all, with the growing realisation of the value of practical teaching, the University had set aside a sum of money for the maintenance of museums and laboratories. The field was now set for the most progressive phase of all and was to be aided by the findings of the Royal Commission of 1872. The year 1871 became memorable for the abolition of the religious tests which led to an influx of medical students in subsequent years. The prosperity of this period had been largely brought about by three great men, whose contributions must be considered in more detail.

George Paget (1809–1892) is well-known as the brother of Sir James

Paget. He read Mathematics at Cambridge, studied medicine at St. Bartholomew's Hospital and in Paris, and graduated MB in 1833. He decided to settle in Cambridge and was appointed Physician to Addenbrooke's Hospital in 1839, a post which he held until 1884. The culmination of his medical career was in 1872 when he was made Regius Professor of Medicine. Throughout his long life he was a successful physician with an extensive practice, though he published little.[35] His main contribution, which was considerable, lay in the field of education. The part that he played with Whewell and others in the foundation of the Natural Sciences Tripos in 1848 has already been mentioned.

Paget's main concern was the value of the Natural Sciences in the education of medical students and he set out his views in a publication some years later. In August 1864 the British Medical Association held its annual meeting in Cambridge and Paget was elected President. His views and his aims were well-stated in his Presidential Address.[36] Outlining what had been achieved over the years, he gave a good picture of how things stood at the time. There were few medical students but he was satisfied with the method of teaching and with the system of examination. The contents of the curriculum was still deficient in Natural History. He pointed out that Cambridge was well-known for Classics and Mathematics but was little thought of as a school of Natural History or Medicine. Students were encouraged by the grants of Scholarships or Fellowships given by the Colleges, but there were practically none in Natural Sciences. When this was rectified, more students could be expected. The function of the University and its Colleges was General Education, and it became a question of choosing the subjects which would be of greatest benefit to the medical student in his later career. He believed that these were the subjects of Natural Sciences for they promoted powers of observation so essential in Medicine. If Medicine was not built on a scientific basis it would simply become empiricism.

In all his endeavours Paget was greatly assisted by another outstanding figure. George Murray Humphry (1820–1896) was born in 1820 and in 1836 became apprenticed to John Greene Crosse (1790–1850), one of the most eminent surgeons of the day who was on the staff of the Norfolk and Norwich Hospital. In 1839 he went to study Medicine at St. Bartholomew's Hospital and in 1841–2 qualified with the MRCS, LSA customary at the time. While at Bart's he attracted the attention of the famous surgeon James Paget, who strongly recommended him to his brother George. It was in this way that Humphry came to Cambridge. There in 1842 he was elected surgeon to Addenbrooke's Hospital at the age of 22 in the face of considerable opposition. He later graduated MB in 1852 and MD in 1857. For the latter he presented a thesis, 'On the formation of clots in the venous system during life',[37] a subject which had interested Virchow at about this time. His skill as a surgeon became recognised and he soon built up a large consultant practice. In spite of this he found time to help Clark with the teaching of Anatomy, to contribute to the development of the Anatomical Museum, and to interest himself in the development of the hospital and the medical school. It would seem that he was trying to prove his favourite paradox, 'If you want a thing done, ask a very busy man to do it; other people have no time'.[38]

By 1870 the teaching of the pre-clinical school had taken shape and there was also an introductory clinical course in the hospital. The year was a memorable one in which Michael Foster (1836–1907) came to Cambridge and revolutionised the teaching of Physiology. There may have been some tuition in the subject prior to this, possibly by Humphry in his Anatomy course, but it would have been relatively minor. Foster was born in Huntingdon and studied Medicine at the University of London whence he graduated MB in 1858. He was precluded from becoming a student at Cambridge because he was a non-conformist and the religious tests were still in operation. On graduation he returned to his home town where he went into General Practice with his father for six years.[39] At University College, London, he had been a favourite pupil of Professor Sharpey, and due to him and to Burdon Sanderson, Foster became interested in Physiology. In 1867 Sharpey persuaded him to return to University College as Demonstrator in Physiology. This post suited him well for he strongly believed that teaching should be conducted from a practical standpoint and his laboratory demonstrations were well-received. From now onwards his progress became very rapid. In 1869 University College made him Professor of Practical Physiology and Histology, and his standing in the scientific world was recognised by his election as Fullerian Professor of Physiology at the Royal Institution in the same year. In 1870 Trinity College, Cambridge founded a Praelectorship in Physiology and Foster accepted their invitation to be the first holder. The remainder of his career was just one long story of success. By 1880, when he became Professor of Physiology at Cambridge, he had built up one of the leading departments in the world. At first his accommodation was limited but new laboratories were provided in 1878. He attracted an amazing number of students including such eminent men as W. H. Gaskell, H. Newell Martin, Sheridan Lee, J. N. Langley, J. Reynolds Green, Sidney Vines, and C. S. Sherrington, all of whom achieved distinction in future years.[40] He was influential in the Royal Society where he was Secretary for 21 years, and in 1901 was elected as a Liberal Unionist Member of Parliament for the University of London. It is small wonder that Cambridge rapidly became world-famous for its Science education.

These three men, Paget, Humphry, and Foster, were the architects and they worked well together. Paget had become a member of the General Medical Council, and on his retirement was succeeded by Humphry. As such they were well able to influence the pattern of medical education as a whole as well as its development within their own university. In this connection, mention should be made of Humphry's Hunterian Oration given in 1879, which gives a good idea of his educational views.[41] For an oration given just over 100 years ago, it has a remarkably modern ring, and could be read with advantage by any modern educator. He naturally stressed the importance of the subjects which should provide a scientific basis for Medicine and Surgery. Having decided what to teach, the next problem was how to teach it. The presentation of the material was all important, for the student must be inspired to want to learn and to enjoy the process. The danger (even at that time!) of the growing volume of factual knowledge was very real and too many facts stifled the process of thought and reflection. He aptly quoted Democritus who said, 'We should strive not after fulness of knowledge but fulness of understanding'. Examinations, a necessary evil, do much to make difficulties for the teacher and he refers to them as 'the despots of education'. To read this oration is to appreciate the quality of the men responsible for the modernisation of the older English Universities.

Some examination changes had been made as for example the introduction of State Medicine into the MD in 1867, and in 1875 the institution of a Diploma in Public Health which was open to anyone on the Medical Register.

During the years 1877–88 further progress was made as a result of the recommendations of the Royal Commission. The University Statutes were rewritten, and the Colleges were requested to contribute to a common fund to defray expenses resulting from the development of university activities. Amongst new professorships, Foster was elected to the University Chair of Physiology in 1880, and Roy became the first Professor of Pathology in 1883 (see also chapter 11). In the same year Humphry, who welcomed the opportunity of teaching Surgery rather than Anatomy, accepted an invitation to become Professor of Surgery, a post without stipend. Five years later the Special Board for Medicine agreed to appoint an assistant and this post was filled in 1892 by Joseph Griffiths, whose stipend was paid by Humphry.[42]

A good general idea of the progress at Cambridge during the 19th century is given by Liveing who contrasts university conditions in 1837 with those in 1897.[43] The teaching staff for Natural Sciences had been greatly expanded from nine professors and three or four others to fifteen professors, two readers, fifteen lecturers, fifteen recognised teachers, and twenty-four demonstrators. The Natural Sciences Tripos had been established and in 1897 there were 100 students who took the examination. Whereas in 1837 there were fewer than 20 medical students, there were now more than at any other single medical school in England. At the outset of this period there was no laboratory accommodation, whereas in 1897 there was no branch of Natural Science which did not have a laboratory suitable for teaching and research. The modern curriculum for medical students had been defined and included some basic clinical instruction. But the men who brought about this transformation never wanted to make Cambridge a full medical school, believing that the local clinical facilities were inadequate and therefore better obtained in a large centre such as London.

With the establishment of the Natural Sciences Cambridge and Oxford were now well-placed for a further phase of prosperity in the present century, and each was fortunate in having an outstanding Regius Professor of Medicine, namely Sir Clifford Allbutt at Cambridge and Sir John Burdon Sanderson at Oxford. Generous financial assistance enabled extension of the premises to be made, and the activity within was evidenced by the remarkable number of outstanding scientific workers who emanated from them. A special word should be said about Physiology. In England this subject had a difficult beginning and lagged behind the Continent in its early days (see chapter 12). Yet by the end of the 19th century, both universities had built up departments which were well-known throughout the world. For this Oxford was indebted to Sir John Burdon Sanderson, and Cambridge to Sir Michael Foster. But a special word should be reserved for University College, London, for it was there, in Professor Sharpey's department of Physiology, that these two men first developed their interest in the subject.

Although outside the period under review there is one later advance in Cambridge pathology which should be mentioned. The Honours Natural Sciences examination at Oxford included Anatomy and Physiology as full subjects, and it may be recalled that Georges Dreyer, the Professor of Pathology, wanted to obtain similar status for his subject. This attempt was not successful and Dreyer was forced to abandon his dream of a Final Honour School in Pathology similar to that already existent in Physiology. A similar attempt was to be made later in Cambridge but with surprising results. Up to this time the only examination in Pathology at the end of the pre-clinical course was the 'Bugs and Drugs', which had to be passed before clinical studies could be commenced. The examination consisted of Pharmacology, with some elementary Pathology and Bacteriology. H. R. Dean (1879–1961) had been appointed to succeed Sims Woodhead as Professor of Pathology at Cambridge at the end of World War I. He wanted Pathology to be made a full subject in the Natural Sciences Tripos Part I, but he encountered some opposition and the proposal was rejected. But surprisingly the authorities were willing to make Pathology a full subject in Part II of the Tripos and to this Dean eagerly assented. This would require an extra year's study and the first course was started in 1924.[44] It proved to be a great success and attracted many students in future years. It was estimated that there were 500 students in all by the year 1961. In 1937 Pathology obtained further recognition by being made a half subject in Part I of the Tripos. The 'Part II' as it came to be called was an important event in the history of pathology, for many students who took this course eventually specialised in the subject.

REFERENCES

1 Green, F. H. H., 'The Universities' Penguin Books 1969, pp. 59, 60.
2 Ibid pp. 59, 60.
3 Rolleston, Humphrey, 'The Cambridge Medical School'. Cambridge University Press 1932, p. 102.
4 Dict. Nat. Biography, Oxford University Press. 1959–60. Vol XXII. Supp 10–12.
5 Sinclair, H. M., in 'Oxford Medicine', ed. Dewhurst, K. Sandford Publications 1970, p. 7.
6 'British Medical Journal'. (1906) i, p. 836.
7 Neuberger, M., Article in 'History, Philosophy & Sociology of Science'. Ed. E. A. Underwood, Oxford University Press 1975 reprint, pp. 263–273.
8 'British Medical Journal'. (1894) i, pp. 245–6.
9 Acland, H. W. & Ruskin, J., 'The Oxford Museum', quoted in 'British Medical Journal'. (1894) i. pp. 245–6.
10 'British Medical Journal'. (1897) i, p. 1597.
11 Dict. Scient. Biography, Vol XI, pp. 513–15. Charles Scribner's Sons, New York.
12 'Lancet'. (1900) ii, p. 1159.
13 Green, V. H. H., 'The Universities'. Penguin Books 1969, p. 233.
14 'British Medical Journal'. (1905) ii, p. 1481.
15 Ibid p. 1482.
16 'Lancet'. (1923) i, p. 307.
17 J. Path. Bact. (1923) 26, p. 138.
18 Ibid p. 139.
19 Sinclair, H. M., in 'Oxford Medicine', ed. Dewhurst. Sandford Publications 1970, pp. 1–13.
20 'Lancet'. (1923) i, p. 307.
21 Bull. Inst. Hist. Med. (1934) II, pp. 259–80.
22 J. Path. Bact. (1925) 28, pp. 702–8.
23 Dict. Scient. Biography. Vol XII. p. 88. Charles Scribner's Sons, New York.
24 MacFarlane, G., 'Howard Florey'. Oxford University Press 1979, pp. 228–32.
25 'British Medical Journal'. (1897) i, p. 1598.
26 Dict. Nat. Biography. Vol IX. pp. 101–2. Oxford University Press.
27 'Cambridge and its Contribution to Medicine'. Ed. Rook, A. pp. 109–10. Wellcome Institute of the History of Medicine 1971.
28 Ibid p. 119. (Article by Williamson).
29 Ibid pp. 110–11.
30 'British Medical Journal'. (1897) i, p. 1598.
31 Ibid p. 1600.
32 Green, V. H. H., 'The Universities'. Penguin Books 1969, p. 236.
33 Dict. Nat. Biography. Vol. XX. pp. 1665–75. Oxford University Press.
34 'Cambridge and its Contribution to Medicine'. Ed. Rook, A. p. 144. Wellcome Institute of the History of Medicine 1971.
35 'British Medical Journal'. (1892) i, pp. 311–12.
36 Ibid (1907) i, pp. 350–1.
37 'Cambridge and its Contribution to Medicine'. Ed. Rook, A. p. 114. Wellcome Institute of the History of Medicine 1971.

38  'British Medical Journal'. (1896) ii, p. 976.
39  Ibid (1907) i, pp. 350–1.
40  'Lancet', (1907) i, p. 398.
41  Ibid (1879) i, pp. 253–6.
42  'Cambridge and its Contribution to Medicine'. Ed. Rook, A. p. 115. Wellcome Institute of the History of Medicine 1971.
43  Liveing, G. D., 'British Medical Journal'. (1897) i, p. 1598.
44  J. Path. Bact. (1962) *83*, p. 591.

# NINE

# The other early British medical schools
# 1700–1830

Oxford and Cambridge have been dealt with in the previous chapter. This chapter will deal with the other older medical teaching institutions of Great Britain, namely those of Ireland, Scotland and London.

## The Irish Universities

In summarising university medical teaching in Ireland, consideration must include the activities of the two Royal Colleges. Indeed, a glance at the number of bodies carrying out this work might give the impression of its being excessive for such a small country. Much of it was rather fragmented, but in spite of this the achievements of the Irish Medical School command one's admiration, particularly when they occurred during periods of political and economic unrest.

Dublin University, frequently referred to as Trinity College, was founded in 1592. It had no medical school till 1711 and in 1785 this was reconstituted as the Dublin School of Physic. The development of the medical faculty followed the pattern adopted at Cambridge and Oxford. In 1656 the University appointed a Regius Professor of Physic, but there was no teaching at the time. This started in 1711 when four lecturers of Anatomy, Botany, Chemistry, and Natural Philosophy were appointed and each gave a lecture in his own subject. In 1724 they all became Professors, and it will be noted that the subjects were essentially the same as those originally founded at the University of Cambridge.

In 1654 the university had allocated a building to house a body known as the 'Fraternity of Physicians'. By a Charter given them by Charles II in 1657 they became 'The College of Physicians in Dublin', and by a further Charter from William and Mary in 1692 this body became 'The King and Queen's College of Physicians in Ireland'. This title was used till late in the 19th century.[1] These two organisations, the University and the College, are mentioned together because throughout the years their medical activities were very similar, and their progress was limited. Their close connection can be realised by two regulations at the time. For election to the Fellowship of the College, the possession of a Dublin University medical degree was essential and conversely anyone taking his university medical degree had to pass an examination by the college before the degree could be conferred. Also in the conduct of the examination for medical degrees, the President and a number of Fellows of the College acted as co-examiners with the university staff.

In 1715 a 'King's Professorship of Physic in the City of Dublin' was established by Royal Charter though it was abolished in 1741 and replaced by three 'King's Professorships of Physic'. Their duties included the teaching of (1) the Theory and Practice of Physic, (2) Surgery and Midwifery, and (3) Materia Medica and Pharmacy.[2] It is not easy to see the relationship between these College and University professors. Doubtless they complemented one another, and probably some gave clinical instruction at the many Dublin hospitals. It is of interest to learn that candidates for the King's Professorships were appointed by examination and that Nathaniel Barry was only 24 at the time of his election.[3]

In 1712, for a degree of Bachelor of Medicine the student was examined in Anatomy, Chemistry, Botany and Pharmacy. For a Doctorate, he had to give an explanation of some of the Aphorisms of Hippocrates, and also be examined in the theory and cure of external and internal diseases. Students usually attended the 'home' university, though a number also took courses at a foreign medical school. Leyden was specially favoured, where Boerhaave was on the staff. His widespread influence had extended to Ireland, for in 1733 three out of the four members of the university medical staff had been his pupils.[4]

The number of medical graduates during the 18th century must have been small. The King and Queen's College restricted the number of Fellows to 14 and it was not until 1814 that it was augmented. The College also offered a licentiate examination for permission to practice medicine but only eleven were awarded over a period of 50 years – namely 1693–1745.[5] At the University matters were not much better for between 1743 and 1773 it awarded only 29 doctor and 27 bachelor degrees.[6]

With the advent of the 19th century and progress in pathological anatomy, the Dublin School advanced steadily and became famous with such names as Adams, Cheyne, Colles, Corrigan, Graves and Stokes. Many of these went to Paris, the Mecca of Medicine in the early 19th century, and came under the influence of Laennec. Stokes, on his return, published the first work in English on the use of the stethoscope. Hospitals advanced, particularly the Meath where Graves and Stokes were on the staff and maintained a profitable friendship.

Trinity College has retained its identity, preserved its traditions, and it still flourishes – a straightforward story over more than 400 years. It was far from being so with the other teaching schools in Ireland, as will be seen. The 'King and Queen's College of Physicians' also still exists, but as 'The Royal College of Physicians in Ireland'. This institution became involved in an unusual legal battle. In London in 1858 the General Medical Council (GMC) had been appointed and a register was compiled of all those persons who were eligible to practice Medicine in Great Britain. A consideration of the qualifications which were accepted makes it clear that only a small number of practitioners would have held the degree of Doctor of Medicine. The question then arose as to whether all the others would be allowed to call themselves 'doctor'. If not, the public would be confused and not know who to consult – perhaps even believing that anyone not possessing an MD degree was a 'quack'. The council decided that anyone having a registrable qualification could use 'doctor' as a courtesy title, but he was not to describe himself as 'Doctor of Medicine' unless he had the MD. In 1860 the King and Queen's College informed its licentiates that they could use the letters MD after their names, and as can be imagined there was some spirited correspondence in the medical press.[7] By this time it had ceased to be a local matter involving Dublin graduates, but involved many throughout the whole of the British Isles. One writer, styling himself 'Veritas', pointed out that the licentiate's diploma stated on it that he was 'entitled to the degree, title and qualification of Doctor of Medicine'[8] The Registrar of the Branch Council of the GMC said that 'no such degree was recognised by the Medical Act and that it was not a registrable qualification'. A leading article in the 'BMJ'.[9] stated that Trinity College, Dublin had questioned the right of the King and Queen's College to confer the MD degree and had called upon them to make it good 'if they could'. Because of some technical difficulties the matter was handed over to the Master of the Rolls. The question was a simple one – did or did not the College have the right to grant degrees in Medicine? The whole matter was settled in early 1864 when the Master said that the judgment was 'the King and Queen's College of Physicians were not legally authorised under this Charter or otherwise to grant a license admitting to the degree of Doctor of Medicine'.

A summary of the development of the other medical schools in Ireland provides an exercise in nomenclature. By 1845 Ireland had but one university, namely Trinity College or the University of Dublin. This was thought to be insufficient and in that year, as a result of an Irish Colleges Parliamentary Bill,[10] it was decided to install three Queen's Colleges at Belfast, Cork and Galway. These were undenominational in order to satisfy protagonists of Catholic Emancipation, a burning question at the time. By 1849 these Colleges were in operation and supplied tuition. The medical degrees were given by a body known as Queen's University in Ireland, but presumably this was simply an office in Dublin, and it took no part in student education. It was assumed that candidates for the examination would have been trained at one of the Queen's Colleges. Many Catholics opposed the scheme and wanted to have a purely Catholic school. As a result, in 1854 they founded the Catholic University of Ireland, comprising six colleges in the country and a headquarters in Dublin.[11] Parliament replied to this by refusing to give the University a Charter, so that it could not grant degrees. Years of discontent followed and the first move to bring about a change was in 1882, though it did not affect the basic issue. The Queen's University in Ireland was abolished and replaced by the Royal University,[12] which again granted degrees to students of the Queen's Colleges but apparently did not associate itself with the Catholic School. The chief benefit seemed to be to facilitate entry into a university and this it did by lowering the standard of the entrance examination, reducing the cost of tuition, and awarding a larger number of prizes and scholarships. Finally, in 1908, a further reorganisation occurred in which the Royal University was dissolved and replaced by two new universities. Queen's College, Belfast, was upgraded to become 'The Queen's University' and a National University was established in Dublin. This latter consisted of three Colleges, one at Cork, one at Galway, and one in Dublin by affiliation of the schools of the Catholic University. These three colleges were all named 'University Colleges' and this reorganisation proved to be comparatively satisfactory and exists at the present time.[13]

The picture would not be complete without some mention of the Royal College of Surgeons, Dublin. This body had developed in much the same way as the corresponding College in London. In the 15th century the Surgeons had shared a guild with the Barbers, and having separated from them later were granted in 1784 by George III a Charter incorporating 'The Royal College of Surgeons in Ireland'.[14] The feature of this body, which makes it unique, was the fact that in its early days and throughout its history it functioned as a teaching as well as an examining body. As far back as 1789 there were Chairs of Anatomy and Physiology, Surgery, Midwifery, and Surgical Pharmacy. By 1830 Professors of Medicine, Chemistry, Medical Jurisprudence, and Botany were added and in 1840 one in Preventive Medicine, the first of its kind in the British Isles. Thus at this time students were really being trained in a way suitable for general practice many years before the Conjoint qualifications became a legal requirement. The only place where a similar training was in existence was Glasgow, under the auspices of the Faculty of Physicians and Surgeons.

In its early days the College of Surgeons granted the following diplomas:

(1) one called the 'letters testimonial' or Licence, and licentiates were eligible for election to the membership.
(2) one for surgeons serving in the Army and of two grades – a Surgeon or a Surgeon's Mate. At a later date there was a similar examination for naval surgeons.
(3) a diploma in Midwifery.

In 1844 a Fellowship was instituted and the grade of Membership discontinued.[15]

To accommodate all these activities, new quarters in St. Stephen's Green were acquired on the site of the old Quakers' Burial Ground and an extension built in 1825. In such developments at this period men like Abraham Colles were the leading spirits. Students do not seem to have been in short supply, as they were in the other schools, and in the early 1800s many were candidates for the Army and Navy, presumably because of the large demands of the Napoleonic wars.

The importance of a Museum for a teaching body was realised and there was an attempt to include in it 'specimens of Natural History and such other sciences as are subservient to Surgery'.[16] There was one unusual development. In December 1829 the College was informed of a gift of £500 from the Lord Lieutenant, the Duke of Northumberland.[17] He intended that the money should be used to purchase wax models of anatomical specimens. In spite of a very critical leading article in the 'Lancet'[18] the money was spent on a number of models made by M. Talrich of Paris which can be seen today, and a model of the sympathetic system purchased in 1836 for £30. The first Museum Curator was John Shekleton, an apprentice of Abraham Colles, who was appointed in 1820, and was very skilful in dissection. John Shekleton was still only in his twenties when he died; he was dissecting a body with an infection resulting from a lithotomy and accidentally pricked himself.

The College maintained its activities as a medical school throughout the 19th century and very recently, in 1976[19], made a further extension to accommodate its large student population of 700 – a remarkable achievement.

No account of the Dublin medical scene of the last century would be complete without a few words about 'private medical schools'. These flourished at a slightly later date than those of London, which were considered in Chapter 2.

From 1804 onwards, some seventeen of these privately-owned schools were founded. They came to an end in 1889 when the last two, the Carmichael and Ledwich Schools, were amalgamated with the School at the Royal College of Surgeons in Ireland. They started at a time when, as previously said, there was a great demand for Army doctors for the Napoleonic wars. It appears that the facilities for practical anatomy and dissection were good in Dublin, and as a result students from all over England and Scotland were attracted. The majority were candidates for the Irish Royal College of Surgeons diploma. The courses came under the control of the College, by whom all teachers had to be approved. They were obliged to make annual returns of the names of the students and of their attendance at classes. Some schools were associated with hospitals, e.g., Jervis Street, Richmond, and Steeven's, while others were the property of individuals or of groups. Amongst their teachers were many of the most distinguished medical men in Dublin.[20]

The first of these schools seems to have been founded by an eminent man, Philip (later Sir Philip) Crampton, who subsequently served four terms of office as President of the Royal College of Surgeons. It consisted of a dissecting room and a lecture theatre. It was closed in 1813 when Crampton became Surgeon General.

The Carmichael School commenced at the Hardwicke Hospital but later became located at the Richmond Hospital, where Adams and Corrigan taught.[21] Its founder was Richard Carmichael, who had been President of the Royal College of Surgeons on three occasions, and was an active member of the Irish medical reform movement. He had hoped that some such body as the British Medical Association might have been formed in Ireland.[22] In 1849 he was tragically drowned when riding home to his country house, but in his will he bequeathed £10,000 to the school. In the same year the School was named after him and continued as such till 1889 when amalgamated with the Royal College of Surgeons School.

The other school which amalgamated in 1889 after a long life was the Ledwich. Dr. J. T. Kirby, who practised both medicine and surgery, founded an anatomical school in 1809 – often called the Peter Street School. It was closed in 1832 when Kirby became Professor of Medicine at the Royal College of Surgeons. In 1836 the premises were taken over by George T. Hayden and opened as a Medical School.[23] This was a great success initially for there were about 80 students who were taught Anatomy (with dissection), Physiology, Materia Medica, Botany, and Midwifery. Later Chemistry, Medical Jurisprudence, and Medicine were added.[24] In the 1840s the attendance fell off, but in 1849 two lecturers in Anatomy were appointed, Thomas Peter Mason and Thomas Hawkesworth Ledwich. There was an immediate and striking improvement but in 1858 Ledwich, who had suffered from asthma and cardiac disease for many years, died. In 1868, at the request of his pupils, the School became known as the Ledwich School. In addition to being an excellent teacher, Ledwich also advocated the use of the microscope. As can be seen the Ledwich had its ups and downs. In 1877,[25] Dublin University refused to accept its certificates following an error in which attendance had been accidentally dated 3 months ahead of time. An explanation of the mistake by the surgeon (Edward Ledwich) was not accepted and this perhaps indicates that rivalries between the teaching bodies ran high.

As in London, there were private tutors, often called 'grinders', who taught a wide variety of subjects purely for the purpose of passing examinations.

There were many important events in the 19th century and one might mention some of these. There was the appointment of a Professor of Hygiene or Political Medicine in 1841, Francis White. With public health very much in the news in 1864 Edward Dillon Mapother (1835–1908) became the first Medical Officer of Health for Dublin. In 1882 the Academy of Medicine in Ireland was founded, there being 150 Fellows at the time. It had a number of sections devoted to special subjects, setting a pattern which the Royal Society of Medicine in London followed some 25 years later. The Irish Academy carried a wide range of membership, there being three grades, namely Fellows, Members and Student Associates.

It remains to mention a group which acted as a licensing board but which took no part in teaching, the Apothecaries. They had been given a Charter by George II in 1745 to form the Guild of St. Luke's. The year 1791 was presumably an important one, for when advertising their examination in 1850,[26] they styled themselves 'Apothecaries Hall 1791'. The examiners seem to have been frequently available for what was almost certainly only an oral examination, for the notice states, 'The Court of Examiners sits every Friday at 2 o'clock'. There were two grades of examination for a license to be (1) an apothecary or (2) an assistant apothecary (confined to practical pharmacy). In 1886, by an amendment to the Medical Act, admission to the Medical Register required a qualification in Medicine, Surgery, and Midwifery. A Conjoint examination was agreed between the Royal Colleges of Physicians and Surgeons. The Surgeons would have admitted the Apothecaries but the Physicians declined. Accordingly, the Royal College of Surgeons formed an independent association with the Apothecaries. But this lasted only until 1894 when the Surgeons withdrew. The Apothecaries then introduced an examination in Surgery, and have since continued granting their licentiateship of the Apothecaries Hall, the LAH, which is registrable.

## The Scottish Universities

Because of the religious restriction imposed by the Universities of Oxford and Cambridge, many English students were obliged to study medicine at the Scottish Schools (chiefly Edinburgh) or at universities on the Continent. Scottish students likewise studied either at home or abroad. The student body at the two largest Scottish Universities (Edinburgh and Glasgow) was considerable for the time. At Edinburgh Professor Alexander Monro, at the end of the 18th century, had 4000 students in his Anatomy class, though the number declined to 200 when his less able son, Alexander tertius, took over;[27] at Glasgow University there were 54 medical students in 1790 and 130 in 1850.[28]

## St. Andrew's and Dundee

Founded in 1411, St. Andrew's was the oldest University in Scotland, but did not develop a complete medical faculty for over 400 years. There is evidence that in the 17th century there was a Professor of Medicine, that he gave some lectures, and that a doctor's degree was first conferred in 1696. After the Reformation there had been a scheme to divide faculties between the Scottish universities so that (a) Medicine would be taught at St. Andrew's, (b) Arts at Glasgow, (c) Laws and Divinity at Aberdeen – but it never materialised. Further progress in development towards a Medical Faculty was hampered by political difficulties which at one time threatened the existence of the University. It had few students compared with the other Scottish schools and its total of 150 compared unfavourably with 300 at Aberdeen, 600 at Edinburgh, and 400 at Glasgow.[29] At the end of the 18th century the University was moribund and only in Medicine did the students bother to take a degree.[30] The relatively favourable position of the Faculty of Medicine at that time may have arisen from the establishment of the Chandos Professorship of Medicine. In 1722 Thomas Simson (1696–1764) was the first to occupy this post. He had studied in Glasgow as well as in Leyden, where he had been one of Boerhaave's pupils. Teaching of Medicine now commenced though it remained haphazard until well into the 19th century. When Robert Briggs was appointed to the Chair in 1811, he taught the Principles of Medicine, Anatomy, and if requested Chemistry.

By 1840 a Chair of Chemistry had been founded and in the same year John Reid (1809–49) was appointed Chandos Professor and taught only Medicine. He had received his training in Edinburgh, was greatly interested in Pathology, and between 1838 and 1841 had been pathologist to the Edinburgh Royal Infirmary. He was a great asset to St. Andrew's and later gave a course on Comparative Anatomy and Physiology. He published several papers and was one of the first to distinguish typhoid from typhus fever. His loss was much felt when he died in 1849 of carcinoma of the tongue at the early age of 40.[31] In future years it became customary for the Chandos Professor to teach Physiology but it was not actually named as a Chair in that subject till 1908.

By 1830 the medical curriculum had been revised and stricter regulations for a degree had been imposed. In 1861[32], the Medical Examination consisted of four parts:

(1)  Translation of a passage from Latin into English, and a Paper on Chemistry.
(2)  Paper on Anatomy and Physiology.
(3)  Papers on Materia Medica, and the Practice of Medicine.
(4)  Papers on Surgery and Midwifery.

In 1874 there was a proposal to found a University College at Dundee, and in spite of some opposition this materialised in 1881. Endowments were forthcoming and Chairs were founded in Chemistry, Botany, Natural History, and Physiology.[33] By an affiliation of the new college with St. Andrew's, a full medical school was at last in sight. This was set up in Dundee in 1897 and during the next year Chairs were created in Medicine, Surgery, Pathology, Materia Medica, Midwifery, and a Lectureship in Forensic Medicine and Public Health. Now the first two years of the medical course were given in University College, Dundee, and the remainder at the University Conjoint School of Medicine in St. Andrews. Clinical instruction was provided at the Royal Infirmary and other medical institutes of the city. St. Andrew's was about to enter a modern era of prosperity, and the class of 60 medical students in 1899 had increased to 134 by 1927–8.[34]

## Glasgow

If St. Andrew's had been noted for its struggle for existence, the opposite was the case in Glasgow. Here the university progressed rapidly as part of the growth and prosperity of the town during the Industrial Revolution. In 1712 the population was only 14,000, but by 1801 it had risen to 83,000, and by 1831 to 200,000.[35] As early as 1599 the Royal Faculty of Physicians and Surgeons of Glasgow was founded to regulate the practice of Medicine, Surgery, and Pharmacy in the West of Scotland. It was the duty of the Faculty to examine and license surgeons, but physicians were required only to produce the diploma from their university. At that time no Scottish Universities granted degrees in medicine so this probably only applied to graduates of foreign universities. In the early 17th century, the Faculty laid down rules for apprentices in Medicine, conducted examinations for proficiency and exacted certain fees if the doctor wished to practice in Glasgow. It was also very active in identifying quacks and unlicensed practitioners. In 1785 the Faculty established a licentiateship permitting country surgeons to practice within a limited area, and at this time many men eminent in Medicine were members of the Faculty.[36] The Faculty had one or two unusual features in that both physicians and surgeons were included under its Charter, and that it undertook treatment of the poor, including visits to their homes, free of charge. This close association of both physicians and surgeons may well be the reason for the reputation of the Medical School in subsequent years as a training ground for general practitioners.

Thus, in these early days, Medicine in Glasgow was chiefly concerned with the practice rather than with the education of the subject. Although the date of foundation of the University is given as 1453 medicine was not taught for a long time. In the meanwhile the Town Council had attempted to attract doctors by offering salaries to those who might come to settle in the town, even as early as 1577.[37] The medical school commenced in 1704 when it was decided to establish a Physic Garden for botanical purposes, and John Marshall, a Glasgow surgeon, took charge of it. Also, the university began to examine candidates for the MD degree, although there was as yet no medical teaching.[38] In 1637 Dr. Robert Mayre had been appointed Professor in the Practice of Medicine, but the Chair lapsed after the death of the holder. A Regius Chair of Medicine was endowed in 1713 and a Chair of Anatomy and Botany founded in 1718. One of the earlier occupants of the latter was James Jeffray (1759–1848), who held the chair of Anatomy for a record period of 58 years.[39]

In 1783 William Hunter died and left his museum, which he had collected in London, to the University of Glasgow. This provided a great stimulus to medical teaching and came at a very opportune time. The earlier occupants of the Regius Chair of Medicine did little teaching until the advent of William Cullen (1710–90) in 1751 at the age of 41. In the absence of an organised university teaching faculty, his education consisted of being apprenticed to a surgeon in Glasgow and later to an apothecary in London,[40] where he met William Hunter. On his return to Glasgow he soon earned a name for himself by lecturing on Chemistry, Botany, Materia Medica, and the Practice of Physic, being second only to Boerhaave as a teacher. With his appointment as Regius Professor of Medicine he can be said to have been the founder of the Glasgow School of Medicine. Cullen went to Edinburgh in 1755 to occupy the Chair of Chemistry and subsequently the Chair of the Institutes of Medicine. One of his pupils, the famous scientist Joseph Black, became Professor of Medicine in Glasgow (1756) and later moved to Edinburgh (1766) to succeed Cullen as Professor of Chemistry.

The first 60 years of the 19th century witnessed a great advance in medical thought and education. In 1802 a Glasgow Medicochirurgical Society for undergraduates was formed and the number of anatomy students increased from 43 in 1790 to 256 in 1860.[41] One advantage in the study of Anatomy was that there was little shortage of bodies. These were thought to have come from Ireland, and there was certainly less hostility to local 'resurrectionists' than in other towns.

In 1794 the Royal Infirmary was opened, thus providing valuable material for clinical teaching of university students.

In 1818 the Crown founded a Chair of Surgery and one of Botany and Chemistry, and in 1839 further Chairs of the Theory of Physic or the Institutes of Medicine, Forensic Medicine, and Materia Medica. In 1831 a laboratory was set up for research in Chemistry, the first in Great Britain. In 1828, the Glasgow Medical Journal was founded.

In 1870 the medical school moved and in 1874 the Western Infirmary was adjacent, a combination patterned on the German University Hospital. The result of this development was to leave the Royal Infirmary, which was rebuilt in 1882, devoid of students for it was some distance from the new site of the University. The final evolution of the Glasgow Medical School is complex and only a brief outline will be given.

In the 19th century two schools of anatomy had sprung up which closely resembled the private schools in Dublin and London. The first of these was the 'College Street School', staffed by a number of private anatomists. There was also a dissecting room and the student attendance was large. But, founded in 1797, it seems to have closed in 1828. In the same way there was the 'Portland Street School', essentially similar and which ran from 1830–1844. With 'Anderson's College' things were different. This had been founded in 1796 from the estate of John Anderson (1726–96), a Professor of Oriental Languages who had had sundry differences with the University authorities.[42] He intended the College named after him to be a rival to the University and his wish was to come true. It commenced by teaching Anatomy and by the middle of the century had achieved striking success, for the number of its Anatomy students was approximately double that in the University department.

The College taught non-medical subjects, and the medical school was conducted separately. It had early success for in 1830 there were 700 medical students. Throughout the century its name was changed several times, being Anderson's College, Anderson's University, and in 1887 Anderson's College Medical School, the name under which it became incorporated. By this time it had moved to a site close to the University and the Western Infirmary. The College now ran a complete medical course and one attraction was published in its prospectus.[43]

'A dispensary is connected with Anderson's College. Students have the privilege of visiting and treating patients at their own homes, being assisted by a specially appointed qualified practitioner.'

The school continued its existence into the next century but changed its name once more to the Anderson College of Medicine in 1913.

There was yet another College which came into existence at the end of the 19th century. It will be recalled that when the Western Infirmary was opened in 1874, the Royal Infirmary, remote geographically, became deprived of its students, and ceased to be a medical school. In 1876 an additional school was set up and called the Royal Infirmary Medical School. Buildings were erected and in 1882, when complete, could accommodate 300–400 students.[44] St. Mungo's College had provided courses in Law, Science, Art, and Medicine outside the University. In 1889 the Royal Infirmary Medical School was incorporated, and continued as the Medical Faculty of St. Mungo's College.[45]

Glasgow, with a century of progress behind it, entered the 20th century with no shortage of medical training facilities. There were now two complete medical schools, one attached to the Western Infirmary and one to the Royal. Additional teaching facilities were available at the extra-academical schools of Anderson's College and St. Mungo's College. The remarkable progress of the University can be realised when we find that in 1859–60 there were 311 students, while in 1929–30 the number had risen to 829 – and this does not include about 500 at the extra-academical schools.[46]

## Aberdeen

The University of Aberdeen was formed in 1860 by the union of King's and Marischal Colleges.

King's College, founded in 1498, had many of the characteristics of a mediaeval university. One unusual feature dating from its early days was the office of 'Mediciner', who might be regarded as a Professor of Medicine (see chapter 7). At that time it was customary for educated persons such as the clergy and landowners to provide medical help for the sick poor, especially those living in remote districts. Such persons, in addition to their own studies, often received courses in Physic, even though they had no intention of practising medicine. This instruction was given by the 'Mediciner' and in a way this could be regarded as the first university recognition of Medicine in Great Britain.[47] There are records of Mediciners at King's College from 1522 until 1844, though there were periods when the appointment lapsed. The first MD degree was conferred as early as 1630 but there was as yet no proper teaching course. In 1632 William Gordon was elected Mediciner and gave some instruction in Medicine and Anatomy. Limited by having only animals to dissect, he petitioned the Privy Council for opportunities to use human bodies, and he was given permission to have two per year.[48] One remarkable 18th century family was that of the Gregories, who had produced sixteen professors in Aberdeen, Edinburgh, and other universities. Three of these had been Mediciners at King's College.

In the meanwhile there had been some developments at Marischal College. It was founded in 1593 but the institution of a Chair of Medicine had been delayed until 1700. The first holder, Patrick Chalmers, had studied at the Universities at Leyden, Paris and Padua and obtained his MD at all three. He was dismissed for Jacobite sympathies and replaced in 1717 by Matthew Mackaile Jr., son of Matthew Mackaile, Sr., an apothecary who had become MD of King's College in 1696. The younger Mackaile, and probably Chalmers too, was a pupil of Boerhaave and therefore anxious to develop clinical teaching in Aberdeen. Thus in 1739 it was decided to found a hospital and the Aberdeen Infirmary opened its doors in 1742. It was a modest start for there were only six beds. James Gordon, who had been appointed Professor of Medicine in 1734, became its first Physician and Surgeon and taught his students daily at the bedside.[49]

One of the earliest physicians to the hospital was John Gregory (1724–1773), who had also studied at Leyden. He first became associated with King's College in 1746 as a teacher of Natural Philosophy and succeeded his brother as Mediciner in 1755. He was most anxious to form a Medical School and his was the first of a number of unsuccessful attempts at this time. With help from Dr. David Skene he gave a course of lectures on Medicine and Midwifery. It was poorly attended and the school never materialised for he left Aberdeen for Edinburgh in 1766.[50] In 1782 Dr. William Chalmers, on becoming Mediciner, announced that he would commence a medical academy for teaching, but nothing resulted. A further attempt was made in 1786, but again it failed. One difficulty was that King's and Marischal colleges were going their own separate ways. Some suggested that they should unite but this was only a bare possibility. Then in 1789 there was hope from an unexpected quarter. Twelve students (one of whom was James McGrigor) founded the Aberdeen Medocochrirugial Society. This was a scientific body composed of academic teachers, physicians, surgeons, and medical students. It was a great success, consolidating those with medical interests, and it became closely attached to Marischal College. In 1818 this College suggested a joint scheme of medical instruction with King's consisting of lectures on Anatomy, Physiology, Surgery, Practice and Theory of Medicine, Materia Medica, Clinical Medicine, Midwifery, and Botany, and strict regulations for a degree were laid down. However there were few graduates, for between 1826 and 1839 King's College produced only four and Marischal twenty-five. This joint association was not a happy one and it was terminated by King's College. If this college had had internal dissension, it had also experienced outside troubles, when in 1831 a crowd, incensed about the dissection of human bodies, burnt down the dissecting room of Moir, the Lecturer in Anatomy, who had to flee for his life.

In 1839 King's College made yet another attempt to set up a medical school, chiefly at the instigation of the Mediciner, Dr. William Gregory. Again, misfortune intervened and the project declined following his departure for Edinburgh in 1844. Some progress was made at Marischal College when the Crown created Chairs of Anatomy and Surgery, and some men of outstanding ability were recruited. These included Allen Thomson (Anatomy), John Macrobin (Medicine), and William Pirrie (Surgery).

The really important year was 1860 when finally, after having so far led an unimpressive existence, the two colleges joined together to form the University of Aberdeen.[51] In 1860 there were Chairs of Medicine, Surgery, Medical Logic and Jurisprudence, Chemistry, and Anatomy. The Crown now added several new Chairs including Botany, Natural History, Physiology, Materia Medica, and Midwifery. This new era in Aberdeen was attended with great success and the student entry which in 1860 had been 145 had risen to 335 by 1880 and has remained at that level. Many outstanding graduates have emerged from Aberdeen but mention can only be made of two. The first of these was Sir Erasmus Wilson, a dermatologist who in 1881 became President of the Royal College of Surgeons of England. In the following year he endowed a Chair of Pathology in the University of Aberdeen. He had wide interests and is remembered for financing the transport of the granite obelisk, Cleopatra's Needle, to London where it stands on the Embankment.

The other Aberdonian to be mentioned was an 18th century graduate of Marischal College named Sir James McGrigor. He is chiefly remembered for his contributions to Military Medicine, and his career is given in chapter 14.

**Edinburgh**

Although Edinburgh University, founded in 1582, was the latest of the Scottish Universities, there had been medical activities in the city before that time.[52] By 1505 the Guild of Barbers and Surgeons was already a well-established teaching body. The Town Council had granted a Charter to the Surgeons in that year and it became ratified by James IV of Scotland in 1506.

The new body, known as the Incorporation of Barber Surgeons, then had the power of examining apprentices to the trade and the granting of licenses. The examination demanded a knowledge of anatomy including the veins used for phlebotomy, and the recognition of some astrological symbols. One body per year was to be available for dissection.

Unfortunately, there are few records of the activities of the Incorporation for the next 200 years. It seems likely that, as in the case of the Barber Surgeons in England, the Surgeons separated. They had their own guild in 1719 and in later times were referred to as the Incorporation of Surgeons.[53] What is perhaps surprising is that there seems to have been little interest in Anatomy in Scotland at this time and no outstanding anatomist at a time when, due to the activity of Vesalius, Eustaceus, Sylvius, Fabricius, Malpighi, and many others, there had been so many advances in the subject on the Continent. It was not until the end of the 17th century that the importance of the subject became realised, and this development came about in a complex and unexpected way.

The university received its Charter in 1582 from James VI of Scotland and by 1583 the buildings were ready. Its foundation was modelled on that of the Academy of Geneva and, being administered by the Town Council, was referred to as 'The Town's College' for about the next 300 years.[54] The Charter permitted the establishment of Faculties of Philosophy and Language, Theology, Laws, and Medicine, but at this stage only Arts and Theology were taught.[55]

At this time, there was a group of physicians who had returned to Edinburgh after studying on the Continent in Leyden and Paris.[56] It included their leader, Robert Sibbald, and also Archibald Pitcairne. Sibbald had been impressed in Paris by the use of herbs for the treatment of disease and had set up a 'Physic Garden'. This had only been achieved in the face of considerable opposition from the Surgeons. It appears that Medicine at the time was extensively practised by 'surgeon-apothecaries', who feared the foundation of a College of Physicians with possible curtailment of their livelihood.[57] Their fears were well grounded for in 1680 Sibbald began to hold conferences of physicians and as a result in 1681 a College of Physicians was formed under a Charter granted by Charles II.[58] Its purpose was 'the vigilant cognizance of all apothecaries' shops in the city and suburbs and the prevention of unauthorised persons practising as physicians'.[59] It therefore had the power of licensing all those who intended to practice as physicians in Edinburgh or its neighbourhood. But it was not permitted to erect a medical school to organise teaching. The examination for licensure consisted of an oral comment on two of the Aphorisms of Hippocrates, and a discussion of two cases provided by the examiners. In 1693, when

Archibald Pitcairne had returned from Leyden, there was added an examination on the Institutes of Medicine. In 1684 Sir Robert Sibbald became the first president of the College. The year 1685 was a momentous one in Edinburgh's medical history, for the Town Council appointed three Professors of Medicine, namely Robert Sibbald, James Halket, and Archibald Pitcairne – and the Faculty of Medicine was launched.[57].

There was very little anatomy teaching taking place, though presumably the Incorporation of Surgeons was dissecting its one body per year. However, Pitcairne realised the growing importance of the subject and, himself a physician, encouraged a colleague, Alexander Monteith, a member of the Incorporation and a noteworthy surgeon, to stimulate interest. As a result, in 1694 Monteith petitioned the Town Council to provide bodies for dissection from the 'house of correction' and also certain unclaimed foundlings.[60] This appears to have been a private venture on his part, and in exchange for this privilege he offered to treat the poor of the city free of charge. A few days later the Incorporation submitted a similar petition. The Town Council granted both requests but stipulated that the Surgeons build an anatomical theatre by Michelmas, 1697, as their part of the bargain. Monteith does not appear to have taught anatomy for long, though he was given a room for dissection, for in 1697 we find him teaching Chemistry in Surgeon's Hall. The Surgeons, however, took it in turn to carry out their dissections, and there is no evidence of any friction between Monteith and the Surgeons for he was elected President of the Incorporation in 1695 and 1696.[61] In 1705 the Surgeons found it more convenient to elect one surgeon, Robert Elliot, to carry out all the dissections, and he was known as the 'Public Dissector of Anatomy'. The word 'public' is misleading and does not mean 'in public', for the Town Council restricted the use of the Anatomical Theatre to apprentices and pupils of Freemen. In addition to his duties as Dissector, Elliot had to inspect 'the condition of the rarities of the College'. By this was meant unusual specimens, and this made him a kind of Museum Curator. Natural history specimens were included for there were 'an egyle (presented by Monteith himself), three scorpions, a chameleon, and an allegatory or young crocodile', and there were a number of books.[62] He was given the title of Professor and thus became the first Professor of Anatomy in the University of Edinburgh. In 1708 Adam Drummond became joint professor, and after Elliot's death in 1716 John McGill replaced him. Teaching of Anatomy by these joint professors seems to have been limited, but in 1720 Drummond and McGill resigned in favour of the brilliant young anatomist, Alexander Monro (primus), and he initiated the golden era of Edinburgh anatomy to which we shall turn later. But it is important to realise that this Chair of Anatomy had been instituted by the action of two bodies. The Surgeons elected the individual and provided also students and accommodation, while the Town Council provided the salary, and thus made it a University Chair.

To follow the further development of the Medical Faculty we must return to the appointment of Sibbald, Halket, and Pitcairne as Professors of Medicine by the Town Council in 1685. They were all Founder Fellows of the recently formed College of Physicians. In 1705 the University awarded its first MD degree, and there was soon to be some evidence of cooperation with the College of Physicians for in 1718 the latter body was invited to appoint one or more of its Fellows to assist as examiners.[63] The course in Medicine was still far from complete but in 1723, when the Anatomy course given by Alexander Monro (primus) was flourishing, the Town Council accepted the following recommendation from the College of Physicians: 'considering the great benefit and advantage that would accrue to this city and kingdom by having all the parts of Medicine taught in this place, decided to appoint a professor to teach the Institutes and Practice of Medicine'.[64] It is doubtful whether the first professor, William Porterfield, gave any lectures at all for in 1726, the Town Council appointed four professors to organise the teaching of Medicine and allied subjects and selected the following:

(1) Dr. Andrew St. Clair to teach the Institutes or Theory of Medicine.
(2) Dr. John Rutherford, the Practice of Medicine.
(3) Dr. Andrew Plummer, and
(4) Dr. John Innes, to share the teaching of Chemistry and Materia Medica.[64]

In the same year these four men petitioned the Town Council for their appointment as Professors. This was granted and now, with the Faculty of Medicine expanded to include Botany, Chemistry, Midwifery, and Pharmaceutical demonstrations, a complete course in Medicine was available to students. With the appointment of Professors in special subjects the old tutorial system was abolished and the transition from College to University became complete.[65]

For this achievement much of the credit must go to John Monro, a distinguished surgeon in the army of King William III.[66] Returning from the wars, he had settled in Edinburgh in 1700 as a surgeon-apothecary, becoming a member of the Incorporation of Surgeons in 1703 and President in 1712. He had served an apprenticeship with a surgeon-apothecary before going to spend 2 years study at the leading medical school of the time, namely the University of Leyden. There he was taught by Archibald Pitcairne and had amongst his fellow pupils Richard Mead, Robert Elliot, and Hermann Boerhaave. The school was unique in that there was clinical teaching, a feature first introduced by Francesco Sylvius (1614–72). In this atmosphere, John Monro conceived the idea of setting up in Edinburgh a medical school which would certainly equal if not outstrip that of Leyden. Apart from his own activities he hoped to bring this about by preparing his son Alexander (primus) to play a leading part as Professor of Anatomy. Alexander Monro (1697–1767) commenced his studies in Edinburgh and in 1717 supplemented these in Leyden where he was one of Boerhaave's pupils. This was followed by a period at St. Thomas's Hospital in London with William Cheselden, a most excellent surgeon and the leading lithotomist of the day. He studied both Anatomy and Surgery and nearly lost his arm following a wound self-inflicted during dissection.[67] In 1719 he became a member of the Incorporation of Surgeons on his return to Edinburgh, and was recognised not only as a very skilful dissector but also an outstanding anatomist. Then in 1720, at the age of 23, he became Professor of Anatomy and gave lectures on both Anatomy and Surgery at Surgeons' Hall. His success was instantaneous and students flocked to him from England, Ireland, and Scotland: in his first ten years he attracted 670. One can well imagine that tuition for this large number entailed much dissection and the acquisition of a good many bodies. It is therefore not surprising to hear that before long there were serious riots in the town in opposition to 'body snatching'. On this account Alexander Monro moved into the university buildings where he felt safer within its walls. He was given a theatre for his work and in 1725 became Professor of Anatomy in the University. There his success continued and twenty years later the number of students had more than doubled.

The record of the Monro family is almost without parallel for it held the Professorship of Anatomy from 1720 until 1846 when John Goodsir (1814–1869) succeeded Alexander Monro (tertius). Alexander Monro (primus) (1697–1767) held it for 38 years; Alexander Monro (secundus) (1733–1817), the most distinguished of the three, held it for 54 years including 4 as joint-professor with his father; Alexander Monro (tertius) (1773–1859), the least eminent, held it for 48 years, 10 of which were as joint-professor with his father. It is always said that Monro tertius did not equal primus or secundus in ability. Laziness seems to have been the trouble and his students were quick to notice that he was reading his grandfather's notes when he came to the passage, 'When I was in Leyden in 1719' – some 54 years before he was born! It was therefore customary for the lecture room to be crowded when this passage was due and when these words were said, showers of peas fell upon his head, but he still made no correction![68] This idea of instituting a joint professorship between father and son ensured that the Chair remained in the family. Alexander Monro (secundus) became Joint-Professor in 1754 at the age of 21, and his father then sent him to Europe for a two and a half year study period. He attended William Hunter's lectures in London, and also studied at Leyden, Paris, and Berlin. He always maintained that his most valuable anatomical training was in Berlin where he not only worked under Johann Friedrich Meckel the younger (1781–1833), but lived in his house.[69]

Thus, the University became renowned in the 18th century for its department of Anatomy, but there were other developments which made it the leading medical school in the British Isles. Medicine continued to be taught but made little progress until the appointment of Robert Whytt (1714–1766) as Professor. A man of great ability who first localised the seat of reflex action in the spinal cord,[70] he taught both the Theory and Practice of Medicine until his death in 1766. In 1755 William Cullen (1710–1790), a most versatile man, had been appointed Professor of Chemistry, following a period in Glasgow where he founded the Medical Faculty. He was an outstanding teacher, gave lectures on Clinical Medicine, and on the death of Whytt took over the teaching of the Theory of Medicine (or the Institutes) while John Gregory became Professor of the Practice of Medicine. Cullen's lectures were unusual for he was the first to abandon Latin and to use English.

At this stage it might be of some interest to consider the meaning of the term 'Institutes of Medicine', which was never used at any of the English Universities. In Scotland it was almost confined to the University of Edinburgh, though it was occasionally used in the other universities. Here, the first professor of the 'Institutes' was appointed in 1726 and the last one was John Hughes Bennett, who retired from the Chair in 1874. In Aberdeen, both Marischal and King's Colleges appointed lecturers in the 'Institutes' between 1819 and 1850 as well as Lecturers in the Practice of Medicine.[71] Glasgow University seems never to have used the term, but divided Medicine between the Theory and Practice of the subject.[72] The University of St. Andrew's also did not use it, for it had one Chair for the whole of Medicine until 1863[73] (see p. 123).

Avicenna (980–1037), the famous Persian physician, produced his well-known work, 'The Canon', which classified all the knowledge of Medicine of the time into five books. The first of these in Part 1 consisted of 'the Institutes of Medicine' which included definition of Medicine, its task, its relation to Philosophy; the elements, juices, and temperaments; the organs and their functions, Anatomy and Physiology.[74] It seems that this approach was followed by the Dutch Schools of the 17th and 18th centuries, for Boerhaave himself published his 'Institutiones Medicae' in 1708 and his 'Aphorisms' in 1709. The use of the term 'Institutes' in Edinburgh is almost certainly due to its close association with Leyden, for we learn that when the Medical Faculty was founded in 1726, St. Clair lectured from Boerhaave's work on the 'Institutes' and Rutherford from his 'Aphorisms'. In the 19th century the term 'Institutes' gradually became synonymous with Physiology.

There was as yet one further step which had to be taken before the Medical School could be called 'complete', namely the provision for clinical teaching. In the 17th century the Royal College of Physicians of Edinburgh had given medicines to the poor and visited some of the sick in their homes. No doubt this was a similar movement to that of the London Royal College of Physicians, which set up a Public Dispensary at the same time. But at the beginning of the 18th century some Fellows of the Edinburgh College hired a small house in Robertson's Close with

133

accommodation for 6 patients.[75] This was in 1729, but in 1736 a Charter was received from George II to build a Royal Infirmary. The foundation stone of this 200-bedded hospital was laid in 1738 and the building completed in 1741. The surgeons had opened a small hospital at about the same time but after a couple of years joined with the Royal Infirmary. In order to staff the new institution it was arranged that Fellows of the Royal College of Physicians and Members of the Incorporation of Surgeons attended the Infirmary by rotation. In 1751 two physicians-in-ordinary, and in 1766 three surgeons, were appointed to the hospital staff. Further adjacent property enabled the hospital to be extended in 1829 and a modern hospital built in 1879.

The relation of the hospital to the medical school was most important and in 1748 John Rutherford (1695–1779) gave a course of clinical lectures in the Royal Infirmary. These were probably the first clinical lectures given in the country and it is likely that he was motivated by the clinical teaching given to him when a student at Leyden. Other professors of medicine followed suit and with the appearance of William Cullen in 1757 the reputation of Edinburgh went on from strength to strength. Cullen lectured for many years and became Professor of the Practice of Physic in 1773.[76]

If the appointment of Professors of Medicine in the University had been straight-forward, the same could not be said for that of Surgery. The first Chair of Surgery was not founded until 1831, more than a hundred years after the Chair of the Institutes. The main reason for this delay was opposition on the part of the Monro family, chiefly secundus. At the time in 1754 when Primus and secundus were made joint-professors they had successfully asked for their titles to be changed. They maintained that as they both had MD degrees the new title should be Professor of Medicine, Anatomy and Surgery. It appears that all three Monros also practised medicine and gave opinions on medical and surgical cases, though they did not operate. Monro secundus had maintained that there was no need for a Professor of Surgery, as he could provide all the information that they required. The earliest lectures on Surgery were given by Mr. James Rae in 1772 with the approval of the Incorporation of Surgeons.[77] In 1776 he had suggested that applications be made to the Crown to establish a Professorship of Surgery in the University of Edinburgh. This was refused by the Lord Advocate, who had been approached by the Principal and medical Professors of the University, saying that such an appointment would be 'useless and very unpopular'. In 1777 Monro secundus applied unsuccessfully to the Town Council to agree that he was Professor of Surgery as well as Anatomy. The turn of the century was to bring about two important events. In 1803 the Town Council founded a Chair of Clinical Surgery to which James Russell, one of the six surgeons to the Royal Infirmary, was elected; in the following year the Royal College of Surgeons instituted a Chair of Surgery whose first occupant was Dr. John Thomson. Monro opposed it but was unsuccessful. In 1806 George III had commissioned and endowed a Chair of Military Surgery, a subject much in vogue at the time, and John Thomson was the first occupant. It was not till 1831 that John William Turner was made the first Professor of Surgery in the University, and at the same time the College of Surgeons' Chair of Surgery was abolished. Although the teaching of Anatomy under Monro tertius declined, Edinburgh retained its high standard due to two excellent extramural lecturers, John Barclay (1758–1826) and Robert Knox (1791–1862). The latter was an outstanding lecturer who attracted over 500 students and it was a tragedy that at the height of his fame he was said to have been involved in the Burke and Hare body-snatching scandal.

The Edinburgh Medical School continued to flourish in the 19th century and in 1807 George III endowed the first Chair of Medical Jurisprudence, held by Andrew Duncan, Jr. (1744–1828). But already, with a student entry of over 400, accommodation had become a problem and the existing buildings were in poor repair. Funds had earlier been raised and in 1789 the foundation stone of 'The New College of Edinburgh' was laid. The architect, John Adam, died suddenly in 1792 and was succeeded by his brothers and a further extension designed by W. H. Playfair was incorporated in the plans. But it was a protracted business because of financial crisis and it was not until 1834 that the 'Adam-Playfair' building was completed at a total cost of £160,000.[78]

Over the previous centuries the tendency for a Professor to cover more than one subject has been noted. Thus Anatomy and Physiology might be combined and the difficulties with the Monros over Anatomy and Surgery were well recognised by the University. All this came to an end in 1829 for it was decided that no Professor or Lecturer would be recognised for more than two branches of education, and in 1839 this was reduced to one.[79]

Throughout the 18th and 19th centuries a steady stream of eminent medical men poured out of the University but space limits us to a cursory mention of the most famous of them.

Edinburgh did not have to wait long to produce a man of distinction, for a year after the establishment of the Medical Faculty John Pringle (later Sir John) came from St. Andrew's to become a medical student. He was destined to become the pioneer in Military Medicine as compared with Military Surgery (see chapter 8).

Sir Robert Christison (1797–1882) became the leading toxicologist of his day. Sir James Young Simpson (1811–1870) was responsible for the introduction of chloroform. William Sharpey (1802–1880) and John Hughes Bennett (1812–1875) became the founders of British physiology. Many migrated to London, including Sir Charles Bell (1774–1842), who ran his famous anatomy school and, after treating casualties from the battle of Waterloo, became surgeon to the Middlesex Hospital. James Syme (1799–1870) and Rober Liston (1794–1847), both pupils of the

Edinburgh anatomist John Barclay, came to University College, London. Liston remained there a life-time, while Syme returned to Edinburgh after only 6 months. Sir William Ferguson (1808–1877) came to King's College Hospital, London, became Surgeon to the Queen and was regarded as the leading operator of the day. Lord Lister (1827–1912), a London graduate, went to Edinburgh to work with Syme, on the advice of his Professor of Physiology, William Sharpey. He stayed for 7 years before moving to Glasgow. Finally, he returned to London after having spent 8 years as successor to Syme in Edinburgh as Professor of Surgery. This is an impressive list, but add to it the names of others who studied in Edinburgh, namely Addison, Bright, Cheyne, Corrigan, Graves, Hodgkin, and Stokes, and the enormous contribution of the school becomes evident.

The level of academic teaching was undoubtedly high, but there was one additional educational feature to which many students paid tribute later. This was the remarkable number of student societies in existence. Of these the Royal Medical is the oldest, having been founded by William Cullen and a few other students in 1737 and receiving its Royal Charter in 1778. As such it is the oldest medical society still in existence in the British Isles. Of others, the Speculative Society, founded in 1764 by six students as a 'school of composition and debate', is a good example. Sir Walter Scott was its secretary at one time (1791–1795) and Richard Bright was a member. In 1833 some of these societies became associated to hold a joint meeting and a debate once a year. They included the Dialectic, the Diagnostic, the Speculative, the Scots Law, and the Philomathic.[80] There were many others and one of some interest was 'The Six Feet Club' founded in 1826; all members had to be six feet tall. Its purpose was 'to practice and encourage gymnastic exercises and games', and there was an annual fete and dinner!

It would be hard to overestimate the contribution of the Scottish Schools to British Medicine. Numerically, Edinburgh and Glasgow were much larger than St. Andrew's and Aberdeen, which might be called 'late developers'. Glasgow owed its success to the growth of the town during the Industrial Revolution, though the University was at one time handicapped by some ill feeling between it and the Faculty of Physicians and Surgeons. No such animosity seems to have occurred in Edinburgh. Edinburgh University, although last in the field, owed much of its success to the stimulating contacts between it and Leyden, and because its hospital for clinical teaching (The Royal Infirmary) was built about 50 years before those in the other university towns. It now remains for us to consider the situation in London and to see how this contrasted with Edinburgh and the Continental Universities.

## The London Schools

In London the situation was totally different, and the question of having a University at all seems only to have been seriously considered in the 1820s. Up to this time, teaching of Medicine and Surgery took place in the large hospitals where students could enroll. They 'walked the wards', might attend occasional lectures, and saw a very limited amount of post-mortem material in the 'dead house'. Those wishing to become surgeons might become apprenticed to a surgeon at these hospitals, on payment of a substantial fee. The real defect of these times was that, up to the 18th century, there were only one or two hospitals which offered a complete course of medical education. The need for tuition was great and as mentioned in chapter 2 a number of private medical schools appeared at about mid-century. These schools, such as Hunter's in Covent Garden (and later in Great Windmill Street), Brooke's in Blenheim Street, Carpue's in Dean Street, and Grainger's in Webb Street, commenced as Schools of Anatomy and flourished in the early part of the 19th century. They had difficulties, for at the time of their foundation there was a shortage of bodies for dissection and some schools looked for help from the 'ressurrection men'. Tuition was given by lectures, and in some cases facilities for dissection were provided. Because of the shortage of bodies, dissections such as those carried out for his brother, William, were performed by John Hunter and preserved in 'spirits of wine', and such collections were the basis of private museums. Joshua Brookes discovered a method of injecting anatomical specimens, and it was said that the museum at his school was second only to that of the Hunters. These schools sprang up in close proximity to the teaching hospitals, the Webb Street School (Grainger's) being convenient to Guy's and St. Thomas's, and the Great Windmill School to St. George's and Middlesex Hospitals. As a result, medical students attended these private schools for courses in Anatomy and Surgery, and some of the teachers might be surgeons on the staff of the adjacent hospital. Some schools like Carpue's retained this function throughout their existence and Carpue was an excellent anatomist and teacher. Other schools such as the Aldersgate Street Medical School (adjacent to Bart's) and the Webb Street School (adjacent to Guy's and St. Thomas's) extended their teaching to other subjects. The Aldersgate Street School taught Anatomy, Physiology, Operative Surgery (including dissection), Medicine, Chemistry, Pharmacy, Materia Medica, Medical Botany, Therapeutics, Midwifery, and Diseases of Women and Children.[81] The Webb School gave courses in Anatomy, Physiology, Principles and Practice of Physic, Midwifery, Diseases of Women and Children, Materia Medica, Chemistry, and Pharmacy.[82] By 1800 or soon afterwards these private schools reached the height of their prosperity but by 1850 they had virtually disappeared. During their heyday they had at times proved serious rivals to the large teaching hospitals, as for example the

Aldersgate Street Medical School which posed a decided threat to neighbouring St. Bartholomew's. The large hospital hastily revised its teaching programmes and was soon able to provide a full medical course. For a time some, like St. George's Hospital, taught all subjects except Anatomy, which the students learned at the neighbouring schools of Lane's or Jermott's. But by 1836 St. George's had established a department of Anatomy and the days of the private schools were numbered. The situation now was that all the voluntary teaching hospitals had their own Basic Science Departments, and they were well-satisfied to continue in this way. It should be pointed out that the generalisations made above applied to most of the London Hospitals between 1750 and 1850, that is to say, St. Bartholomew's, St. Thomas's, the Westminster, Guy's, The London, the Middlesex, and St. George's. Charing Cross, St. Mary's and the Royal Free belong to a later period. Two of the London schools not yet dealt with differed from the others, namely King's College and University College.

By the early part of the 19th century the need for education was very great. In the previous century the Dissenters, resentful of the religious restrictions imposed by Cambridge and Oxford, founded a number of academies throughout the country as, for example, the Warrington Academy, which provided courses similar to those given at the Universities. With the advent of the Industrial Revolution there was a demand for scientific information and as a result a number of Philosophical Societies, such as the Lunar Society, were founded. They aimed at bringing together industrialists and men of science so that there could be a free exchange of ideas and the industrialists could benefit from hearing of the latest advances in science. With the increasing complexity of Industry, there was a demand for men with both scientific and technical training. Add to this the enormous increase in population and it becomes obvious that the Universities of Cambridge and Oxford were totally unable to fulfil the educational demands, even if they were to adopt a more liberal policy in their terms of entry. The idea of founding universities throughout the country gained ground in order to assist dissenters and sons of the middle class. Durham and other sites were proposed, but the London University, with which we are concerned, was first in the field. Since 1812 dissenters, radicals, and secularists had been considering such a foundation but this did not really take shape until the poet Thomas Campbell visited Germany in 1820 and in 1825 wrote a letter to the 'Times', giving his plans for a 'great London University'.[83] He was also supported by Isaac Lyon Goldsmid, a financier, and Henry Broughman, a politician.[84] Campbell had been very much impressed by the progress of the University in Berlin, founded in 1809, a subject that we shall return to later. A Council was appointed to raise money and establish the new university. The setting up of a theological faculty immediately produced difficulties because there was great disagreement as to the type of religious instruction, especially as so many dissenters were concerned. As a result it was decided not to teach Theology at all and this was the signal for the opponents of the scheme to refer to it as the 'radical infidel college'.[85] For this reason this University has always been free from religious tests of entry. In 1827 a plot of ground was obtained in Gower Street and the foundation stone laid on the 30th April. A list of professors was drawn up and University College opened in 1828. Charles Bell, who was attached to the Middlesex Hospital, agreed to become Professor of Anatomy and Morbid Anatomy after a breakdown of negotiation with Johannes Meckel (junior) of Halle, who had been invited to occupy the Chair and to bring his museum with him.[86] Charles Bell gave an inaugural lecture which from all accounts was an outstanding success.

But in the meanwhile the opponents of the College had not been idle and had urged on Sir Robert Peel, the Prime Minister, that the University of London was inadequate, chiefly because of its lack of spiritual and moral education. They therefore suggested that a new college called King's be founded and a site for it was chosen beside Somerset House in the Strand. Once more religious difficulties arose and a compromise resulted. The Principal and the Professors had to be members of the Church of England (except in the cases of Oriental Literature and Modern Languages). While the system of entry was almost as free as at University College, all students had to attend a course of religious instruction. On 1st October 1831 the doors of King's College were opened.[87] Ultimately in 1836 the Charter of Incorporation was granted to a University of London, at which both King's College and University College were able to present their students for degrees.

The new colleges had appeared in the face of considerable opposition not only from certain sections of the public but also from the other medical schools, and from the Royal College of Surgeons which feared that its precincts would be invaded. They even suggested that the University Degree should not be recognised as a qualification to practice. But the Colleges in their initial years faced an even greater problem in regard to their medical faculty. It will be remembered that one of the difficulties of the London teaching hospitals was their lack of departments of basic science subjects. Now the new colleges were in the precisely opposite difficulty of having basic science departments, but no attached hospitals for their clinical teaching. In the case of University College it seems likely that the basic science departments were patterned on those in the University of Edinburgh, for many of the earlier professors had come from that school, as for instance, Charles Bell, Anthony Todd Thomson, and John Conolly. The students of University College went either to the Middlesex Hospital or to an adjacent dispensary for their clinical work, but this was by no means satisfactory. Accordingly, it was decided to build a North London Hospital, and the foundation stone was laid on a plot of ground opposite the College. The hospital was opened in 1834 and in 1837 it was named University College Hospital.

King's College obtained its Charter in 1829 and opened on the 1st October 1831. The building had been designed to blend with the hand-some facade of the adjacent Somerset House and was not completed until 1834. In 1831 the College commenced with a department of Liberal Education which soon became the Department of General Literature and Science.[88] A Medical Department followed and in 1838 and 1847 depart-ments of Engineering and Theology were added. It seems likely that the Medical Department was founded in 1833 for we know that John Simon went to King's College for Chemistry as a first year student in October of that year. There must have been an Anatomy Department for he carried out dissections there as a first year student and in 1838 he became a demonstrator in that department. There do not appear to have been any clinical facilities for he went to St. Thomas's Hospital for surgical lectures because he was apprenticed to Mr. Joseph Green, a surgeon at that hospital. In order to provide a hospital linked with the College, in 1840 a workhouse building near Clare Market, adjacent to Lincoln's Inn Fields, was taken over. But if the beginnings had been modest, King's was soon to gain prominence in Surgery when William Fergusson was joined by Joseph Lister, and by William Bowman who soon became one of the landing ophthalmic surgeons.

REFERENCES

1 Underwood, E. A., 'Boerhaave's Men'. Edinburgh University Press, p. 71.
2 Ibid p. 80.
3 Ibid p. 81.
4 Ibid p. 79.
5 Ibid p. 144.
6 Widdis, J. D. H., 'Schools of Surgery'. Williams & Williams Co., Baltimore 1949, p. 9.
7 'Lancet'. (1861) ii, pp. 366, 389, 414, 439, 490.
8 'British Medical Journal'. (1862) i, p. 296.
9 Ibid (1860) ii, p. 674.
10 Gash, N., 'Sir Robert Peel'. Rowman & Littlefield 1972. p. 479.
11 'Lancet'. (1907) i, p. 1249.
12 Ibid (1882) ii, pp. 1322–3.
13 Ibid (1908) i, p. 1087.
14 'British Medical Journal'. (1976) i, pp. 1264–6.
15 Widdiss, J. D. H., 'Schools of Surgery'. Williams & Williams, Baltimore 1949. p. 44.
16 Ibid p. 61.
17 Cameron, C. A., 'History of the Royal College of Surgeons in Ireland'. Fannin & Co. Dublin 1916, p. 329.
18 'Lancet'. (1829–30) ii, pp. 13–19.
19 'British Medical Journal'. (1976) i, p. 1264.
20 Widdiss, J. D. H., 'Schools of Surgery'. Williams & Williams, Baltimore 1949, p. 86–7.

21  Ibid p. 88.
22  Ibid p. 80.
23  Ibid p. 89.
24  Cameron, C. A., 'History of the Royal College of Surgeons in Ireland'. Fannin & Co., Dublin 1916, p. 670.
25  'British Medical Journal'. (1976) i, p. 1264.
26  'Lancet'. (1950) ii, p. 436.
27  Comrie, J. D., 'Hist. Scottish Med.' Bailliere, Tindall & Cox 1932, p. 495.
28  Ibid p. 514.
29  Green, V. H. H., 'The Universities'. Penguin Books 1969, pp. 87–8.
30  Ibid p. 91.
31  Hist. Scottish Med. Vol II, pp. 577–8.
32  'Lancet'. (1861) i, pp. 149–50.
33  Hist. Scottish Med. Vol II, p. 581.
34  Ibid p. 583.
35  Ibid p. 513.
36  Ibid Vol I, pp. 350–1.
37  'History of Scotland'. Vol I, p. 345.
38  Ibid p. 358.
39  Ibid Vol II, p. 519.
40  Guthrie, D., 'A History of Medicine'. Thomas Nelson & Sons Ltd 1945, p. 222.
41  Hist. Scottish Med. Vol II, pp. 514–8.
42  Ibid p. 515.
43  'British Medical Journal'. (1882) ii, p. 487.
44  'History of Scotland'. Vol II, p. 663.
45  'British Medical Journal'. (1889) ii, p. 556.
46  Hist. Scottish Med. Vol II, p. 661.
47  Ibid Vol I, pp. 367–8.
48  Hist. Scottish Med. Vol I, pp. 380–1.
49  Ibid Vol II, pp. 460–1.
50  Ibid Vol I, pp. 384–5.
51  Ibid pp. 391–3.
52  Guthrie, D., 'A History of Medicine'. Thomas Nelson & Sons, Ltd 1943, p. 153..
53  Hist. Scottish Med. Vol I, p. 354.
54  Underwood, E. A., 'Boerhaave's Men'. Edinburgh University Press p. 88.
55  Gemmeli, J., 'Edinburgh University: a Sketch of its Life for 300 Years'. James Gammeli, Edinburgh 1884, p. 17.
56  Ibid pp. 19–20.
57  Ibid pp. 20–21.
58  Underwood, E. A., 'Boerhaave's Men'. Edinburgh University Press p. 89.
59  Chambers, R. W., 'Gazetter of Scotland'. Thomas Ireland Jr. Edinburgh 1832, Vol. I. p. 381.
60  Gemmeli, J., 'Edinburgh University: a Sketch of its Life for 300 years'. James Gemmeli, Edinburgh 1884, p. 34.
61  Struthers, J., 'Historical Sketch of Edinburgh Anatomical School'. Maclachlan & Stewart, Edinburgh 1867. pp. 9–11.
62  Hist. Scottish Med. Vol. I, p. 253.
63  Underwood, E. A., 'Boerhaave's Men'. Edinburgh University Press p. 102.

64  Hist. Scottish Med. Vol. I, pp. 295–6.
65  Gemmeli, J., 'Edinburgh University: a Sketch of its Life for 300 Years'. James Gemmeli, Edinburgh 1884, p. 19.
66  Underwood, E. A., 'Boerhaave's Men'. Edinburgh University Press pp. 95–7.
67  Hist. Scottish Med. Vol. I, p. 294.
68  Gemmeli, J., 'Edinburgh University: a Sketch of its Life for 300 Years'. James Gemmeli, Edinburgh 1884, p. 74.
69  Struthers, J., 'Historical Sketch of Edinburgh Anatomical School'. MacLachlan & Stewart, Edinburgh 1867, pp. 27–8.
70  Guthrie, D., 'A History of Medicine'. Thomas Nelson & Sons, Ltd 1945, p. 231.
71  Hist. Scottish Med. Vol. II, pp. 550–1.
72  Ibid pp. 538–40.
73  Ibid p. 578.
74  Billroth, T., 'Medical Sciences in the German Universities'. Macmillan Co. 1924, pp. 9–10.
75  Hist. Scottish Med. Vol. II, p. 449.
76  Ibid pp. 453–4.
77  Struthers, J., 'Historical Sketch of Edinburgh Anatomical School'. MacLachlan & Stewart, Edinburgh 1867, p. 86.
78  Gemmeli, J., 'Edinburgh University: a Sketch of its Life for 300 Years'. James Gemmeli. Edinburgh 1884, pp. 66–70.
79  Struthers, J., 'Historical Sketch of Edinburgh Anatomical School'. MacLachlan & Stewart, Edinburgh 1867, p. 83.
80  Gemmeli, J., 'Edinburgh University: a Sketch of its Life for 300 Years'. James Gemmeli, Edinburgh 1884, pp. 95–6.
81  'Lancet'. (1829–30) i, p. 15.
82  Ibid. (1830–31) ii, pp. 30–32.
83  Merrington, W. R., 'University College Hospital and its Medical School'. Heinemann 1976, pp. 2–30.
84  Green, V. H. H., 'The Universities'. Penguin Books 1969, p. 104.
85  Green, V. H. H., 'The Universities'. Penguin Books 1969, p. 105.
86  Merrington, W. R., 'University College Hospital and its Medical School'. Heinemann 1976, p. 7.
87  Green, V. H. H., 'The Universities'. Penguin Books 1969, p. 107.
88  Kent, W., 'An Encyclopedia of London'. J. H. Dent & Sons 1937, p. 415.

# TEN

# English and Welsh provincial medical schools 1824–93

For many centuries the universities of Cambridge and Oxford held a monopoly of higher education in England. Yet the possibility of founding additional universities was mooted at a relatively early time. In 1612, Sir George Buck even referred to Gresham College as 'the University of London'.[1] Such a title was over-ambitious and certainly premature, and the future of this body lay in the foundation of the Royal Society. Some thirty years later William Dell, the Master of Caius College, Cambridge, suggested that it would be advantageous to have 'Universities or Colleges, one at least in every great town or city in the nation'.[2] This idea never materialised and it was almost two hundred years before another English university was founded.

The limitations of the two older English institutions were considerable for the students were invariably sons of the wealthy and entry was confined to members of the Anglican Church. It is therefore not surprising that during the 18th century a number of educational establishments arose which were largely sponsored by Dissenters. Such 'academies' were originally used to educate ministers of religion, but they subsequently gave courses in language, literature, history, mathematics, philosophy and other subjects. It was an attempt to provide Nonconformists with education such as was given at Cambridge and Oxford, though the approach was more liberal, scientific, and utilitarian. But although they undoubtedly filled an educational need their existence was relatively short. Even the best known of them, the Warrington Academy, was only open between 1757 and 1786. More important at the time were the Literary and Philosophical Societies. They were founded by Dissenters and by men grown wealthy through the Industrial Revolution, and many of their members had received their education at one of the Academies. The dates of formation of these Philosophical Societies in the future provincial university towns were:

1781 Manchester
1793 Newcastle
1812 Liverpool
1819 Leeds
1822 Sheffield

Their main interest was in science and in particular its application to local industry, which naturally varied from place to place. It was about another century before the northern provincial universities came into being, but it was a period of great activity. With population increase and the growth of towns, the need for skilled labour became even greater.

143

Both scientists and technologists were in demand and this reflected the insufficiency of available education. In this connection, brief mention should be made of the Cambridge Extension Lectures. In 1866, the idea came from a Cambridge don, James Stuart, who organised a series of public lectures on scientific and allied subjects. They were held in large towns, mostly in the industrial north, where they were attended by large crowds of working-class men and women. Their success, though local, was considerable and they greatly contributed to the formation of local colleges which were later incorporated in the universities.[3] Finally, a wealthy managerial class had developed and their generosity, coupled with the civic pride of townspeople, was to do much towards bringing the local university into being.

## The Provincial Medical Schools

In Scotland, the Medical Schools grew up allied to the universities. By contrast, in London they necessarily developed in association with hospitals, for there was no university till 1827, and it was to be many years before the university would be accepted as an educational body by these medical schools. The provincial medical schools (excluding Cambridge and Oxford) appeared throughout the 19th century and were likewise attached to hospitals, but with the important difference that as they expanded they stimulated the creation of new universities. Such developments were a product of the Industrial Revolution and the rapid growth of large cities.

At the beginning of the 19th century, there were several private provincial schools which gave tuition in Anatomy and Surgery and were essentially similar to the private schools of London at an earlier date. These were followed by schools which ran courses in most medical subjects. This development was the direct result of the passing of the Apothecaries' Act in 1815. It proved to be a great step forward in medical education, for it gave the Company the responsibility for laying down a pattern of training for their apprentices and of conducting an examination to test their proficiency. The Apothecaries attacked these tasks with such commendable enthusiasm that by 1835 a suitable curriculum had been designed, and the first written examination was held in 1839.[4] In order to be admitted to the Company's examinations, 'Certificates of Attendance' at approved medical schools had to be presented. The provincial apprentice faced a problem, for distance and expense precluded his attendance at a London School, to say nothing of the fact that it was probably already overcrowded. To meet this deficiency in medical education, a more complete type of medical school, referred to above, arose in some large towns.[5] It will be noted that nearly all of these schools which survived in later years were founded in the 10-year period 1824–34 (see Table).

144

# TABLE

| TOWN | MEDICAL SCHOOL FOUNDED | FOUNDATION OF COLLEGE OF ARTS AND SCIENCES | AMALGAMATION OF MEDICAL SCHOOL AND COLLEGE | UNIVERSITY CHARTER GRANTED |
|---|---|---|---|---|
| Manchester | 1824 | 1851 Owen's College | 1873 | Victoria University 1880 |
| Birmingham | 1841 | 1880 Mason College | 1892 | Birmingham 1990 |
| Sheffield | 1828 | 1879 Firth College | 1883 | Sheffield 1905 |
| Leeds | 1831 | 1874 Yorkshire College College of Science | 1884 | Leeds 1902 |
| Newcastle-upon-Tyne | 1834 | many colleges | – | Durham 1837 Newcastle 1963 |
| Bristol | 1833 | 1876 University College | 1879 | Bristol 1909 |
| Liverpool | 1834 | 1882 University College | 1884 | Liverpool 1902 |
| Cardiff | 1893 | 1893 University College | 1893 | University 1931 |

In general, the pattern of development of these centres was similar. Later in the century, with the increasing demands for education, there arose colleges devoted to the Arts and Sciences. Their foundation was often motivated by civic pride and supported by benefactions from local industrialists whose names were given to the establishments (see Table). Later still, the Medical School amalgamated with the College to form a university, for which a charter had to be obtained if degrees were to be conferred. There were many local differences and some facts about the University of Durham must be considered before dealing with the other individual universities.

## Durham and Newcastle

Of the modern universities, London in 1827 was the first to appear and was rapidly followed by Durham in 1834. The latter was intended as a university of the North which would provide teaching facilities which Cambridge and Oxford could not provide. The stimulus for this foundation came from the Cathedral which at that time was very wealthy and it was feared that these resources might be diverted by ecclesiastic reformers of the day.[6] To found a college seemed to be a desirable way to spend some of these funds. The number of students was not large and consisted mostly of those reading Theology or Arts, though there were a few studying Engineering. The Whig government of the time delayed the granting of a University Charter till 1837 as it wanted to be assured that the institution would be open to Dissenters.[7]

The complexity of the relationships between Durham and Newcastle is reflected in the history of the Medical School. This will be dealt with briefly for a good, detailed account is at present available.[8] In Newcastle's early days, education must have been foremost in some people's minds, for the Literary and Philosophical Society had been founded in 1793,[9] and at a meeting in 1831 Thomas Michael Greenhow (1792–1881) gave a paper, 'On the expediency of establishing an academic institution of the nature of a College or University'.[10] Medical education commenced in 1832 when six local practitioners gave instruction to 8 or 9 students, one of whom was John Snow who was later to become distinguished for his work on anaesthetics and on the transmission of cholera. It is generally agreed that the true start of the Medical School was in 1834, the same year in which the University of Durham was founded.[11] There were 26 students and lectures were given at the Barber Surgeons' Company's Hall. One great difference of the Newcastle School of Medicine, compared with the other northern schools, was its growth within a university framework from its early days. When founded in 1834 the school was called 'The Newcastle School of Medicine and Surgery'. But in 1852 it became included in the University of Durham and was renamed 'The Newcastle-upon-Tyne College of Medicine in connection with the University of Durham'. It seemed likely that this union might strengthen the University, whose fortunes were at a low ebb. During the next 20 years, the demand for more scientific education led to the foundation in 1851 of a College of Physical Science to provide instruction in the application of science to Mining and Agriculture. Progress was satisfactory and in 1880 a Chair of Mining was endowed. By the end of the century a number of small colleges had appeared[12] and in 1904, when the original College was being extended, it was renamed Armstrong College. The existence of a university in one town and a considerable number of its colleges in another gave rise to endless difficulties and it was not until 1937 that any kind of solution was reached. In that year the University constitution was re-written, and as a result the Newcastle School of Medicine and Armstrong College were merged into King's College. This became a constituent college of the University of Durham, and students received degrees from the latter.[13] This was still rather unsatisfactory for it meant that a medical student would do all his training at Newcastle and then be granted a degree from a University town which he had rarely visited. It was not until 1963 that the final chapter was written and Newcastle was given independent university status.[14]

## Manchester

In Tudor times Manchester was a small market town and its character remained unchanged until the Industrial Revolution. It was then that the cotton industry produced a phenomenal transformation and the population which was about 40,000 in the 1780's, had increased to 142,000 by 1831. It was the first of the industrial towns of the Midlands and the North, and its university was the first of the 'red-brick' universities in those areas. These early years, until about 1830, were ones of great prosperity and wealth poured into the town. As it grew with prodigious speed, it produced two groups of people, namely, a small group of men, grown wealthy, and a large group of working men living under rather squalid conditions. The plight of the latter became accentuated during the years of depression which followed the 'boom years'. The 1840s were years of great distress and the appalling living conditions of the poor, surrounded as they were by cotton mills, became known generally throughout the country. The gap between the rich and poor was so great that there was no sympathy between them. Also, Manchester was not incorporated as a local authority until 1838 and therefore before that year there was no local government which might have investigated and possibly alleviated the suffering of the poor. With the advent of unemployment in the years of depression it is small wonder that the town became known for rioting and social discontent. The passing of the Reform Bill in 1832 had ushered in a period of activity in public health matters and the reports which came from Manchester were an added stimulus for reform.

But in spite of so much discontent, the town was one of great vitality and there was a powerful middle-class group that promoted its cultural and intellectual activities. The 'Halle' orchestra had made the town famous in the world of music and the Literary and Philosophical Institute, founded in 1781, was still very active. One of the outstanding successes of the century was the foundation of the university.

The first step was the foundation of a Medical School. In Manchester there were two original schools of Medicine. In 1824 Thomas Turner founded the first 'complete' school. It was the first medical school in the provinces, excluding Cambridge and Oxford. Its certificates were recognised by the College of Surgeons of Edinburgh and by the Society of Apothecaries, but not by the London College of Surgeons. It was named the 'Manchester Royal School of Medicine'. In 1826 Joseph Jordan, who had been giving Anatomy lectures since 1814, expanded his course and founded another school which he called the 'Manchester Medical Institution'. This was closed in 1834 and in spite of the subsequent appearance of two small schools, the only one which survived was Turner's Royal School.[15]

At the time of the depression, the cotton industry was suffering from foreign competition. It had also fallen behind in its technology. Accordingly, there was a demand for better education both in science and in technology. In 1846 a wealthy Manchester merchant, John Owens, died and left £97,000 to provide youths with instruction in all branches taught at the English universities. It was emphasised that such education should be free from all religious tests. In 1851, a College named after the donor was opened in a modest building with two Professors as staff, namely Mr. Frankland (Chemistry) and Dr. W. C. Williamson (Natural History). It prospered from the start and even in 1856 there was some discussion about amalgamating Owens College with the Royal School of Medicine. This did not come about until 1873 when the College was preparing to move into what are described as 'palatial' new buildings. This came about in 1874 when there had been considerable expansion of the courses available, and the Manchester public had shown much generosity in providing endowments. At the same time an adjacent building was obtained for the Medical School which now had 112 students registered and was able to provide space for biological laboratories and for museum accommodation.[15]

Clinical teaching was given at various hospitals of which only a few need be mentioned. The Royal Infirmary had been opened in 1755 when it incorporated a dispensary and, in 1765, a lunatic asylum. It grew over the years into a General Hospital and by the end of the 19th century had about 300 beds. In 1790, St. Mary's Hospital appeared and when it was greatly extended in 1855, it became a special institution for diseases of women. Another special hospital, for children's diseases, was established at Pendlebury in 1875 with 163 beds; a bazaar held at the time provided £21,000. In the earlier days the dispensary movement was prominent and six of these establishments were scattered throughout the city. Of special note is the Ancoat's Dispensary which was founded in 1828 and had a hospital, still well known, added to it in 1875.[15]

It was a period of great activity and in 1880 a university charter was granted for the Victoria University of Manchester. There were some restrictions in conferring degrees but in 1883 a supplementary charter removed them, so that the new university could confer degrees in medicine and surgery.

The relation of this institution with the medical schools of Leeds, Liverpool and Sheffield must be explained. The Leeds Medical School was founded in 1831 and in 1887 was joined to the Yorkshire College of Science which had been in existence since 1874. In Liverpool there was a Medical School in 1834 and a University College in 1882, the two becoming united in 1884. These two bodies at Liverpool and Leeds were not given their own University Charter immediately but, with Owens College, became constituent colleges of the Victoria University, Manchester. Their students could thus receive their degrees from Manchester until 1902, when Leeds and Liverpool were granted their own University Charter with the right to confer their own degrees. Sheffield was less fortunate. A medical school had been founded in 1828, but at one time there seem to have been two schools, though only one – the 'Medical Institution' – survived.[16] In 1879 a University College was founded, thanks to generous financial assistance from a local steelmaster, Mark Firth, and named after him. Its main purpose was to provide technical instruction and to prepare students for matriculation at one of the national universities. Four years later the Medical School and Firth College became amalgamated. In 1895 application was made for affiliation with the Victoria University. This was refused and it was not until 1905 that a University Charter was granted.[17]

The new Victoria University now flourished and the medical student entry of 1883 was double that of 1874. In 1881 the University Court raised the status of Materia Medica and Pathology by appointing Professors in those subjects. Julius Dreschfeld, a physician, became the first Professor of Pathology and held the post until 1891, when he became Professor of Medicine at Owens College and was succeeded by Sheridan Delepine (see chapter 11). During this period, Pathology became established as a separate discipline and in 1895 received additional lecture rooms and laboratories for practical student instruction in pathology, physiology, bacteriology, and hygiene. It was fast becoming one of the leading departments of pathology in the land.

# Liverpool

The growing need for medical care was indicated by the opening of the Royal Infirmary in 1749 and by the foundation of three dispensaries in the succeeding years. By 1823 a new Infirmary was established. During this period the importance of education, both general and medical, was realised. A group of doctors had organised a Medical Library in 1778 and in 1812 the Liverpool Literary and Philosophical Society was formed. Two years later a group of citizens founded a society to promote interest in Literature, Science, and the Arts, and in 1817, when granted a charter, it became known as the Royal Institution.[18] It promoted a series of lectures, some of which were on medical subjects and given by doctors. This led to the foundation in 1834 of a medical school, which was given accommodation in the Institution. Most important of all was the fact that the new school became approved by the Apothecaries Company and by the Royal College of Surgeons of London. The regulations of these two bodies soon became more stringent and this led to a reorganization of the Liverpool school. Thus, in 1844, it was transferred to the Royal Infirmary and became known as 'The Liverpool Infirmary School of Medicine'.[19] As such, it gradually expanded though it was handicapped by lack of space until 1882, when it became merged with University College.

One unique feature of the growth of Liverpool was its involvement in the slave trade. This has been excellently described by Sheperd[20] and only a few important points will be mentioned here. The African slave trade flourished throughout the 18th century and its ships operated from London, Bristol, and Liverpool. The latter was geographically preferable and came to attract most of the trade. Trinkets and other products of industrial England were taken to West Africa where African natives were bought with the proceeds. These were then taken to the West Indies where they were auctioned. On the return journey the ships carried raw materials such as cotton for use in the mills of Lancashire. This trade became a major factor in the growth of the town. But by this time many persons became aware of the appalling conditions and high mortality of the slaves on board ship. By 1787 an anti-slavery movement had been started by a group of Quakers. Two acts of Parliament in 1788 and 1789 decreed that a surgeon must be carried on a slave ship and that such men should be examined for proficiency. This test was much less exacting than those normally given by the Apothecaries Company and by the Royal College of Surgeons. Permission to hold these examinations was given to the Royal Colleges and to a number of hospitals throughout the country, but the vast majority were conducted at the Royal Infirmary at Liverpool. Over the seventeen years up to the abolition of slavery in 1807, this institution examined 643 candidates, of whom 151 were unsuccessful. Apart from the conduction of this examination, clinical staff of the Infirmary organised a series of lectures for students and it is tempting to conclude that this did much to stimulate medical education in the town in those early days.

When the first Holt Professor of Pathology was appointed in 1894, the Liverpool College was without university recognition and very much in the shadow of the Victoria University, Manchester, to which it was affiliated. The new incumbent, Rupert William Boyce (1863–1911), occupied the Chair till his death, by which time the College had attained university status and included a first-class department of Pathology. Of Irish extraction, he had studied medicine in Heidelberg and Paris and had graduated from University College, London. His scientific ability was soon apparent when his researches with Victor Horsley on the pathology of the nervous system earned him the Fellowship of the Royal Society when not yet 30 years of age. At about the same time he also wrote a 'Text-book of Morbid Histology' and was part-author of 'A handbook of Pathological Anatomy (Museum Pathology)'.[21] When he moved to Liverpool in 1894, he was to live through a most important period of university development during which he was to reveal his unusual ability as an organiser and administrator. He was quick to see the needs of the growing city and the special lines along which Pathology should be developed. Like Delépine in Manchester, he faced public health problems and one of his first actions was the creation of a School of Hygiene which carried out routine municipal work as well as providing training in the subject. His department of Pathology also performed bacteriological work in connection with his post as Bacteriological Analyst to the city.[22] Laboratory accommodation was meagre until 1898 when the Thomson-Yates laboratory was opened in the University College Medical School. But Boyce's outlook was always a broad one and he was thinking of the development of the University College as a whole or even the city itself. His peculiar ability in finding financial resources was to prove a great asset, and his father-in-law, a wealthy ship owner, gave him generous assistance. It was at this stage that, aided by another rich ship owner, he was able to develop his real interest, for which he is always remembered, namely Tropical Medicine. His choice of subject was not surprising, for in a busy port like Liverpool quite a number of tropical diseases made their appearance from time to time.

It all started in 1898 when Mr. Joseph Chamberlain, the Colonial Secretary, influenced by the tropical diseases expert, Dr. Patrick Manson, issued a circular. It proposed the establishment of a School of Tropical Medicine in London, partially subsidised by the Government. It would provide special instruction in the subject for doctors selected for the Colonial Medical Service or for those who proposed to practice in tropical countries.[23] Boyce immediately saw its importance, but felt that such a centre would be ideal for Liverpool because of its geographical location and its connection with the tropics. He quickly consulted his wealthy friend, Sir Alfred Jones, and on the 22nd April, 1899, the two men, as twin founders, saw the Liverpool School of Tropical Medicine and Hygiene opened by Lord Lister. The London School followed and was opened on 3rd October, 1899, and it is interesting to note that other similar institutes soon followed in Paris, Hamburg, Belgium and the United States of America. In charge of the Liverpool Institute in 1899 was Ronald Ross. Originally appointed as Lecturer, in 1902 he became Professor of Tropical Medicine, a post which he held till 1912. Both Institutes flourished and by the end of 1913 the Liverpool institute had sponsored 31 research expeditions to tropical countries. For Boyce it was a period of tremendous activity. In addition to building up a good department of Pathology, he was actively working for university recognition for the Liverpool College. In addition, he still found time to travel with many of his research expeditions and he became very interested in yellow fever. All of this could not have come at a better time for although there had been previous developments in Tropical Medicine, there were a remarkable number of advances which came to light between 1894 and 1914.[23] They concerned such diseases as malaria, filariasis, yellow fever, trypanosomiasis, ankylostomiasis, and kala-azar. Boyce's numerous activities necessitated periods of absence from his department and he was fortunate in having a very competent deputy. Ernest Edward Glynn (1873–1929) had been a student at Cambridge and Liverpool. He was soon interested in Pathology and became a University Fellow in the subject. In 1901 he became Physician to the Liverpool Hospital for Consumption, and also Pathologist to the Royal Infirmary. In 1904 he became Physician to the latter. He was closely attached to his old teacher, and acted as deputy for him during periods of absence. In 1906 Boyce's activities were curtailed as a result of a stroke, though following a good but slow recovery he courageously continued working till he died in 1911. Following this disaster, Glynn resigned all his clinical appointments to act as Deputy Professor. In 1910 he became Associate Professor and succeeded his old master as Holt Professor of Pathology in 1912, a post which he held until 1927. During the life-time of Boyce, Glynn had played a very important part in the development of the Pathological Department. It will have been noted that no mention has been made of any teaching activities by Boyce. This is not surprising when we consider his multiple contributions. He was quick to stimulate his assistants and to encourage research but he probably had little time for student tuition. This gap was undoubtedly filled by Glynn, who was an excellent teacher and very popular with students. With a good background of Clinical Medicine he was well-equipped to give classes in Pathological Anatomy which were well attended even on Saturday mornings. In addition he was very interested in Bacteriology and Dental Pathology. When the Pathological Society of Great Britain and Ireland was founded in 1906 he was one of its original members.

Boyce had built up an excellent department of Pathology in a remarkably short period of time which included, amongst others, departments of Bacteriology, Bio-chemistry, Comparative Pathology and Cancer Research, to say nothing of his Institute of Tropical Medicine, now known world-wide.

## Leeds

Parallel with the development of Manchester and the cotton industry on the west side of the Pennines, there was a later growth on the east and related to wool. As a result, two large towns, namely Bradford and Leeds, appeared. Leeds was the older city of the two, having received its borough charter as far back as 1626. By virtue of a number of industries, including wool, leather, pottery, glass, and mining, it had grown to a city of 152,000 population in 1841 and to 172,000 by 1851. By contrast Bradford was a purely woollen town which in the above periods had grown particularly rapidly from 34,000 to 103,000.[24] In Leeds there was some concern for the provision of education for in 1826 John Marshall, the President of the Philosophic and Literary Society (founded in 1819) raised the possibility of a university for the town. In that same year there were signs of medical teaching and hopes that a Medical School would be a great stimulus in the further growth and development of the town.

Medical care first became organised when in 1767 the General Infirmary was established. It had only 27 beds but by repeated expansion there were 150 beds by 1859. During this period other hospitals, some special, had arisen though for present purposes it will be necessary to mention only the Leeds Public Dispensary, founded in 1824 and providing only out-patient care.[25]

Medical education started with some occasional courses in Anatomy, given between 1800 and 1809. The first regular instruction in the subject was given in 1826 by Charles Thackrah to his six apprentices. It will be recalled that Thackrah was a practitioner in the town and a pioneer of Industrial Medicine. This private school was intended to provide instruction for students taking the Diploma of the Royal College of Surgeons of London, but unfortunately this body refused Thackrah's application for it to become recognised.

A group of medical men reorganised and extended the course and when it became approved in 1831, it was the beginning of the Leeds School of Medicine. Classes were held at the Public Dispensary which included tuition in all medical subjects and was attended by about a dozen pupils. It was an immediate success and when additional accommodation became necessary it was moved to a large house next to the Infirmary.[26] As in other provincial schools medical education had started in association with a hospital.

Throughout the rest of the century the town continued to prosper though it viewed with some concern the developments in Manchester, its rival on the other side of the Pennines. Nearer home another rival had appeared in the very rapidly-growing Bradford. In some provincial university towns such as Liverpool, philanthropy played a large part in their advancement. This was not so in Leeds, which owed its ultimate success to the development of a strong sense of civic pride amongst its citizens, a quality greatly fostered by the rivalry with Bradford. It is for this reason that some events in the latter town will need to be briefly mentioned.

Both towns faced the public health problems of a growing city, but with the introduction of improved hygienic measures, improvements were on the way. But in the population growth there was a unique feature in Bradford, namely the influx of a number of foreign merchants who housed themselves in an area which became known as 'Little Germany'. In 1864 the town had a foreign-born Mayor, Charles Seman, who came from Dantzig.[27] This enclave did much for the town; it stimulated a number of cultural societies and showed its concern for education by being instrumental in the rebuilding of Bradford Grammar School. In the early half of the century neither town had been conspicuous for the architectural beauty of its buildings and it was Bradford which moved first to redress this deficiency. Following a public meeting in 1849 it was decided to build a large hall, the cost being borne by the sale of shares to the populace. The foundation stone was laid in 1851 and the building was completed without delay. It was a massive building known as St. George's Hall, which would hold 3,000 people and featured an unusual type of gas-lighting. Locally it was acclaimed as the best known example of concert building in the country and it undoubtedly added to the beauty of the town. More important still, it facilitated civic and cultural activities, and of course augmented 'civic pride'. A new park – Pell Park – had been given to the public and more buildings followed, including a new Town Hall in 1873.

The events in Bradford had not gone unnoticed in Leeds where, during the 1846–8 period, a number of attractive buildings had been erected. But there was nothing to compare with St. George's Hall, Bradford. It is noteworthy that at the time of the Opening Concert special trains had been run from Leeds and Manchester so that the Hall had been well-publicised. Accordingly, following a number of public meetings it was decided that a Town Hall should be built in Leeds and financed by the Town Council.[28] There was an atmosphere of great enthusiasm as indicated by the formation in 1851 of 'A Leeds Improvement Society to suggest and promote architectural and other public improvements in the town'. At the same time the Philosophical and Literary Society had become very active, following a previous period of decline. A site was purchased for the new hall and the foundation stone laid in August, 1853. As time went on there were many alterations and modifications of the original plan. Labour problems caused delay and in January 1857 the building stopped altogether. The question of having a tower caused an enormous amount of discussion and in 1857 there were plans to install a clock and bell. Finally it was completed in 1858 and the 7th September was chosen as the opening date. The cost had been £122,000, or £80,000 more than the original estimate. Queen Victoria and the Prince Consort attended the opening ceremony which was combined with an exhibition of local manufacturers and a Musical Festival to raise funds for the General Infirmary.

This atmosphere of civic enthusiasm did much to influence the design of the new and handsome General Infirmary. It will be remembered that in 1859 there were 150 beds and now more accommodation was essential. In 1862 a new site was purchased and George Gilbert Scott (later Sir George), who had recently designed St. Pancras Station, was chosen as architect. The Foundation Stone was laid in 1864 and the building completed in 1868. It was built on the 'French pavilion' style similar to that of the new St. Thomas's hospital at Lambeth. The architectural style was Italian Gothic.[29] The opening ceremony seems to have been rather unusual. It consisted of a National Exhibition of works of Art and was held in the new infirmary in a large central hall formed by covering an open court with a permanent roof of iron and glass.[30] The ceremony was performed by the Prince of Wales in May, 1868, but the building was not opened as a hospital till a year later, namely 22nd May 1869.

At this time Leeds was feeling the effects of a trade depression and also some strong competition from the Continent. The need for the training of scientists and technologists was realised and in 1874 a Yorkshire College of Science was founded at Leeds. This was amalgamated in 1884 with the Medical School, and as already mentioned, following affiliation with the Victoria University, Manchester in 1887, the College was given independent university status in 1902. Two years later the first full time Professor of Pathology was appointed, namely, Albert Sidney Gruenbaum (1869–1921), who held the Chair for the next 13 years.

The earlier history of Pathology in the town is difficult to trace. We learn that the original course designed for 1832 consisted of a series of lectures on all medical subjects. Those on Anatomy, Physiology, and Pathology were given by two prominent surgeons, Thomas Pridgin Teale senior, and Joseph Prince Garlick.[31] The progress of the school was such that in 1864 there were about sixty students. But adequate accommodation was lacking and in 1865 a new medical school was built. It was located close to the Infirmary but it is noteworthy that there was no laboratory of Pathology or Physiology, and presumably tuition in these subjects was limited. This would explain the statement made by Professor J. B. Hellier who joined the school in the early 1870s and stated that 'the local teaching was very defective in many points, especially in the early subjects and Physiology'.[32] Over the next ten years the Medical Course was extended as indicated in the prospectus for 1883.[33] There was extensive tuition in various aspects of Clinical Medicine and Surgery at the General Infirmary and other hospitals. Basic subjects were taught at the School but there are no details. Pathology is now mentioned but only that 'there are Anatomical, Pathological, Chemical, Botanical, and Materia Medica Museums'. Students could also use the Museum of the Literary and Philosophical Society on payment of a nominal fee.[33] The year 1884 was an important one for it saw the amalgamation of the School of Medicine and the Yorkshire College of Science. It provided additional accommodation for the Medical School for instruction in Chemistry, and Botany was moved to the Yorkshire College. It is not known who taught Pathology at the time but it may have been a Physician, for in many schools it had been customary to appoint an Assistant Physician who was also Pathologist until he became promoted to Full Physician. There were certainly some who had an interest in the subject for both A. G. Barrs and J. B. Hellier had joined the Pathological Society of London in 1881 and 1878, respectively.[34] But in 1884 the staff of the Infirmary had been reorganised and the three Physicians replaced by two Physicians and two Assistant Physicians, the latter being A. G. Barrs and E. H. Jacob. This was a major development for Jacob was to carry out the teaching of Pathology for the next ten years and to raise it to a new level. As part of developments of the subject, we learn that in the same year a Department of Pathology and Morbid Histology had been established and this title was maintained until 1896–7 when it became changed to Pathology and Bacteriology.[35]

Ernest Henry Jacob (1849–94) was a classical scholar who had not commenced his medical studies till aged 23 when he went to Oxford University and St. Thomas's Hospital. He moved to Leeds where he soon became a practising physician who was on the staff of the Leeds House of Recovery and the Leeds Public Dispensary. In 1881 he became Demonstrator and subsequently Lecturer in Physiology in the School of Medicine. From that time onwards his heart and soul were in teaching. When the school became united with the Yorkshire College in 1884, he was appointed Professor of Pathology, a post which he retained for the rest of his life. During this time, in addition to teaching Pathological Anatomy and Practical Histology, he was Assistant Physician from 1884 and Full Physician to the Infirmary from 1892. It was a great loss to Leeds when he died at the early age of 44 from meningitis complicating middle ear disease.[36] The teaching of the subject was now taken over by Birch, the Professor of Physiology. It was sad that Jacob was unable to see the opening, later in 1894, of a new school of medicine to which he had made a substantial contribution.

By contrast with 1883, the prospectus of the School now advertised the extensive laboratories for Pathology and Physiology, to say nothing of the fine museums of Anatomy and Pathology. But if there had been progress in Pathology in the medical school, the subject as a whole remained fragmentary for some time. There was a need for a clinical laboratory to serve a large hospital such as the Infirmary and it may be recalled that Matthew Stewart was appointed Clinical Pathologist in 1910. Lack of unity was evident when in 1905 Oskar C. Grumer became

Honorary Pathologist to the Public Dispensary. In 1906 he resigned and was replaced by George W. Watson.[37] From then on a number of successors followed and it is only necessary to mention one, namely J. Godwin Greenfeld, who stayed only four months prior to proceeding to the National Hospital, Queen Square, where he became the leading neuropathologist in the country.[38] It was to be many years before unity in Pathology was achieved in Leeds.

The problems which Albert Sidney Grünbaum (1869–1921) faced on his appointment as the first University Professor in Leeds in 1902 can well be imagined. The town badly needed a coordinated service of Pathology and of course public health pathology was a high priority. It is interesting to note that the title of the Chair was Pathology and Bacteriology at a time when the latter subject was only just being recognised as independent. It must have been pleasing to Grünbaum for he had a special interest in Bacteriology as applied to Clinical Medicine. For his medical education he had gone to Cambridge University and St. Thomas's Hospital where, due to the teaching of C. S. Sherrington, he showed early interest in the physiology of the nervous system. After graduation he spent time in Gruber's laboratory in Vienna working on a quantitative assessment of antibodies in cases of typhoid fever in the wards of the great Austrian physician, Nothnagel. He delayed publication of his serological test for the disease and in the meanwhile Widal described it and the test has continued to bear his name. There was much controversy at the time and many felt that Grünbaum should have had a share in the discovery. In these early years he devoted himself largely to immunology. In 1897 his MD thesis was entitled 'Some practical and theoretical points concerning serum diagnosis'. By 1903 his views had become broader when, as Goulestonian Lecturer, he spoke on 'Theories of immunity and their clinical application'.[39] In spite of this he still maintained contact with his teacher, Sherrington, who in 1895 had been appointed Professor of Physiology at University College, Liverpool. He was accompanied by Grünbaum who became his Demonstrator in Physiology prior to being appointed Lecturer in Experimental Medicine. During the years at Liverpool he developed many interests. Still devoted to infectious diseases, he took the Diploma in Public Health in Manchester. In addition he gained clinical experience in a post of Assistant Physician, became Lecturer in Boyce's Institute of Tropical Medicine and in 1903 was made Director of Cancer Research.

He was now well-equipped to take over the University Chair of Pathology at Leeds, and his 13 years in the post were extremely busy. He continued his researches on cancer and other subjects but also played an active role in university life. He was Dean of the Medical Faculty for eight years and Honorary Librarian to the Medical School for five. His interest in teaching resulted in his well-illustrated 'Essentials of Morbid Histology'. This work did much to improve practical aspects of the subject. He was made Honorary Pathologist to the Infirmary, but at a time when there was a full-time Clinical Pathologist. His period of office was interrupted by the 1914–18 War, when he became Consulting Bacteriologist to Northern Command. A sensitive man, it was at this time that, with anti-German feeling rife, he changed his name to Leyton by deed of poll. In July 1917 he had a severe stroke and resigned his Chair in December. He recovered sufficiently to become Director of the Clinical Laboratory at Addenbrooke's Hospital, Cambridge, but died in 1921.

He did much at Leeds to establish a modern department of pathology, though it did not become unified until the time of his successor, Matthew Stewart. In paying tribute to him, Sherrington pointed out that it was unusual to find a man who spent much of his time in laboratory work and technique, yet who had as his main aim the advancement of Clinical Medicine.[40]

## Birmingham

During the Victorian period the population of Birmingham rose from 70,000 to 500,000. Like other large towns of this era, it faced problems in public health resulting from overcrowding and poor living and working conditions. Yet each town had also its own special problems determined by its social and economic conditions as well as by its particular industries. To illustrate this point, comparisons of Manchester and Birmingham have been frequently made. Manchester, built up on a single industry, cotton, was advancing in the early part of the century. Large numbers of relatively unskilled workers were employed to work in factories by a small number of wealthy men, the mill owners. This economic gap between employers and employees became serious, for the workers were living in conditions of appalling poverty. Labour troubles soon followed and socialism thrived. Birmingham developed later towards the end of the century and prospered from a very large variety of small industries such as light engineering, machine tools, hardware, bicycles, and many others. The work force was relatively skilled and was employed by men who owned small workshops. As a result, 'men' and 'masters' were more closely associated and much in sympathy with one another. The political climate which developed was one of middle-class liberalism rather than socialism.[41] It has been pointed out that of all the large industrial towns, Birmingham was the only one not located on or near to a major river. This, however, was to be no disadvantage for by the later part of the century the railways had largely eliminated transport by water.

Medical care was first organised in the 18th century and in Birmingham the General Hospital was opened in 1779 with 100 beds. Several extensions followed over the succeeding years and by 1870 when the town had grown considerably there were about 270 beds. Other developments occurred and for our purposes it is of interest that at this time there was 'a pathological department and an excellent mortuary'.[42] At this time another general hospital named 'The Queen's Hospital' had been in existence for almost 30 years. In 1873 it was enlarged to accommodate about 200 in-patients, and again we learn that it contained 'a mortuary and a pathological theatre'. The hospital picture of the time was completed by a number of small special institutions.

Brief mention must be made of the growth of the city before turning to the origin of the School of Medicine. Growth had been slow in the 1850s, but it became very rapid in the 1870 and 1880 decades. Its early organisation seems to have been good for it was described, perhaps with some exaggeration, as 'the best governed city in the world'.[43] In this growth period a strong middle class had emerged which was supported by many of the working class. The part played by civic pride in the development of Leeds has been mentioned, and the part played by local rivalry with Bradford stressed. In Birmingham pride played much the more important role, strengthened by the many improvements in the town produced by municipal reform. The Liberals were gradually gaining power but there was as yet need of a leader. This came in the form of a young 18-year-old man who moved from London to Birmingham in 1854. After a short and successful business career, Joseph Chamberlain turned his attention to Local Government and became a Town Councillor in 1869. In 1865 the Birmingham Liberal Association had been founded and Chamberlain with his Radical views was a forceful member. Surprisingly, it co-operated well with, and received support from, the Socialist Reform League. In 1873 he became Mayor and held office till 1876. He introduced many improvements and, in contradiction to his predecessors, he was not reluctant to borrow and expend money for a worthy municipal cause. Two outstanding changes were the taking of Gas and Water out of the hands of private individuals and putting them under the control of Local Government. The power that he wielded was considerable, supported as he was by the Nonconformists, a group which had been prominent in the town since the 17th century.[44] There were also the Quakers, strongly represented on the Town Council, including Alderman White, who assisted Chamberlain in launching a Birmingham Improvement Scheme. In 1876 Chamberlain became a Liberal Member of Parliament and was a prominent national politician for the rest of his life.

There had been a remarkable transformation in all aspects of the life of the town, and in 1873 Chamberlain laid the foundation stone for a new set of municipal buildings. The Improvement Scheme was directed towards housing conditions and involved the first Medical Officer of Health, Dr. Alfred Hill. He had been appointed in 1872, just 25 years after the first Medical Officer of Health in England, namely Duncan of Liverpool. Health was a major consideration in this decade for there had been a severe smallpox epidemic in 1874. Five years later, Birmingham set up its first Health Committee.[45]

Throughout the century, as in other large towns, there was the need for education and it is now time to consider the evolution of the University. The foundation date for the School of Medicine is usually given as 1841, but it seems that there was some instruction being given some years before. In 1828 an opening speech to the 'Birmingham School of Surgery and Medicine' by Dr. L. Pearson was quoted in the 'Lancet'.[46] A list of patrons is given but there is no list of teachers. Clinical tuition was to be given at the General Hospital and it seems likely that the course was an incomplete one, similar to those quoted in relation to other schools of medicine. In 1837 there was in existence a School of Medicine organised by a local surgeon, Mr. Sands Cox.[47] With the opening of Queen's Hospital, clinical facilities became available and the course was reorganised. In 1845 a Royal Charter was granted and the Medical School became known as 'Queen's College'. Subsequent developments were to prove rather complex. Queen's College progressed in the succeeding years and was more than a medical school when departments of Arts, Law, Engineering, and Architecture were added. The events of later years were less happy for there appears to have been a period of mismanagement associated with financial difficulties. An enquiry was held and a subsequent Act of Parliament laid down provisions for the administration of the College. But in the meanwhile there had been other happenings. In 1851 a second medical school attached to the General Hospital had appeared under the name of Sydenham College. This achieved moderate success until it became merged with Queen's College in 1868, as it was felt that one medical school was sufficient for the town. Now clinical teaching was available at two general hospitals and mention is made of a 'valuable museum' which had been assembled at Sydenham College.

With the town nearing its peak of development, the demand for technical and scientific education became ever greater, and it was now that Josiah Mason came to the rescue. He had been brought up in poor surroundings and as a child had sold cakes in the streets of Kidderminster. Possessed of a flair for business, he eventually made a fortune by the manufacture of steel pens and electroplating.[48] He subsidised institutions for the poor and in 1879, on his 80th birthday, laid the foundation stone for a scientific college to which he subscribed £75,000. It was opened in 1880 by Thomas Huxley under the name of Mason College but in the following year Josiah Mason died. Progress now became rapid for in 1882 students of Queen's College attended Mason College for lectures in Chemistry, Physiology, Botany, Physics and Comparative Anatomy. In 1892 the Queen's College school of medicine was merged into Mason College and called the 'Queen's Faculty of Medicine'. This transfer entailed the extensive provision of buildings and much financial support. Accommodation seems to have been generous and amongst many facilities is mentioned a museum of Pathology. At this early stage of bacterial knowledge it is interesting to read that 'a large bacteriological classroom is in course of construction, in which not only will the students be taught, but work will be performed on behalf of the Public Health Committee, who have shown a wise public spirit in the arrangements they have made with the college'.[47] In 1897 a newly-built General Hospital was opened with the provision of 340 beds.

But during the next few years the aim foremost in people's minds was the establishment of a university, and it was now that Joseph Chamberlain was to play a large part in fulfilling this desire. The Royal Charter was granted in 1900 and at the first meeting of the Medical Faculty on the 1st October, mention was made of the 'new pathological laboratory and bacteriological research laboratory'.[49]

The first occupant of the Chair of Pathology in the new university was R.F.C. Leith (1854–1936). His scientific life was spent in two cities – in Edinburgh from 1885 till 1899 and in Birmingham from 1899 till 1919, when he retired. Graduating from Edinburgh in 1885, he became interested in Pathology, largely no doubt due to W. S. Greenfeld, who was Professor at the time. In a matter of a few years he became successively Pathologist to the Royal Infirmary, Lecturer in Pathology in the School of the Royal Colleges, and Assistant Physician to the Royal Infirmary.[50] It should be noted that as in Leeds and Liverpool, the title of the new chair in Birmingham was 'Pathology and Bacteriology'. Leith appears to have had all his training in Edinburgh and not to have spent time on the Continent as was customary in those days. It would have been a broad training with an emphasis on the relation of Pathology to Clinical Medicine. He was also very interested in Bacteriology and was referred to as 'that well-known bacteriologist'.[51] He was probably very well suited for the Birmingham post which he occupied for 20 years until his retirement, for he was an excellent teacher and a good all-round pathologist. He was well known in pathological circles and was President of the Section of Pathology at the B.M.A. Annual Meeting in Birmingham in 1911.

## Sheffield

If there was a shortage of rivers in Birmingham, the opposite was the case in Sheffield, which was located near the Don and its four tributaries, the Loxley, Porter, Rivelin and Sheaf. The district had therefore a source of water power for forging and grinding, and there was also coal and iron in the neighbourhood. As a result a steel centre developed and was early known for its cutlery, though we do not know exactly when this started. For many years the area was known as 'Hallamshire' and we learn of the incorporation by Act of Parliament in 1624 of the Company of Cutlers.[52] Until late in the 18th century Sheffield was a relatively small town and cutlery was a cottage industry. Its subsequent growth included two phases. The earliest one was due to the appearance of a number of small workshops, and in this way came to resemble a number of small independent towns. This is reminiscent of the mode of growth in Birmingham, though its subsequent municipal developments were quite different for Sheffield had no social and economic leader such as Joseph Chamberlain. The later growth phase occurred in the late 19th century with the advent of heavy industry in the town. By now it had become the centre of the steel industry and was supplying materials for armoury, guns, firearms, and railway equipment. With this phase of phenomenal growth it had now become the largest city in Yorkshire.

But the earlier period had seen some remarkable discoveries which undoubtedly contributed to the business prosperity of the town. In 1740 a new type of hard steel had been developed and in 1742 Thomas Bolsover accidentally discovered how to plate copper with silver and thus created the Sheffield Plate industry.[53] In 1769 James Vickers of Sheffield discovered 'Britannia Metal', an alloy of tin, antimony, and copper. It had a silvery appearance not unlike pewter and became famous for its use in teapots, jugs, and other tableware.[54] Lastly, in 1840 Mr. John Wright, a Birmingham surgeon, discovered electroplating. He was a native of the Sheffield district and prior to taking up surgery had been an assistant to Dr. Shearwater of Rotherham.[54]

In the midst of its great Victorian prosperity, a disaster struck the town. The Dale Dyke reservoir had been constructed in the winter of 1863–4 and held a large volume of water. Following some inclement weather in March, 1864, a rift occurred in the embankment with resultant heavy flooding of the valley of the Loxley river. The water rushed down into part of the town, causing extensive damage and the loss of 260 lives. It is said to have been well described by Charles Reade in his novel, 'Put yourself in his place'.[55]

By the end of the century there had been much modernisation of the city including a fine set of municipal buildings and a Town Hall which was opened by Queen Victoria in 1897. The city's population was now approaching half a million.

Hospital care in the town was provided in 1797 when the Infirmary was opened. Throughout the 19th century additions were made and by its centenary year it had 225 beds and was known as the Royal Infirmary. Sheffield Royal Hospital originated in 1828 as a 'self-supporting dispensary'. Out-patient care only was provided until 1860 when 61 beds were available and the name changed to 'Public Hospital and Dispensary'. Finally, in 1895, it was re-named once more as the Sheffield Royal Hospital and had accommodation for 165 in-patients. Special hospitals such as the Jessop Hospital for Women and the Children's Hospital were founded in 1864 and 1876, respectively.

As with other provincial universities the School of Medicine in Sheffield was bedevilled by the existence of two separate groups. Prior to 1828 a local surgeon, Hall Overend, assisted by his son Wilson, had made a collection of specimens illustrating Human and Comparative Anatomy. It was housed in a building connected with his residence and was used to teach students who were apprenticed to him. In 1828 a Sheffield physician, Arnold (later Sir Arnold) Knight, and others decided to found a medical school in the city and Mr. Overend seconded the proposition. But a quarrel broke out as to whether or not the museum should be used for the school. As a result Dr. Knight founded 'The Medical Institution' in July, 1829. But before it was opened, Dr. Wilson Overend and a Dr. Thompson obtained a license for the Museum and opened it as 'The School of Anatomy and Medicine' in October, 1829. So Sheffield had two medical schools until 1835 when the problem was solved in a surprising way. At this time and following the Burke and Hare murders in Edinburgh, there were strong feelings about 'body snatching'. Mr. Overend felt that it was undesirable to have his museum in close proximity to his house. His fears were not without reason, for in January 1835 the Museum was sacked and completely destroyed by an angry mob. The 'Medical Institution' then proceeded on its own though there are few details about its progress.[56] There seems to have been no outstanding change before 1883.

The Cambridge Extension lectures proved to be very popular in Sheffield and the need for scientific and technological training was expressed by a local Member of Parliament. He even hoped that there would ultimately be a university in the town. In 1874 a successful steelmaster of the town, Mark Firth, became Mayor. Realising the need for a College, he purchased a site and financed a building which was opened in 1879 as Firth College.[57] He wanted it to extend the range of instruction whenever the technical resources for this should be available, so as to include a system of technical education for the due qualification of the artisans of the town 'and to prepare students for matriculation at one of our national universities.'[58]

In 1888 the Medical School moved into new quarters and in 1897 became the medical department of University College, Sheffield through incorporation by Royal Charter with Firth College and the Technical School.[59] In 1895 it had been decided to apply to the Victoria University of Manchester for affiliation as had been granted to Leeds and Liverpool. But this proposal was rejected, and a University Charter for Sheffield delayed until July, 1905.

Pathology was taught in the medical faculty of University College and as was customary at the time instruction was given by physicians. Dr. Duncan Burgess lectured on the subject from 1897 until 1899 when he became Professor of Medicine. In 1898 Arthur J. Hall was made Demonstrator in Pathology and Museum Curator.[60] In the following year he was appointed Professor and in the years 1899–1906 he made a very substantial contribution to the subject. The Pathological Museum was almost entirely due to his activity. He played a great part in raising the standard of the Medical School and became Professor of Medicine in the new university from 1916 until his retirement in 1931.

In 1907 Louis Cobbett became the first occupant of the full time Chair in Pathology at the University. As a student at Cambridge, he had taken the Natural Sciences Tripos in 1884. The atmosphere of Cambridge at the time was a most stimulating one and Cobbett's interest was aroused by a course in Medicine and Surgery given by the respective Professors of the two subjects, namely Sir George Paget (1809–1892) and Sir George Humphry (1820–1896). After clinical studies at St. Thomas's Hospital he graduated in 1891. By 1893 he decided to turn to Pathology and returned to Cambridge where he worked for Professor C. S. Roy, first as Demonstrator of Pathology and later as John Lewis Walker Student. Already he was then being attracted to Bacteriology, for his first paper (with W.S. Melsome) was 'On local and general immunity' and the title of his MD thesis in 1899 was 'On the nature of the action of antitoxin'. Diptheria particularly commanded his attention, possibly because of the outbreaks of that disease in Cambridge and Colchester. He visited the Pasteur Institute in Paris and later made and tested diptheria antitoxin for Messrs. Burroughes Wellcome.[61] Now known as a Bacteriologist, he played a significant part as Scientific Investigator to the Royal Commission on Tuberculosis in 1902. In 1906 he seemed well suited to occupy the Chair of Pathology and Bacteriology at Sheffield. But the adjustment from Cambridge to Sheffield proved too great for him and after only one academic year he resigned the post and returned to his beloved Cambridge, where in 1908 he became lecturer in Pathology. In some ways Cobbett's decision was a great loss for Sheffield, for he had many qualities desirable in a Professor. He was fond of students, was a very good teacher, and was also a man of wide interests. On the other hand, it might be argued that a new university department of Pathology would be better served by someone with a wider viewpoint of the subject.

As successor to Cobbett, James Martin Beattie (1868–1955) was appointed in 1907. Born in New Zealand, he had graduated in medicine from Edinburgh University in 1894. After sundry house-appointments, he advanced to University Tutor in Clinical Medicine. Now deciding to specialise in Pathology, he became Senior Assistant to Professor W. S. Greenfield, Lecturer in pathological bacteriology, and Assistant Pathologist to the Royal Infirmary.[62] Such a period, namely 1901–7, spent in Greenfield's laboratory, was just about the ideal training in General and Applied Pathology that any young man could wish to have. Beattie applied himself industriously to his new post in Sheffield and in 1908, with W. E. Carnegie Dickson, he published his volume on General Pathology; in the following year the volume on Special Pathology appeared. In addition to his duties as Professor at the University he was also Honorary Bacteriologist to the Royal Hospital and to the Royal Infirmary. For a period he was also Dean of the medical faculty. By 1912 all seemed to be progressing well in the Pathology department and the university must have been well satisfied by their choice of Professor. But suddenly in that year Beattie resigned his Chair to go to Liverpool as Professor of Bacteriology in the University and Bacteriologist to the city. The university must have regretted Beattie's decision for he had served them well, and it appears that Beattie himself had some misgivings about leaving Morbid Anatomy and Histology. As had been said, there were many new developments in Liverpool at the time, and with these he must have been well-satisfied, for he held the post for 22 years, until his retirement in 1934.

## Bristol

The history of Bristol is much longer and more complex than that of the provincial cities already dealt with, but in spite of this a brief summary will be attempted. Her beautiful natural harbour and her well known woollen cloth made her a trading centre from the 14th century or even earlier. Situated in the West Country, her ships avoided contact with Hanseatic League vessels operating in northerly or easterly waters. Until the 16th century most of the trade was with Europe, Ireland and the Near East, and its volume made Bristol the second largest port in England. In the succeeding years the pattern of trade changed and became directed towards Africa and the New World. In 1497 John and Sebastian Cabot sailed from Bristol on their well known voyage to North America, and in 1551 Sebastian became one of the founders of the Bristol Merchant Venturers, a society still in existence. In its early years it did much to encourage Bristol ships to embark on voyages of trade, exploration, and colonisation, mostly to North America and the Caribbean. The activity of the ports of London, Bristol, and Liverpool in connection with the slave trade in the 18th century will be recalled. Throughout the century the activity of Bristol declined in this and other aspects of trade and finally gave second place to Liverpool which was rapidly advancing. There were several reasons. Navigation on the river Avon for larger ships was becoming more difficult and there had been a shift in the national economy due to the Industrial Revolution and the discovery of coal fields in the North and the Midlands. Also, for sailing to Africa, Liverpool was better placed geographically than was Bristol. Ships sailing from the former followed the North Irish coast, thus avoiding the English Channel which was a hunting ground for pirate vessels and privateers.

Improvement did not occur until the port of Bristol was reorganised and enlarged and there was much opposition to the early plans. It was not till about 1880 that developments proceeded. The Avon was satisfactorily dredged and the large port of Avonmouth was built on the Bristol Channel with adequate docking facilities. The final chapter, namely the introduction of the aircraft industry, belongs to the 20th century.[63]

The 18th century has been known as one of great hospital development and between 1721 and 1745, five new general hospitals had been founded in London. By 1789 thirty similar institutions made their appearance in the Provinces in England. The first of the latter was the Winchester County Infirmary in 1736 and in 1737 Bristol opened its Infirmary. Four physicians and two surgeons were appointed, and one of the former had been a postgraduate student of Boerhaave's at Leiden.[64] A second hospital, the General, was founded in 1832. These two hospitals grew with the city and by 1894 the Royal Infirmary had 264 beds and there were 200 in the General.

The early days of the Medical School bear some resemblance to those in other Provincial centres. In the early 1800s, some surgeons gave classes in Anatomy and dissection in their private houses and Dr. J. C. Prichard, a well-known local physician, gave some lectures on Medicine.[65] But about 1830 it appears that this private venture became associated with the Infirmary, for we learn that this institution had been recognised by the Royal College of Surgeons for the teaching of Anatomy. It is further stated that for some periods of the day the deadhouse was turned over for dissection and instruction given by members of the staff. When the General Hospital was founded in 1832 it started a school of Medicine in which its pupils were in a sense apprenticed to the medical staff.[66] So once more there were two Medical Schools based on the two hospitals. Happily this did not last long for in 1833 it was decided to merge them into one school. The founders were Dr. Riley and Mr. Henry Clark, and a full programme was drawn up. There were lecturers for Surgery, Chemistry, Chemical Toxicology, Materia Medica, Therapeutics, Theory and Practice of Medicine, Midwifery, Diseases of Women, Anatomy, Physiology, Anatomical dissections, and Botany. For that time it seems an ambitious undertaking. It is noteworthy that Pathology is not listed, but it may have been included in the Theory of Medicine. Although the original accommodation was limited it seems that the tuition was satisfactory.

As in other centres there was considerable pressure for scientific education, partly due to the enthusiastic reception of University Extension lectures. In 1876 a University College was founded and by 1903 there had grown up a number of specialised Institutions such as the Agricultural and Horticultural Research Station at Long Ashton, set up by the National Fruit and Cider Institute. In 1889 the Government had given grants of money to some of the University Colleges, but the one at Bristol only survived through the generosity of the Wills family, who had introduced the tobacco industry into the town.[67]

The year 1892 was a vital one for it witnessed the amalgamation of the Medical School and University College. By now there was a modern curriculum and one notes that Pathology and Morbid Anatomy are included. The Medical School also possessed a teaching museum for Pathology which was fostered by Dr. Swayne and Mr. Greig Smith.

In 1894 the British Medical Association held its Annual Meeting in the Bristol suburb of Clifton.[68] A glance at the programme shows that at the time Pathology was attracting much attention. A special Pathological Museum exhibit was made from a selection of the most interesting specimens from the museums of the main hospitals and it is stated that 'it is hoped that a special feature will be made of Bacteriology'. Progress continued and eventually in 1909 Bristol was given full university status.

In 1906 the Bristol University College (as it was then) established a Chair of Pathology and Isaac Walker Hall (1868–1953) was appointed to it. He was also made the first honorary Pathologist and Bacteriologist to the British Royal Infirmary. He had graduated in Medicine in 1899 at the Victoria University of Manchester, and for the next year he worked in Leipzig, Stockholm, and Wiesbaden. Returning to Manchester in 1900, he supplemented his initial training by becoming Demonstrator in Physiology and in 1901, Lecturer in Pathology. The next five years in Lorrain Smith's department gave him good general pathological experience with the result that in 1905, with G. Herxheimer, a practical laboratory handbook entitled 'Methods of morbid histology and clinical pathology' was produced. The title is interesting for at the time the term 'clinical pathology' was rarely used, but it indicates that Walker Hall was interested in the practical application of his subject to clinical medicine. One aspect of this was bacteriology and he showed early interest in it by papers on typhoid, abortus fever, and plague. When Bristol was granted independent university status in 1909, he became the first Professor of Pathology. In the following year he was given laboratory space in the university which was very limited. In spite of this he was able to carry out all the clinical pathology required as well as the Public Health bacteriology not only for Bristol but also for the surrounding areas where no pathological services were available. At the same time he carried out his teaching duties and has been described as a 'delightful lecturer'. In retrospect, one might hazard a guess that he developed the first university department of Clinical Pathology.

Although not relevant to our present purpose it might be added that when he retired in 1933 he became Director of the new university department of Preventive Medicine. By his skill and with the co-operation of the Medical Officer of Health, a close link was forged between the University and the City.

## Cardiff

The University of Wales was late on the scene and a product of the 20th century. A small theological college, St. David's, Lampeter, had been founded in 1822 but made little progress. Following discussions on the desirability of providing university education, three further colleges were established: in 1872 at Aberystwyth, in 1883 at Cardiff, and in 1884 at Bangor. In none of these was there any sign of a medical faculty. In 1893 University College, Cardiff instituted Chairs of Anatomy and

Physiology and a Lectureship in Materia Medica. With the growth of the neighbouring King Edward VII hospital, which was re-named Cardiff Royal Infirmary, clinical facilities became available, and Chairs of Pathology, Medicine, and Surgery were appointed.[69] Now for the first time students could obtain a full medical course, but had to obtain their degrees from the University of London. It was not until 1931 that a University Charter was granted to the School. Its subsequent progress was rapid and in the next fifty years the number of professional departments increased from six to thirty.

REFERENCES

1 Green, V. H. H., 'The Universities'. Penguin Books 1969, p. 98.
2 Ibid p. 99.
3 Ibid p. 115.
4 Copeman, W. S. C., 'The Worshipful Society of Apothecaries of London, 1617–1967'. Pergamon Press, London 1967, pp. 66–7.
5 Anning, S. T., 'History of Medicine in Leeds'. W. S. Maney & Son Ltd., 1980, pp. 135–6.
6 Briggs, A., 'Victorian Cities'. Penguin Books 1968, pp. 107–8.
7 Green, V. H. H., 'The Universities'. Penguin Books 1969, pp. 107–9.
8 Bettenson, E. H., 'The University of Newcastle-upon-Tyne'. University of Newcastle-upon-Tyne 1971.
9 Briggs, A., 'Victorian Cities'. Penguin Books 1968, p. 47.
10 Hume, W. E., 'The Infirmary, Newcastle-upon-Tyne'. Andrew Reid & Co., Newcastle-upon-Tyne 1951, p. 42.
11 Bettenson, E. H., 'The University of Newcastle-upon-Tyne' University of Newcastle-upon-Tyne 1971, p. 13.
12 Green, V. H. H., 'The Universities'. Penguin Books 1969, pp. 111–2.
13 Ibid p. 132.
14 Ibid p. 135.
15 'British Medical Journal'. (1897) i, 1610.
16 Champan, R. W., 'The Story of a Modern University'. Geoffrey Cumberlage, Oxford University Press 1955, p. 107.
17 Ibid p. 191.
18 Sheperd, J. A., 'A History of the Liverpool Medical Institution'. Liverpool Medical Institution 1979, pp. 45–6.
19 Ibid pp. 170–1.
20 Ibid pp. 16–21.
21 'Lancet'. (1911) ii, 59–60.
22 'British Medical Journal'. (1911) ii, 53–4.
23 Trans. Roy. Soc. Trop. Med. & Hygiene. 1929–30. *23*, p. 217.
24 Briggs, A., 'Victorian Cities'. Penguin Books 1968, p. 86.
25 Anning, S. T., 'History of Medicine in Leeds'. W. S. Maney & Son Ltd, 1980, pp. 2–29.
26 Ibid pp. 147–8.
27 Briggs, W., 'Victorian Cities'. Penguin Books 1968, pp. 152–3.
28 Ibid p. 158.

29  'Illustrated London News'. (1869) *52*, p. 512.
30  Ibid *53*, 196.
31  'British Medical Journal'. (1897) i, p. 1607.
32  Anning, S. T., 'History of Medicine in Leeds'. W. S. Maney & Son Ltd 1880, pp. 149–50.
33  'British Medical Journal'. (1883) ii, p. 491.
34  Trans. Path. Soc. London, 1897, List of members.
35  Shimmin, A. N., 'University of Leeds, the first Half Century' Cambridge University Press 1954, p. 211–12.
36  'British Medical Journal'. (1894) i, pp. 611–12.
37  Anning, S. T., 'History of Medicine in Leeds'. W. S. Maney & Son Ltd 1980, p. 97.
38  J. Path. Bact. 1959, *75*, p. 577.
39  Ibid 1922, *25*, pp. 109–12.
40  'Lancet'. (1921) ii, pp. 825–6.
41  Briggs, A., 'Victorian Cities'. Penguin Books 1968, p. 34.
42  'British Medical Journal'. (1897) i, p. 1602.
43  Briggs, A., 'Victorian Cities'. Penguin Books 1968, p. 36.
44  Ibid p. 201.
45  Ibid pp. 225–6.
46  'Lancet'. (1828) i, pp. 104–6.
47  'British Medical Journal'. (1897) i, pp. 1604–5.
48  Green, V. H. H., 'The Universities'. Penguin Books 1967, p. 101.
49  'British Medical Journal'. (1900) ii, p. 1120.
50  Ibid (1937) i, p. 50.
51  'Lancet'. (1937) i, p. 114.
52  'British Medical Journal'. (1907) ii, p. 1689.
53  Encyc. Americana. 1979, Vol. 24, pp. 688–9.
54  'British Medical Journal'. (1908) ii, pp. 32–3.
55  Ibid (1907) ii, p. 1692.
56  'Lancet'. (1928) i, pp. 26–7.
57  Chapman, A. W., 'Story of a modern University'. Geoffrey Cumberlage, Oxford University Press 1955, p. 14.
58  Green, V. H. H., 'The Universities'. Penguin Books 1967, pp. 115–16.
59  'British Medical Journal'. (1907) ii, p. 1695.
60  Chapman, A. W., 'Story of a modern University'. Geoffrey Cumberlage, Oxford University Press 1955, p. 158.
61  J. Path. Bact. 1947, *59*, pp. 695–702.
62  Ibid 1956, *71*, pp. 544–7.
63  Encyc. Americana. 1979, Vol. 4. p. 558.
64  Underwood, E. A., 'History, Philosophy & Sociology of Science'. Article by Neuberger. Geoffrey Cumberlage. Oxford University Press 1953. reprint 1975, pp. 263–273.
65  'British Medical Journal'. (1897) i, p. 1606.
66  'Lancet'. (1933) ii, p. 186.
67  Briggs, A., 'Victorian Cities'. Penguin Books 1968, p. 182.
68  'British Medical Journal'. (1894) i, pp. 1209–10.
69  Green, V. H. H., 'The Universities'. Penguin Books 1967, pp. 113–14.

# ELEVEN

# The first Pathologists from 1830

In 1830 the importance of Pathology in relation to Clinical Medicine was well recognised, though the full time Pathologist did not appear until the end of the 19th century. Such progress as had been made in the subject was largely due to the work of the French school and consisted almost solely of Pathological Anatomy. Now, progress developed in several different ways, and the first logical step was the application of microscopical studies to anatomical lesions, namely Pathological or Morbid Histology. For this to occur, technical improvements in the microscope were necessary and it will be remembered that Joseph Jackson Lister (1786–1869), the wine merchant and father of Lord Lister (1827–1912), designed an achromatic microscope in the early 1830s. In medical circles in Great Britain the new instrument was not accepted with any great enthusiasm and any advances made in Histology were mostly due to physiologists who were pioneering a new subject. It is interesting to note that at the end of the century in most English medical schools Histology was taught to medical students by Physiologists, whereas it would have been much more logical to teach it as an extension of Anatomy.

To carry out the new developments, laboratory accommodation became essential. Anatomical and histological studies were later in demand after advances in surgery which followed the discovery of anaesthetics and asepsis. It became customary to appoint a Curator to work in the laboratory. As such he was made responsible for the collection of suitable specimens for inclusion in a pathological museum. Microscopy was also applied to the examination of body fluids such as urine, blood, pleural and ascitic fluids and this work was done in a 'clinical section' of the laboratory. By the middle of the century, certain chemical tests were applied to these fluids, and towards the end bacteriological and haematalogical techniques necessitated additional laboratory space. The need for experimental animal studies became recognised by physiologists, though once the pathologist came on the scene, he too realised their importance in the development of his subject. After this brief outline of developments in Pathology it will be necessary to examine them in more detail.

## London and Edinburgh

In the London teaching hospitals of 1830, there was only one man, namely Thomas Hodgkin (1798–1866), who could be called a full time pathologist, for in 1825 he had been appointed Lecturer in Morbid Anatomy and Curator of the Pathological Museum at Guy's Hospital.

As such he carried out the autopsies, and the reports were of a much higher standard than those from other hospitals where no such person had been assigned these duties. Instead, they might be carried out by a student-dresser, a house surgeon, or even the surgeon himself. Handling such a large amount of pathological material, Hodgkin was well placed to augment the museum collection. In succeeding years the post of Curator became universal for by the end of the century every teaching hospital and some of the larger non-teaching institutions had a Pathological Museum. In looking at the careers of such Curators, one notes that most held the position for only a short period, often prior to their appointment to the hospital clinical staff. This system had a two-fold advantage for it served to fill in an interim period and at the same time provided good basic experience in Pathology for those who would subsequently be practising either Clinical Medicine or Clinical Surgery. It may be recalled that Hodgkin held his Curator's post until 1837, waiting for a vacancy on the clinical staff. When his application for the post of Assistant Physician was rejected he was so disappointed that he gave up Pathology for the rest of his life. He thus became lost to Pathology as of course were those who successfully obtained clinical appointments. This system of using Pathology as a stepping stone to a clinical career was partly responsible for the long delay in the recognition of Pathology as a special subject. In Germany it was quite different, for the young pathologist at the University centre was committed to a career in the subject, and was trained for it by the Professor. With the rapid acceptance of Pathological Histology it is easy to understand the large number of pathologists which emerged from these 'schools' at the German Universities. By contrast, in England there were individuals interested in the subject but no schools where they were trained.

As already mentioned microscopy was not taken up immediately by medical men. There was interest in the subject, but by a number of different types of scientist (see Quekett Club and the Royal Microscopical Society, Chapter 5). But in spite of these there are two exceptions which must be noted.

John Hughes Bennett (1812–1875) was apprenticed to a Maidstone surgeon and at this early age showed his interest in Pathology by carrying out some autopsies during this apprenticeship. He completed his medical training at the University of Edinburgh in 1837 and subsequently spent two years working in Paris and an additional two years in the leading German universities.[1] Influenced by the Continental methods, on his return to Edinburgh in 1841 he gave a public course of lectures on Histology. In addition he gave private courses on the 'Practical manipulation of the microscope'. He was intensely interested in Anatomy, Physiology and Pathology, but in 1842 was unfortunately unsuccessful in his application for the Chair of General Pathology at the University. However, he retained his interest in Pathology when in the above year he was appointed Physician to the Royal Dispensary and

Pathologist to the Royal Infirmary. In 1848 he was made Professor of the Institutes of Medicine at the University. He advocated the methods of Practical Medicine which he had learned at the Polyclinics in Germany, and was continually emphasising the value of the microscope in its application to Medicine. Many students were influenced by this approach to medicine, not least Burdon Sanderson, who acted as his demonstrator.[2] It is ironical that such a pioneer of pathology never held a Chair in the subject.

In contrast with Hughes Bennett and his widespread training, Lionel Smith Beale (1828–1906) stayed in London for almost the whole of his long life. Like Bennett he had a great interest in the microscope. He commenced his medical career by being apprenticed to a Surgeon-Apothecary in Islington before matriculating at London University in 1847.[3] His next two years were spent at Oxford working as an assistant to Henry Ackland in the Anatomical Museum. It may have been here that he first developed his interest in the microscope for Henry Ackland (later to be Sir Henry and Regius Professor of Medicine at Oxford) had received special tuition on the use of the microscope when a medical student at St. George's Hospital.[4] Beale worked hard and passed his MB London University examination in 1851, but never went on to take the MD. In 1853, when only 25, he became Professor of Physiology at King's College, London, and by this time had established his own laboratory where he carried out experimental work, and taught Morbid Histology and Physiological Chemistry. He was a prolific writer and amongst many publications wrote 'The Microscope in Medicine'. In 1869 he became Professor of Pathological Anatomy and Physician to King's College Hospital. In 1876 he became Professor of Medicine, and at this time gave up lecturing in Pathological Anatomy. Strangely enough in this year he became Curator of the museum, an appointment which as previously indicated was usually held by a much younger man. But Beale had been a practical pathologist all his life and this latest appointment which he held till 1888 allowed him to remain in contact with his favourite subject. He was compelled to resign his Chair of Medicine in 1896 when he suffered a cerebral haemorrhage.

These two men were very important for they were laboratory pioneers and the story of Pathology in the 19th century, particularly the second half, was one of laboratory development. It became essential for each of the new branches of Pathology which were coming into being. Hughes Bennett used it for histology of blood, tissues, and for experimental work. Beale used it for histology and examination, chemical and otherwise, of body fluids. But at the centre of all their work stood the microscope. Sir John Simon, responsible for developing Public Health in England, requested a laboratory at St. Thomas's when he was appointed Lecturer in Pathology soon after graduation. He used this for many years for studies which were chiefly experimental and related to the natural history of disease. He influenced many of his Medical Officers of Health, especially Burdon Sanderson, who advocated the experimental approach to Pathology throughout his lifetime. Such work was not easily performed for at mid-century laboratory accommodation was scarce until the establishment of research institutes of which The Brown Institute in 1871 was the first (see Chapter 16). Beale's first laboratory in 1851 was in his house in Care Street and Burdon Sanderson had a private laboratory in Howland Street some 15 years later. By the end of the 19th century laboratory space (very necessary then for the rapidly growing science of Bacteriology and Immunology) was not nearly so scarce. Yet in 1898 we find Burdon Sanderson in a lecture making a plea for laboratory accommodation in every university department of Physiology and Pathology.

A few words must now be said about the early University Chairs of Pathology. In this matter Continental Europe was ahead of Great Britain for in 1819 J. F. Lobstein (1777–1835), a native of Giessen, was elected to the Chair of Pathological Anatomy in the University of Strasbourg, a French town at that time. His book, which was never finished, dealt with the correlation of clinical symptoms and morbid anatomical lesions, but it also emphasised the need for animal experiment.[5] A further such appointment followed in 1836 when Jean Cruveilhier (1791–1873) became Professor of Pathological Anatomy at the University of Paris. He had been a pupil of the surgeon Guillaume Dupuytren (1777–1835) and it was due to his master that the Chair was created.

It is often said that the first chair of Pathology in Great Britain was at the University of Edinburgh, when John Thomson was appointed in 1831. He had previously been Professor of Military Surgery at the University and Professor of Surgery at the Royal College of Surgeons, Edinburgh. When he came to occupy this third chair, the famous anatomist, Robert Knox, promptly referred to him as 'the old chair maker'. In the same year Robert Carswell (1793–1857) was appointed to a Chair of General Pathology at University College, London, and it could well be argued that this was the first. In 1827 the newly-formed University College had appointed its professional staff. Amongst these was Johann F. Meckel the younger (1781–1833), the famous pathologist and comparative anatomist at the University of Halle. He was invited to be Professor of Pathology and as part of the deal he was to bring his museum with him. There were also financial considerations in regard to the museum and the result was that Meckel and University College could not come to terms. Accordingly, in 1828 the Chair was offered to Robert Carswell. At the time he was working in Paris on his celebrated 'Atlas of Pathology' which appeared in 1837. In order to finish his drawings of specimens supplied to him by Magendie and Louis, he stayed in Paris and only returned to London to take up his appointment in 1831.

In subsequent years many Chairs of Pathology were founded in Europe and it is said that by mid-century there were twenty in Germany, ten in Austria, and nineteen in Italy.[6] In Great Britain things were very different and no further Chairs of Pathology were founded for 40 years or more. One thing that the Edinburgh and London Chairs had in common was that they were part-time.


## Edinburgh – part-time Professors

In Edinburgh, the early holders of the Chair were:[7]

| | |
|---|---|
| 1831–1842 | John Thomson |
| 1842–1869 | William Henderson |
| 1869–1881 | William R. Sanders |
| 1881–1912 | William S. Greenfield |
| 1912–1931 | James Lorrain Smith |

In Edinburgh, Pathology was first taught by the Professor of Anatomy and later by the Professor of Clinical Surgery. When Thomson was appointed Professor of General Pathology he was also a Consultant Physician and Surgeon. In addition, he found time to play a large part in the founding of the Museum of the Royal College of Surgeons. Henderson was an authority on the cardiovascular system and a Physician to the Royal Infirmary. He was also one of the early advocates of the use of the microscope in Medicine. Unfortunately he came to believe in Homeopathy and was forced to resign his post at the Infirmary. Attempts were made by his colleagues to remove him from his Chair of Pathology but they were unsuccessful. Likewise Sanders was a Physician and because of a very busy practice he found little time in his later years for teaching Pathology. Under Greenfield, a University College London graduate, the Department of Pathology in Edinburgh really blossomed. In addition to General Pathology it was broadened by the introduction of experimental and surgical sections. The amount achieved by Greenfield was remarkable, and particularly so when one remembers that he was also a Professor of Clinical Medicine with charge of beds in the Royal Infirmary. Because of this he could be termed 'part-time' but there is no doubt that his heart was in Pathology. When he vacated the Chair of Pathology, his beds were handed over to the Professor of Medicine, and his successor, Lorrain Smith, assisted by a Professor of Bacteriology, a new appointment, became the first full-time Professor of Pathology in Edinburgh.

The sequence of events at University College London bore some resemblance to those described at Edinburgh. There must even have been a strong Edinburgh influence for of the first professors appointed, namely Charles Bell (Surgery), A. Todd Thomson (Materia medica and Pharmacy), Robert Grant (Zoology and Comparative Anatomy), and John Conolly (Nature and treatment of disease), all had studied there. The London University opened in 1828, and throughout the remainder of the century seven Professors of Pathology were appointed to University College.[8]

## The first Pathologists from 1830

| | |
|---|---|
| 1831–1840 | Robert Carswell |
| 1840–1848 | Walter H. Walshe |
| 1849–1861 | Sir William Jenner |
| 1861–1867 | Wilson Fox |
| 1867–1887 | H. Charlton Bastian |
| 1887–1896 | Sir Victor Horsely |
| 1896–1906 | Sidney H. C. Martin |

Following this group, A. E. Boycott was appointed as the first Graham Professor of Pathology in 1919 of the University of London and became the first full-time Professor in University College.

In studying the lives of these early professors of Pathology, a number of questions come to mind. Firstly, if they were part-time, what other duties did they perform? As we have seen, the duties of the Edinburgh group were mainly clinical. In University College, as will be seen, there was more diversity. Secondly, where was training and further experience in Pathology obtained? The Edinburgh professors seem to have remained in Scotland whereas the London group went further afield. Thirdly, what was the exact title of the Chair of Pathology? In some instances it was a Chair of General Pathology, whilst in others it was one of Pathological Anatomy. However, their main duties were initially the provision of a lecture course on the principles of the subject and thus 'General Pathology'. It was not until the time of Greenfield that a Practical Course in Pathology was provided for students.

Some details of the University College group will be of interest. Robert Carswell was a physician as well as Professor of Morbid Anatomy. He was also an excellent artist as evidenced by the illustrations in his well known Atlas. He undoubtedly obtained much of his interest in Pathology in Paris where he worked with F. Magendie and P.C.A. Louis. It is unfortunate that in 1840 at the early age of 47 he gave up Pathology and spent the rest of his life as physician to the King of the Belgians.[9] The entry of Walshe into Medicine was fortuitous. Born in Dublin he went to Paris in 1830 to study philology. There he met Oliver Wendell Holmes who was a medical student, and he decided to change his career. He worked with Louis at the La Pitié. As a result of this contact with the French school he became advocate of the use of percussion and auscultation. He later had experience at La Charité with the surgeons Alexis Boyer (1757–1833) and P. J. Roux (1780–1854).[10] After graduating from Edinburgh in 1836 he was appointed Professor of Pathology in 1841 in succession to Carswell. Again a clinical association is apparent for in 1848 he gave up Pathology and became Professor of Medicine to replace C. J. B. Williams.

Although essentially a physician, William Jenner had studied Pathology at University College for four years following his MD graduation in 1844. His enthusiasm for observing post-mortem appearances enabled him to distinguish typhus form typhoid fever. In 1849 he was appointed Assistant Physician to University College Hospital and

175

Professor of Pathological Anatomy. In 1854 he became full Physician but held his Chair in Pathology till 1861. For years he ran a lecture course on Pathological Anatomy, emphasising the structural changes of disease, together with microscopical appearances.

Jenner's successor as Professor of Pathological Anatomy, namely Wilson Fox, seems to have been the first one to receive a definite training in the subject. Graduating MB from University College in 1854 he worked with Walsh as a physician's assistant and may well have developed an interest in Pathological Anatomy. Following a year at the Royal Infirmary Edinburgh he spent a year working in the medical schools of Paris. This was followed by a year in Vienna where Rokitansky was still in charge of Pathology, and two years in Berlin working with Virchow. With this extensive training in Pathological Anatomy it is surprising to read that on his return to England he became Physician to the Royal Staffordshire Infirmary (1859). His health lapsed but he recovered and in 1861 became Professor of Pathological Anatomy at University College. He must have had considerable ability for in applying for the post he had obtained very strong support from Virchow.[11] He carried out some interesting experimental studies on pyaemia, but in 1867, like others, he deserted Pathology, to become Holme Professor of Clinical Medicine and a Fellow of University College.

Charlton Bastian was a very different character. He graduated MB from University College and MD in 1866. His ability was recognised at an early age for he was made FRS when only 31. He showed an early interest in Pathology when appointed Lecturer in Pathology and Assistant Physician to St. Mary's Hospital, London. Later in the same year (1867) he became Assistant Physician to University College Hospital and Professor of Pathology. He became interested in nervous diseases and was a neurologist of some repute.[12] He occupied the Chair till 1887 when he became Professor of Medicine, and does not appear to have made any significant contribution to the pathology. The most surprising feature of his life was a growing interest in the doctrine of spontaneous generation. In spite of overwhelming opposition he retained his support for this theory with remarkable tenacity to the end of his long life.

Another University College graduate, namely Victor Horsley, was destined to change the character of the Pathological Department. He passed his MB examination in 1881 and three years later was appointed Professor-Superintendent of the Brown Institute. This suited him well, for he believed that 'disordered function' was much more important than 'disordered structure'. For investigations from a physiological angle, the experimental approach was essential, and for such research an animal institute such as the Brown was ideal. The student lectures given by Burdon Sanderson had done much to stimulate his interest in Physiology.[13] He stayed three years at the Brown Institute during which time his research included localisation of cerebral function, the thyroid gland and rabies. His efforts in obtaining compulsory muzzling of dogs was responsible for the eradication of the disease from Great Britain. While at the Brown Institute he became Assistant Surgeon to University College Hospital in 1885. He left the Institute in 1890 and in 1893 became Full Surgeon to University College Hospital and Professor of Pathology, a post which he held till 1896. Not only an excellent general surgeon, he became the leading neurosurgeon of the day. In spite of all his activities he found time to influence the study of modern pathology and appreciated the contributions being made by the newer branches such as biochemistry, bacteriology, and haematology. It was a tragedy when he died of heat-stroke in the Middle East during World War I.

The last part-time Professor of Pathology at University College with clinical responsibilities was Sidney Martin. After graduating in 1883 he spent time studying in Vienna. His interest in Pathology grew with his early appointments. In 1885 he became Pathologist, Curator of the Museum and Medical Tutor to Middlesex Hospital; also, Pathologist and Registrar to the City of London Hospital for Diseases of the Chest. In 1890 he became Assistant Physician at both University College and the Brompton Hospitals. In 1903 he published his textbook on General Pathology and in 1906 became Professor of Pathology.[14] He was a great advocate of the experimental method in Pathology and therefore most suitable to continue the lines which Horsley had laid down.

Due to disorganisation during the First World War it was not until 1919 that A. E. Boycott was made the first full-time Professor of Pathology at University College.

The first full-time Professor of Pathology in Great Britain was not appointed till 1882. Before this is detailed, mention must be made of the academic appointments of Lionel S. Beale, who has been already mentioned. In 1853, at the age of 25, he became Professor of Physiology at King's College, London. In 1869 he resigned this post to become Professor of Pathological Anatomy and also Physician to King's College Hospital. In 1878, on the retirement of Dr. George Johnson, he resigned his Pathology Chair and became Professor of Medicine.[15] Pathology seems to have been an important subject at King's College although the Chair which Beale occupied was only part-time. Throughout the century there were regular appointments of the post of Museum Curator, there were lectures in the subject, and in 1887 the First Professor of Bacteriology, Edgar M. Crookshank, was elected to a chair of Bacteriology and Comparative Anatomy.

Consideration must now be given to the first full-time University Professors of Pathology.

## Aberdeen

When D. J. Hamilton was appointed Professor at the University of Aberdeen in 1882, he became the first full-time holder of a Chair of

Pathology in the British Isles. Such was the growth of the subject that by 1906, the year in which the Pathological Society of Great Britain and Ireland was founded (see chapter 6), nine more Chairs had been instituted.

In 1878 Sir Erasmus Wilson, a well-known dermatologist, who had become wealthy through a number of business speculations, financed the transportation from Egypt to London of a granite obelisk since known as 'Cleopatra's Needle'. Three years later he endowed the first Chair of Pathology in the University of Aberdeen; and in 1882 Dr. David James Hamilton became its first occupant and later proved to be a very worthy choice. Born in Scotland, he graduated from Edinburgh University where he had been a pupil of Professor Sanders, to whom he was indebted for his early interest in Pathology. This he was able to pursue as Resident Medical Officer for two years at Liverpool Northern Hospital with charge of the Pathological Department. His ability soon became obvious when in open competition he won the Triennial Astley Cooper Prize of £300 at Guy's Hospital. This enabled him to spend two years on the Continent in the pathological departments of Munich, Strasbourg, Paris, and Vienna. There he worked with such eminent men as Rokitansky, von Recklinghausen, Koch, Hoppe-Seyler, and Virchow, whom he greatly admired. On his return he worked in Edinburgh with Professor Sanders.[16] Here he organised a course in General Pathology and greatly raised the standard of teaching. When Sanders died in 1881 there were many who saw in Hamilton his natural successor, but in the end a brilliant young pathologist called W. S. Greenfield was given preference. Hamilton did not have to wait long for his opportunity, for in 1882 he was appointed the first Professor of Pathology at Aberdeen, a post which he held for twenty-six years. With his valuable Continental experience he built up his department into one of the best in the country. He was chiefly noted for his teaching ability of both General Pathology as well as its practical application to Medicine and Surgery. He ensured the close co-ordination of these two aspects by giving lectures on them on alternate days. His 'Text Book of Pathology' became the standard work in the English language, until Ziegler's German work was translated by Sir Donald MacAlister.[17] His teaching was supplemented by a fine collection of museum specimens which he housed in Marischal College. Pathology was taught in its widest sense and he emphasised the value of the experimental approach. He realised the value to Public Health of the bacteriological advances of the time, including the diagnosis of typhoid and diptheria. He was also interested in animal diseases and his research led to his discovery of the bacillus which caused 'louping-ill' in sheep.

In 1880, Alexander Ogston had been appointed senior surgeon to the Aberdeen Royal Infirmary.[18] He was later to become Regius Professor of Surgery in the University and his twenty-six years of activity exactly coincided with those of Hamilton. More important still, Ogston had

178

bacteriological interests which led to his discovery of his 'micrococci' in acute abscesses. In these early days views on septicaemia and pyaemia were so confused that the Pathological Society of London held a prolonged inquiry into the subject in 1879. Koch had published his small book on 'Aetiology of Traumatic Infective Diseases' in the previous year.[18] Ogston examined 100 abscesses and found that whereas cocci could be found in acute abscesses, more were present in 'cold abscesses'. He published three papers in 1880, 1881, and 1883 and described his micrococci.[19] Those that grew in chains he, like Billroth, called 'streptococci', those that grew in clumps 'staphylococci', on the suggestion of W. D. Geddes, the Professor of Greek at Aberdeen. Ogston's contributions were considerable for he had shown that pyaemia and septicaemia were not blood diseases, and that blood was merely a vehicle by which a local lesion could in some cases become generalised. With these two great figures, Ogston and Hamilton, Pathology in Aberdeen got off to a good start.

## Cambridge

Cambridge University was next to follow and Charles Smart Roy (1854–1897) was appointed as the first Professor of Pathology in 1884. There had been lecture courses on both General and Systematic Pathology throughout the 19th century and these were usually given by the Professor of Medicine. In 1877–80 a Royal Commission on Cambridge and Oxford was sitting with a view to drawing up some new University Statutes. It was presented with a memorandum signed by 138 graduates of Cambridge engaged in the study or practise of medicine. It urged the recognition of Pathology as one of the foremost subjects and, as a result, in 1883 three new professorships in Physiology, Pathology, and Surgery were created.[20] The new Professor of Pathology's training and his subsequent interests were very different from those of the conventional Pathological Anatomist and certain details must be given. Born in Scotland, Roy was educated at St. Andrew's, and subsequently at Edinburgh University from which he graduated MD in 1878. He had in 1875 been Resident Physician at the Edinburgh Royal Infirmary prior to taking up a post at the Brown Institute, where he worked under John Burdon Sanderson. This period was interrupted for a short time when he served as surgeon in the Turkish Army in the Turco-Serbian War, and his operative skill was to prove most valuable in his later experimental work, as was his remarkable ability at designing laboratory apparatus. He spent about two years on the Continent where he had training in pathology with Virchow and von Recklinghausen. But already he was showing a preference for physiology, no doubt as a result of his studies at the Brown Institute, and these were fostered by his work in the Physiological Institute in Strasbourg under Goltz, in Berlin under Du

Bois Reymond, and in Leipzig under Cohnheim.[21,22] He returned to England as a confirmed experimentalist and in 1880 logically became the first George Henry Lewes student under Michael Foster, the Praelector of Physiology in Trinity College, Cambridge, and the leading English physiologist of the day. In 1882 he became Professor Superintendent of the Brown Institute, a post which he held till his appointment at Cambridge.

The new professor was given very meagre accommodation, consisting of two and a half rooms and a staff of one 'boy'. In spite of this he attempted to develop the teaching programme of the department by giving lectures in General Pathology with courses in Morbid Anatomy, Histology, Bacteriology and Experimental Medicine. When these proved to be unsuccessful he launched his Long Vacation Course, meant to attract students who had passed their second MB and were waiting to start their clinical training at one of the London hospitals in the autumn. By now it was clear that Roy's teaching ability appealed only to advanced students or to assistants engaged on research projects. He attracted many outstanding young men during his tenure, including such names as J. G. Adami, A. A. Kanthack, J. Lorrain Smith, Louis Cobbett, and many others.[23] He sponsored much research work amongst his staff, and his collaborative work with Adami must be mentioned. It extended over a period of ten years commencing with work in Cohnheim's laboratory and being continued at the Brown Institute and finally at Cambridge. When ready for publication in the Philosophical Transactions, it consisted of a 100-page article on 'Contributions to the Physiology and Pathology of the Mammalian Heart'.[24] The authors considered their study of importance because previously similar studies had been done only on amphibian organs.

Cambridge was to be unlucky in the health of its early professors. When just over 40, Roy became ill and was able to do little work thereafter, finally dying suddenly at the age of 43. Towards the end of 1897, Alfredo Antunes Kanthack (1863–1898) became Roy's successor but held the post for only 13 months, dying in December 1898 at the age of 35.

In 1896, during Roy's terminal illness, Kanthack was appointed Deputy head of the department and was given the impossible task of also running his department at St. Bartholomew's by frequently travelling between Cambridge and London.[25] As a result, when he became Professor at Cambridge, the department was rather disorganised. Due to his teaching ability the department made great progress during his short period of office. His preparatory training for the post had been very different from that of Roy and Hamilton. Born in Brazil, where his father was British Consul in Bahia, he came to Europe when aged six and was educated in Germany. In 1882 he attended Liverpool College and graduated in 1882 from St. Bartholomew's Hospital, London. He then spent a year in Berlin with Koch, Krause, and Virchow, where he learned the importance of the clinical approach to Pathology. He returned to Bart's to become a Resident in Obstetrics, and during this time served on a Leprosy Commission. This took him to India where he saw two specimens of Madura foot. With these and a study of other specimens obtained from the London hospital museums he published a paper on this unusual subject.[26] At this stage his interest in clinical medicine was such that he even contemplated practising as a physician in Liverpool.[27] But in 1892 he was appointed Director of the Pathological Department at Bart's and so returned to London. This post suited him well with its wide approach for he was lecturer in both Pathology and Bacteriology as well as Curator of the Museum. Clinical material flowed into his department and his teaching flourished. The department at Bart's provided a striking contrast to Roy's experimental laboratory and would, no doubt, have been the pattern which Kanthack would have adopted on his appointment to the Chair at Cambridge at the end of 1897. His first concern was the teaching programme which showed an immediate change. His methods appealed to his students and he expended much energy on the Long Vacation Course instituted by Roy. It was shortly after this that his health deteriorated and he died in 1898, just before the end of the year. He was much loved and respected by students and staff and one instance of his great kindness should not be left untold.

One day in about 1950, the present author was visited in his laboratory at Bart's by an 85 year-old pathologist, Ernest H. Shaw. He related how, when he left school, he was given the post of a library messenger at Bart's. On his visits to the laboratory Kanthack took a fancy to the boy and later took him on as a laboratory assistant. When appointed to Cambridge, Kanthack took three persons with him, namely T. S. P. Strangeways (who became a well-known pathologist), Ernest H. Shaw, his laboratory assistant, and his 'laboratory boy', W. A. Mitchell. When Kanthack died, he made financial provision in his will for Shaw to study Medicine, and he ended up as Pathologist in the Great Northern Hospital.[28] Small wonder that on that day in 1950, Ernest Shaw came back to see the library in the Pathological Department dedicated to and named after his old master.

In contrast with Kanthack, German Sims Woodhead (1855–1921) occupied the Chair at Cambridge for 22 years. A brief study of his career will illustrate the many directions in which Pathology was developing at the time and also the changes which occurred in Cambridge. Born in Yorkshire, he commenced his medical career in Edinburgh in 1873 and graduated in 1877. He has been described as a good but not brilliant student,[29] though he had many other attributes. An excellent sprinter, he won an English International Cap for Rugby Football, was a good organiser, and was socially very acceptable to all those around him. He spent some time on the Continent at Vienna, and also worked with Koch in Berlin, and with Pasteur in Paris. He first became interested in

Pathology when he joined a voluntary practical class in the subject run by Dr. D. J. Hamilton. From 1881 till 1887 he worked under Professor Greenfield and during that time published his Practical Pathology (1883), and his Practical Mycology (1885), written with his friend, A. W. Hare. He was now very well known in Edinburgh and became the first Secretary of the Pathological Club in 1886. As a result of his training, he came to regard Pathology as a subject essentially related to the practical requirements of Medicine.[30] At this time in Edinburgh there was a remarkable medical man called John (later Sir John) Batty Tuke who in 1856 sailed to New Zealand where he became Senior Medical Officer to the colonial troops in the Maori War. After many thrilling adventures he returned to Edinburgh, where he devoted himself for many years to studying and treating mental disorders.[31] He became very influential through his close association with the Royal College of Physicians of Edinburgh and for years he represented the University in Parliament. He became aware of the growing need in medicine for research and he was responsible for the foundation of the Research Laboratory by the Royal College of Physicians in 1887. Woodhead was well known to Tuke and it was therefore no surprise that he was appointed the first Superintendent of the new laboratory. It was a new venture but he soon equipped his rooms for physiological and chemical work as well as for pathological anatomy and examination of body fluids. Young men were not slow to take advantage of laboratory accommodation which in those days was scarce. Woodhead did not stay long for in 1890 he became the first Director of the Laboratories of the Conjoint Board of the Royal College of Physicians (London) and the Royal College of Surgeons (England) (see chapter 16). It might be thought that this new post in London would be similar to the previous one in Edinburgh, but there were many differences. Pathology was lagging behind in London and there were as yet no professorial departments in the London schools. Many of the young men who requested space for research were young clinicians. Woodhead found that there were other demands for space, which he supplied, such as the bacteriological testing for diptheria, and the production of diptheria antitoxin for the Metropolitan Asylums Board. With his supervisory and administrative duties he found little time for personal research but he managed to publish several papers. In addition, he found time to produce a second edition of his Practical Pathology and to start the Journal of Pathology and Bacteriology (see chapter 6). On the basis of scientific work which he did for the Royal Commissions of 1890 and 1894 on tuberculosis, he came to be regarded as an expert on this subject. Mention should be made of his association with the 'Lancet', for he had been special correspondent when in Edinburgh. In 1851 Thomas Wakly, the editor of the 'Lancet', decided to issue reports on the microscopical and chemical analyses of foodstuffs, the project being designated as 'The Analytical Sanitary Commission'.[32] The first reports concerned water, bread, vinegar, spices, potted meats, vegetables, jellies, jams, lard and butter – even tobacco and opium were included! Such reports appeared in an irregular manner until 1893, when the 'Lancet' announced the existence of 'The "Lancet" Laboratory'.[33] Because of a large number of requests for analysis it had been decided to build 'an excellent laboratory on the premises of 'The "Lancet"'. The journal described the equipment available and furnished the results of examinations of commercial preparations put out by drug houses. Private analyses would not be done and any work carried out would be at the expense of the proprietor. These examinations would be devoted 'wholly to matters relating to public health and the analyses of drugs and articles of food so far as they are considered to be of interest and concern to the medical reader.[34] From further reports it is clear that there were also statistical studies and others relating to public health.[35] There is little said about the staffing of the 'Lancet' Laboratory but we do know that the director was Mr. Vasey and it appears that Woodhead and he made a valuable study on the standardisation of disinfectants.[36] It looks as if Woodhead may have acted in an advisory or supervisory capacity. Lastly, when these analyses of food products were reported, the name of the manufacturer was given and a comment made on the value of it.

It seems obvious that by this time Woodhead was running a very diverse kind of laboratory and quite unlike a conventional pathological department. His versatility was to be tested further when in 1899 he was chosen to succeed Kanthack as Professor of Pathology at Cambridge University. At that time, Pathology was at a low ebb, and Woodhead's idea of a University department linked to a hospital for clinical pathology, as at the Royal Infirmary in Edinburgh, was not a practical proposition. Addenbrooke's Hospital had been opened in 1766 but no student teaching had been instituted during its first 50 years. Even throughout the rest of the 19th and into the first half of the 20th century, there was insufficient clinical material for the purpose. As a result, it became customary for medical students to study the basic sciences at Cambridge and then attend one of the large London hospitals for their clinical work. This resulted in the average student leaving Cambridge at an early stage in his career and preparing for his Final Examination (which included Pathology) by studying in London. Occasionally a few of the better students might return to Cambridge for a further year, usually to carry out a research project, and this was the kind of man who had been well-catered for in Roy's laboratory. The accommodation for laboratory work was nevertheless totally inadequate, and Woodhead immediately set about drawing up a scheme for building a medical school which would include adequate space for Pathology.[37] Progress was rapid and the new building was opened by Edward VII in March, 1904. Two of the Professor's assistants at the time were T. S. P. Strangeways, who had been brought from Bart's to Cambridge by Kanthack, and G. H. F. Nuttall, who came to Cambridge in 1899, and these three taught on a Long Vacation course (instituted by Roy) for students preparing for their final MB examination. In later years Nuttall became the Quick Professor of Biology and founder of the 'Journal of Hygiene' while Strangeways carried out valuable studies on tissue culture in a small laboratory which subsequently bore his name.

With his enthusiasm and teaching ability, Woodhead reorganised the General Pathology course which had so far been purely scientific, and tailored it to the needs of the average student of medicine. The institution of an elementary examination in Pathology taken after his course and before the clinical years was then followed by an examination in Pathology as part of the Final MB. Once this was achieved, the Long Vacation course was abolished. From the students' point of view, the teaching of Pathology in Cambridge was very satisfactory, but it did not appeal to some of the members of the other Basic Science departments, who felt that only the purely scientific side of the subject should be taught. It is generally agreed, however, that Woodhead's approach, even if undesirable, had been done exceedingly well. It seems likely that he had some powerful support for his teaching policy, including Sir Clifford Allbutt, the Regius Professor of Physic. In 1914, the John Bonnett pathological laboratory at Addenbrooke's Hospital was opened and the Regius Professor performed the ceremony. In his speech he advocated the close co-operation between clinician and pathologist. It appeared that in 1898 he and Kanthack had attempted to set up a clinical laboratory in the hospital but had been overruled by the board. Now with great satisfaction he saw his earlier dream fulfilled.[38]

The amount of work that Woodhead achieved was remarkable, for in addition to building up a modern pathology department he was occupied in work for The Royal Commission on Tuberculosis, of which he was a member in 1902; he instituted studies disproving a remarkable statement made by Koch in 1901, namely that 'the bovine tubercle bacillus was not pathogenic to man';[39] he aided and encouraged P. C. Varrier Jones in setting up the Papworth Village Settlement for the treatment of convalescent cases of tuberculosis.[40] Lastly he carried out a number of active duties during the First World War.

Woodhead had transformed the Cambridge department during his 22 years in office, and now the feature of its Professors seems to have been longevity, for his successor, H. R. Dean, was to occupy the Chair for 40 years and to die in 1961 at the ripe old age of 82.

## Manchester

Sheridan Delépine was the first Professor of Pathology in the Victoria University of Manchester, but it will first be advisable to recall something about the earlier development of both the University and Pathology. The Royal Medical School had been founded in 1825, and in 1851 Owen's College had appeared. In 1872, by fusion of these two schools, the Victoria University came into being. In these early days, a young Bavarian called Julius Dreschfeld (1845–1907) came to study science and mathematics at Owen's College. He returned to Germany and graduated in Medicine from Wurzburg where he had been much influenced towards Pathology and Physiology by von Kölliker and Von Bezold. In 1869 he qualified with the LRCP Diploma and became a physician in Manchester. In 1891 Dreschfeld was appointed Professor of Medicine at Owen's College. He was noted for his interest in Pathology and in 1875 he was asked to supervise the pathological section of the medical museum of the College and to prepare a catalogue. He became lecturer in Pathology, and in 1881, Professor. During this time, he organised one of the first pathological laboratories in the country and his success was phenomenal. By 1891 the number of students attending his classes rose to 11.[41] Thus, when the Department of Pathology was established in the University, there was no lack of interest in the subject.

Sheridan Delépine (1855–1921), of European parentage, was educated in France and Switzerland, graduating B.Sc. from the University of Lausanne. In 1877 he came to Edinburgh to study medicine and graduated in 1882.[42] At first a demonstrator in Anatomy, he later became a demonstrator in Pathology under Professor Sanders and Dr. D. J. Hamilton. In 1882 he moved to London where he became a private assistant to Sir Andrew Clark. He carried out pathological work and also engaged himself in research with his chief. Amongst several observations, his conclusions on the histology of the liver could well stand today, e.g., 'what was looked upon as the central duct of an acinus is really the peripheral channel, the usually described peripheral channels being really central ducts'.[43] Also while in London he had been appointed Curator of the Museum and Demonstrator of Pathology, St. George's Hospital, and subsequently Pathologist and Lecturer on Physiology and Pathology in the Medical School. The school at St. George's was a large one at the time and Delépine obtained ample experience of both Practical Pathology and of teaching. By 1891 he was ready to take charge of a department of Pathology and it is interesting at this stage to note that the first Chair at Manchester was named 'of Pathology and Bacteriology'. Delépine had his opportunity, and during the next 10 years the department flourished and its standard of teaching became known as one of the best in Great Britain.

But over the years Delépine changed his viewpoint, placed as he was in an industrial area where public health problems abounded. He still provided stimuli for the research of his young assistants but he was carrying out an increasing number of tests related to Public Health and Hygiene. He felt that the volume of this work was too great to enable him to do justice to his teaching of Morbid Anatomy and Histology. Fortunately the University saw the great value of his new work and as a result a Chair of Public Health and Bacteriology was established for him. He designed new laboratories which were opened in 1905.[44] By now Delépine had 13 qualified Assistants and was carrying out work for about 100 sanitary authorities. Courses had been organised in Bacteriology for such diverse groups as students for the Diploma in Public Health, chemists, veterinary students and teachers in Dairy and Agricultural schools. Delépine had developed a first-class department, but he had done even more, for he made his Bacteriology department the chief centre in England for Public Health Bacteriology. The Manchester Diploma in Public Health was the first to be established in England.[45] Such great names as Topley and Wilson emerged from this department; and Topley succeeded Delépine, but in 1927 he moved to the Chair of Bacteriology and Immunology at the newly-founded London School of Hygiene and Tropical Medicine, and the Manchester influence was soon felt in London.

A successor to Delépine's Chair of Pathology was then sought and in 1904 James Lorrain Smith (1862–1931) was elected Professor of Pathology. He came to Manchester from Belfast where he had been first Lecturer (1895) and then Professor of Pathology (1904) at Queen's College, Belfast. He stayed in Manchester till 1912, when he succeeded W. S. Greenfield in the Chair of Pathology at Edinburgh. Lorrain Smith's career had been both interesting and varied. Born in Dumfriesshire, he graduated in Medicine in 1889 from the University of Edinburgh where he had earlier shown particular ability in Philosophy. As a student he was attracted to Physiology by Noel Paton and to Anatomical Pathology by Greenfield, but a series of circumstances directed him towards research in the former subject. As a postgraduate student he worked at Oxford with Professor J. Burdon Sanderson, already well known for his physiological approach to medicine, and was associated with Professor J. S. Haldane in some problems of respiratory physiology. He became the John Lucas Walker Scholar, working under Professor C. S. Roy at Cambridge, and spending a short time in Strasbourg with von Recklinghausen and in Copenhagen with Christian Bohr.[46] The work of these early years might have led him into physiology but he grew more and more concerned with problems of Pathology which had a physiological basis, an approach which was fostered when he became Demonstrator in Pathology in Roy's department, and subsequently Lecturer at Queen's College, Belfast and Honorary Pathologist to the Royal Victoria Hospital. There he continued his researches and published an important paper on blood volume in chlorosis and pernicious anaemia.[47] It was a busy period for Lorrain Smith, for the Irish Universities had been in disarray for some years. Now they were soon to be reorganised and Queen's College, Belfast became 'The Queen's University in Ireland'.[48] The Belfast authorities, well pleased with his achievements, advanced him to Professor in 1904, but later in the year he moved to Manchester. Here he became the first Proctor Professor of Pathology and Honorary Pathologist to the Royal Infirmary. The foundation of a separate Chair of Bacteriology was a wise decision which enabled him to concentrate on the teaching aspects of his subject. He began by building up a pathological museum with properly catalogued specimens, and taught students by case studies and clinicopathological correlation, a method which he fully developed later in Edinburgh.[49] Most pathologists so far concentrated on either research or teaching, but Lorrain Smith believed that both could be done together and felt that his teaching helped him with his research and vice versa. His research now followed the question of fatty degeneration and, aided by C. Powell White, he studied the technical demonstration of fats and fatty acids, including especially staining by Nile Blue Sulphate. Throughout all these years he preserved his philosophic approach to the whole subject and his breadth of vision made his viewpoint that of a biologist. It was during his stay at Manchester that he became recognised as one of the leaders in Pathology. By the time he moved to his final Chair in Edinburgh (1912), he was a fitting successor to as great a man as Greenfield. As a final work, it should be remembered that he, with Robert Muir, was largely responsible for the founding of the Pathological Society of Great Britain and Ireland (see chapter 6). His contribution to Pathology had thus been substantial.

## Glasgow

The next Chair of Pathology to be established was at Glasgow in 1893, and its first occupant was a graduate of the University, namely Joseph Coats (1846–1899). In a nutshell, his contribution put Pathology in Glasgow 'on the map', a great achievement which required much patience and perseverance. Born in Paisley, he graduated in Medicine from Glasgow University in 1867. In his early days he had been house surgeon to Lord Lister at the time when the latter was working out his antiseptic system. At this time Pathology had scarcely emerged in the town. At the University it was taught only as part of the Institutes of Medicine. There was a pathologist at the Royal Infirmary who carried out a number of autopsies, some medicolegal work and, in addition, some general practice. It is obvious that he had no time to teach students the important application of Pathology to Medicine.[50] It would be interesting to know why, in such inauspicious surroundings, Coats decided, soon after graduation, to spend two years in Germany. There he was fortunate to come under the influence of the great physiologist Carl Ludwig in Leipzig, and the well known pathologist von Recklinghausen in Wurzburg. With this good basic training, he was well-suited to become Pathologist to the Royal Infirmary in Glasgow on his return. In 1874 there was an important development, for Coats was appointed to be Pathologist to the new Western Infirmary, and Lecturer in Pathology at the University, where this subject had now become separated from the Institutes of Medicine. Coats must have thought that his dream was about to become true. Yet, such were the difficulties that it was almost another 20 years before the Chair of Pathology was established (1893). After his appointment to the Chair he was able to pursue, with courage, tact, and determination, his ambition to form an Institute of Pathology which would be the first of its kind in Great Britain. Through the joint action of the management of the Western Infirmary and the University, this was opened in 1896.[51] Coats is always remembered for his Institute but his contribution was much greater. He was greatly respected as a teacher, probably because of his great sincerity rather than his outstanding eloquence. He believed in Pathology and set out to convince all his students of the importance of his subject in all branches of medicine. He was not a prolific writer but he achieved prominence through his Manual of Pathology, first published in 1883, and by his Lectures to Practitioners in 1888. Regrettably, Coat's tenure of office was all too short, for he died in 1899.

He was succeeded by Robert (later Sir Robert) Muir who held the Chair for 37 years, finally retiring in 1936. During this time the Glasgow School of Pathology became the leading one in the country. An excellent teacher, Muir inspired not only undergraduates but also the young assistants in his department. In all, 21 of these came to fill Chairs of Pathology and Bacteriology. He became recognised as the leading pathologist in the British Isles and practically every conceivable honour came his way during his 95 years. There is much more that could be said though for our present purposes we are only concerned with his earlier years at St. Andrew's (see below).

## St. Andrew's

The Chair of Pathology at St. Andrew's was established in 1898 and Robert (later Sir Robert) Muir became its first holder. Born in Scotland, he studied Medicine at the University of Edinburgh, graduating MA in 1884 and MB.CM in 1888. Following a research project in Professor Greenfield's department of Pathology, he became assistant to the Professor and Pathologist to the Royal Infirmary (1892). A few years later he was appointed to a new Lectureship in Pathological Bacteriology.[52] In 1897 he published with James Ritchie of Oxford a 'Manual of Bacteriology', which remained the standard text for some years. Coming to St. Andrew's in 1898, he stayed only a year. Muir appears to be the first of these pathologists not to have had some training at the well known German laboratories. However he could not have had a better master than Greenfield and his subsequent record speaks for itself.

Robert Muir was succeeded in 1899 by Lewis Robertson Sutherland who occupied the Chair until 1930. Little is known about him except that he was interested in Comparative Anatomy, especially the skeletons of birds. It seems that there were few advances in Pathology at St. Andrew's during these years and developments were delayed until the arrival of Daniel Fowler Cappell in 1931.

## Dublin, Royal College of Surgeons

In chapter 9 the growth of the Irish universities up to and including the 19th century was outlined. There had until the end of this period been little or nothing said about the emergence of pathology. The universities as they stand today are the University of Dublin (Trinity College), University College Dublin (including Queen's College Cork and Queen's College Galway), and The Queen's University, Belfast. An additional medical school for undergraduates has existed in the Royal College of Surgeons in Ireland for many years.

The last-named school was the first to recognise Pathology as an independent subject by establishing a Lectureship in 1878. This was held by Stewart (later Sir Stewart) Woodhouse (1846–1921) for a short time, but in 1889 it was elevated to a Chair. The first holder was Thomas (later Sir Thomas) Myles (1857–1937), a leading Dublin surgeon who was on the staff of the Richmond Hospital at the time. He had graduated from Trinity College, Dublin, and in 1885 became a Fellow of the Royal College of Surgeons in Ireland. In 1889 he graduated MD and by this time was regarded as one of the outstanding figures in Irish surgery. His post in Pathology was a part-time one and consisted of lectures and classes at the Royal College. For this he was well-suited for he was an excellent lecturer and his ability as a teacher went back to his younger days when he was a very popular 'grinder'. It is likely that he taught pathology as applied to surgery for we have no record of his having any training in pure pathology. With Pathology rapidly advancing, like the honest man he was, he felt his limitations, for Professor P. D. J. Holland told me that when he resigned the Chair in 1897 he declared in his letter of resignation that 'the science of Pathology had developed to such an extent that a clinician is no longer a fit person to occupy a Chair in this subject'.

Those responsible for the appointment of his successor must have taken these words to heart when in 1898 they selected Arthur Hamilton White (1868–1915). He was educated at King's College, London and at the Royal College of Surgeons School in Dublin from which he became licensed to practice medicine in 1893. In contrast with Myles he had a fairly extensive training in Pathology. First of all, he had worked with Victor Horsley at University College, London and with Kronecker in Berne. He also visited Vienna and Freiberg, and by this time had done some research work on the nutrition of the frog's heart. On returning to Dublin he became Pathologist to the Meath Hospital where he had been a pupil. He was a good research worker who was conscientious and meticulous, though he was less successful as a teacher of junior students. It is sad to relate that his career was dogged by ill-health which finally forced him to resign his post in 1915. He should always be remembered as the first full-time pathologist in Ireland. A brief word about his successors might not be out of place. In 1915 William Boxwell (1875–1943), a grandson of the famous physician, William Stokes, followed. Once more, there was a change in the approach of the teaching. Boxwell was clinically orientated, and when appointed he insisted that he should be allowed to continue his clinical work at the Meath Hospital. He was a good teacher and also published with his friend, Francis Purser, a book entitled 'Introduction to the practice of medicine'. The present holder of the Chair, Professor P. D. J. Holland, has maintained the high standard of his school and in 1981 achieved the distinctions of being President of the Royal College of Physicians in Ireland and President of the Association of Clinical Pathologists.

## Belfast, The Queen's University

In 1845, as a result of the Irish Colleges Parliamentary Bill, Queen's College Belfast came into being. In 1878 a Medical School was formed but it was not until 1908 that university status was granted and with it the power to confer degrees.

In the earliest days Pathology may have been taught with Physiology but in 1895 a Lectureship in Pathology was established and James Lorrain Smith appointed (1862–1931). The choice could hardly have been better, for he had had excellent training. His undergraduate pathology he learned from Greenfield in Edinburgh, and in his early postgraduate years he had become interested first of all in Physiology when working with Burden Sanderson in Oxford and later in Pathology while in Cambridge with Roy. This was supplemented by some Continental experience in Strasbourg and Copenhagen. As a result he was well-equipped to build up an academic department of Pathology with emphasis on the experimental method and this he proceeded to do. It should be added that in order to enable him to maintain a clinical association he had been made Honorary Pathologist to the Royal Victoria Hospital. The authorities must have been well-satisfied with the results for in 1904 he was made Professor of Pathology to Queen's College, but in the same year, he accepted the Chair of Pathology at the Victoria University of Manchester.[53,54]

His successor would require unusual versatility in the future development of the department for in 1908 the College had been given enhanced status as 'The Queen's University of Belfast'. The teaching programme was to include pathology, bacteriology, and medical jurisprudence; there would also be responsibility for the pathology for two large hospitals. Once more the choice was a happy one and William St. Clair Symmers

(1863–1937) was appointed. Symmers had been born and brought up in South Carolina, but had received his medical education at Aberdeen, from which he graduated in 1887. In his earlier years he was attracted to Pathology and had the opportunity of working with that fine teacher, D. J. Hamilton, Assistant Pathologist at the Royal Infirmary, Aberdeen. He gained further general experience in a similar post at the General Hospital in Birmingham. But at this time he had become interested in Bacteriology, and after nine months study at the Pasteur Institute in Paris, he became Assistant Bacteriologist to the British Institute of Preventive Medicine (later re-named the Lister Institute, see chapter 16).

In 1897, he was for the next seven years to obtain some unique experience as Professor of Pathology and Bacteriology at the Government Medical School in Cairo and Pathologist to the Government Hospital. Amongst many achievements, he set up a department for the production of cattle plague serum, and built up a large teaching museum consisting of about 600 specimens which he prepared and mounted himself.

He came to Belfast in 1904 for his new post which he held until 1929 when he retired. In 1908 he became the first Professor of Pathology in the new university. He tackled his new tasks with great enthusiasm and in a few years the department expanded with laboratories for pathology and bacteriology. His ability as a speaker stood him in good stead whether in the lecture room or giving evidence in forensic cases. He was respected by his colleagues chiefly on account of his wide general knowledge, and his unfailing courtesy endeared him to all. He was active in research, published a number of papers, and greatly inspired students and graduates. The Queen's University of Belfast thus developed a modern pathology department in the early years of the 20th century due to the work of two outstanding early pathologists with widespread knowledge in their subject.

## Dublin, Trinity College

The earlier history of Trinity College, founded in 1592, has already been given (see chapter 9). Although there is mention of a Professor of Anatomy in the early 18th century, there is no reference to Pathology and Physiology till much later. In 1863 John Mallet Purser (born in 1839) graduated MB from the College and in 1869 was appointed Professor of Anatomy and Physiology at the Carmichael School. With the nomination of R. C. Mayre as another Professor in these subjects, Purser is said to have devoted most of his time to Physiology and Pathology. Then on the 13th February 1874 we learn that he was elected Professor of the Institutes of Medicine in the School of Physic – the name given to Trinity College in 1785.[55] Thus, Pathology would have been taught at that time as part of the 'Institutes'. In 1895 it became a separate subject for the first time when a Lectureship was established. In 1876 a very remarkable student had entered the College, namely Alexander Charles O'Sullivan (1858–1924), who was a classical scholar and an outstanding mathematician. He turned to Medicine and by the time of his graduation had developed an interest in Pathology, thanks to his teacher, John Purser. He spent two years gaining experience in pathological research at Vienna and Freiburg, and on his return to Dublin became the first lecturer in Pathology referred to above.[56]

He held the post till 1922 and was therefore responsible for Pathology at Trinity College through its formative years. He stimulated interest in research but seems to have been reluctant to publish his own work. He was very highly rated by his colleagues and certainly considered to be one of the leading men in Irish medical circles. During this period he had for a short time in 1919 the assistance of Adrian Stokes (1887–1927), Professor of Bacteriology and Preventive Medicine, an outstanding man who became Professor of Pathology to Guy's Hospital, London, in 1922. His early death from yellow fever in Lagos was a great tragedy.[57] One problem remains, namely why did the College delay the upgrading of Pathology from Lecturer to Professor for 27 years when they had a most suitable man available? It was ironical that the College with the oldest tradition should be the last to recognise Pathology. However, in 1922 O'Sullivan was elevated to the Chair of Pathology, but held it only for two years, for he died of septicaemia five days after cutting himself when carrying out a post-mortem.

## Dublin, University College

Founded as the Catholic University Medical School, it had gone through troubled times before being re-named University College in the National University of Ireland in 1908. It is therefore surprising to learn that Pathology was recognised as a separate discipline as early as 1891. In that year the first Professor of Pathology, Edmond Joseph McWeeney (1864–1925) was appointed. He was only 27 at the time and was one of the few persons who had been trained in Pathology and Bacteriology. McWeeney had graduated from the Catholic University Medical School in 1887 and subsequently studied under Koch in Berlin and in Rokitansky's laboratory in Vienna. On his return he was well-suited for the job which he held for 34 years though he was greatly handicapped by suffering from paralysis agitans. He faced the problem of building up a modern pathology department with little assistance and poor equipment. Nevertheless, he worked hard and kept in touch with advances in his subject. He was a member of the BMA for many years, was elected a member of the Pathological Society of London in 1896 and was a signatory of the letter in 1906 suggesting the formation of the Pathological Society of Great Britain and Ireland. He had been a brilliant student, and throughout his life had many interests, especially in fungi and plant diseases. He spoke well and was an acceptable lecturer. His appointments to several hospitals in Dublin, and his post of bacteriologist to the Local Government Board, kept him in touch with the practical application of his subject to medicine in general. He laid the foundations of a good department in its formative years but lacked the facilities for its full development.

REFERENCES

1  'British Medical Journal'. (1875) ii, pp. 473–4.
2  Ibid (1905) ii, p. 1481.
3  Ibid (1906) i, p. 836.
4  'Lancet'. (1900) ii, p. 1158
5  Castiglioni, 'History of Medicine'. Alfred A. Knopf, 2nd Ed. Translator, E. B. Krumbhaar. 1947, p. 692.
6  Ibid p. 797.
7  Currie, A. & Duvall, E., 'The first hundred years of the Development of Pathology, (1831–1931)'. University of Edinburgh 1981, pp. 5–10.
8  Merrington, W. R., 'University College Hospital and its Medical School'. Heinemann 1976, pp. 5–6.
9  Ibid p. 7.
10  'Lancet'. (1892) ii, pp. 1535–8.
11  Ibid (1887) i, pp. 1011–13.
12  Ibid (1915) ii, pp. 1220–4.
13  'British Medical Journal'. (1916) ii, p. 162.
14  'Lancet'. (1924) ii, p. 680–1.
15  'British Medical Journal'. (1906) i, pp. 836–7.
16  Ibid (1909) i, pp. 631–3.
17  Ibid (1909) i, p. 730.
18  'Lancet'. (1929) i, p. 309.
19  Bullock. W., 'History of Bacteriology'. Oxford University Press 1938, pp. 149–50.
20  Rook, A., 'Cambridge and its Contribution to Medicine'. Wellcome Institute of History of Medicine 1971, pp. 120–1.
21  'British Medical Journal'. (1897) ii, p. 1031.
22  'Lancet'. (1897) ii, p. 1954.
23  Rook, A., 'Cambridge and its Contribution to Medicine'. Wellcome Institute of History of Medicine 1971, pp. 123–4.
24  'Philosophical Transactions'. (1898) *183*, pp. 199–298.
25  J. Path. Bact. (1900) *6*, p. 89.
26  Ibid (1892) 1, p. 142.
27  'British Medical Journal'. (1898) ii, pp. 1941–2.
28  Rook, A., 'Cambridge and its Contribution to Medicine' Wellcome Institute of History of Medicine 1971, p. 127.
29  J. Path. Bact. (1922) *25*, pp. 118–37.
30  Edin. med. J. (1922) *28*, p. 132
31  Ibid (1913) ii, p. 431.

32  Sprigge, S. S., 'The Life and Times of Thomas Wakley'. Robert E. Kriege Publishing Co. 1974, pp. 460–1.
33  'Lancet'. (1893) i, pp. 29–30.
34  Ibid (1893) i, p. 176.
35  Ibid (1894) i, pp. 34–5.
36  Ibid (1922) i, p. 51.
37  Rook, A., 'Cambridge and its Contribution to Medicine'. Wellcome Institute of History of Medicine 1971, pp. 129–30.
38  Ibid pp. 263–4.
39  Ibid p. 133.
40  Ibid p. 134.
41  'Lancet'. (1907) i, pp. 1819–20.
42  Ibid (1921) ii, p. 1080.
43  J. Path. Bact. (1921) 25, p. 114.
44  'Lancet'. (1905) i, pp. 326–7.
45  J. Path. Bact, (1944) 56, pp. 451–77.
46  'Lancet'. (1931) i, p. 943.
47  Trans. Path. Soc. London. (1900) 51 quoted in Ref. 46.
48  'Lancet'. (1908) i, p. 1087.
49  'British Medical Journal'. (1931) i, p. 774.
50  Ibid (1899) i, pp. 317–19.
51  J. Path. Bact. (1900) 6, pp. 89–93.
52  'British Medical Journal'. (1969) i, pp. 976–7.
53  'Lancet'. (1931) i, pp. 943–4.
54  'British Medical Journal'. (1931) i, pp. 773–7.
55  Cameron, S. A., 'History of the Royal College of Surgeons of Ireland'. Fannin & Co. Dublin 1916, p. 304.
56  'Lancet'. (1924) i, p. 467.
57  'British Medical Journal'. (1927) ii, pp. 615–17.

# TWELVE

# The birth of Physiology and Experimental Medicine 1820–90

At the beginning of the 19th century an interest in function rather than structure developed and resulted some years later in the establishment of Physiology. It is only fair to point out that before this time there had been a few individuals who showed interest in function but at the time this did not amount to a movement. Vieq d'Azyr (1748–94) although classed as a comparative anatomist was greatly interested in function and was thus also a comparative physiologist.[1] His views linked him with Cuvier who also worked in Paris.[2] In England John Hunter (1728–93) stood alone, well ahead of his time. Trained in Anatomy by his brother William, he became a surgeon. However, his outlook was always that of a naturalist. At the time there were a number of private anatomical museums and Hunter was a great collector. But his collection was biological in nature and included human, animal and even plant specimens. The material from man and animals was arranged to form a comparative collection in which function was regarded as all-important and which included a number of physiological experiments.[3] Hunter's outlook was therefore experimental and he had no use for theoretical and abstract thinking. The latter approach became prevalent and was developed in the late 19th and early 20th centuries in Germany by a group of men known as the 'Nature Philosophers'. As already mentioned the empirical or clinico-pathological method had resulted in medical advances in France. But this piecemeal approach had no appeal to the German mind, which was idealistic and therefore anxious to develop a system which would explain all natural phenomena, and as can be imagined many systems were proposed, all of which probably contained a grain of truth.[4] Following the unhappy days of the Napoleonic domination a wave of idealism swept the country. There was considerable intellectual activity and the University of Berlin was founded in 1810. But the whole picture of the time is very complex and confused, chiefly because of the different schools of thought. Although Schelling (1775–1854) is said to have been the founder of the Nature Philosophy School, its most lively spirit was Lorenz Oken, who had been much influenced by the philosophical writings of Immanuel Kant and Goethe.[5] His aim was to construct a classification of animals similar to that of Linnaeus for plants. He is probably best remembered for his theory that the skull was formed from three modified vertebrae. This attracted many adherents and was only disproved by T. H. Huxley as late as 1858.[6] The Natural History School soon followed that of Nature Philosophy. It was founded by Johann Schönlein (1793–1864) and attempted to name and classify diseases.[5] This period of systems and schools of thought did much to delay the progress of German Medicine and it was not until Johannes Müller and his pupils founded the Rational School that the seeds of Physiology were sown.

For more than the first half of the 19th century the British School continued its anatomical study of disease by clinicopathological correlation, carried out by a number of eminent physicians and surgeons. Hand in hand with social and legal reform came the public health movement initiated by Chadwick and Southwood Smith and later further developed by John Simon (see chapter 13). Much was learned about epidemic disease even though the actual causation was as yet unknown. However, by the time Simon had almost completed his work, he had realised that there was a crying need for more information about disease, and this would entail research in experimental medicine (see chapter 13).

On the Continent enthusiasm for anatomised structure in disease waned, and a movement developed towards the study of disordered function which entailed the use of animal experiments. The leading figure in this trend was the French physiologist, Francois Magendie (1783–1855) who had rejected the vitalistic theory out of hand and now began to study experimental medicine. As early as 1816 he published his 'Précis de Physiologie' and in 1821 he was elected to the Academie des Sciences. In 1830 he succeeded Laennec as Professor of Medicine at the Collège de France where he opened a physiological laboratory. By 1822 he had confirmed the observations of Sir Charles Bell (1811) on the sensory and motor roots of the spinal nerves.[7] Pierre Flourens (1794–1867), a contemporary of Magendie, who held a Professorship at the Museum and at the College de France, discovered the function of the semicircular canals, and also the anaesthetic properties of chloroform in the same year as James Young Simpson (1847). The next few years were to see the appearance of an outstanding French physiologist, namely Claude Bernard (1813–1873). He started his career as a playwright, but took up medicine in 1834 and in 1839 worked under Magendie at the Collège de France. In 1855 he succeeded Magendie and in 1865 wrote 'Introduction à l'étude de la médecine expérimentale'. His work embraced a wide range of subjects. By his studies on glycogen and the liver he was able to demonstrate that the body not only broke down but could build up complex chemical substances. He revealed the digestive power of pancreatic juice and also the vasomotor mechanism by which the blood supply to various parts of the body could be regulated. He is probably best remembered for his concept of the regulation of the 'internal environment of the body'. Thus by the latter decades of the century France occupied a prominent place in Physiology. Amongst a number of workers on the central nervous system are included Brown-Séquard (1817–94) (the successor to Claude Bernard), Duchenne de Boulogne (1806–75), Broca (1824–80), Charcot (1825–93), Pierre Marie (1853–1940) and others.[7]

If at the beginning of the 19th century German medicine had fallen behind, it was soon to make up for lost time. With the appearance of Johannes Müller (1801–58) a remarkable phase of progress was initiated. He was not only the greatest German physiologist of his time, but also a great medical naturalist. Having studied medicine, he occupied the Chair of Anatomy and Physiology at Bonn (1830) and subsequently went to Berlin to succeed Rudolphi in 1833. His most important research work was on the mechanism of the special senses. When he published his 'Handbook of Physiology' in 1834–40, 'the results of comparative anatomy, chemistry and physics were for the first time systematically brought to bear on physiological problems'.[8] He did not make any discovery himself but the number of excellent students whom he inspired is extremely impressive. He was a voluminous writer and was a firm believer in Vitalism throughout his life. His pupils included Du Bois Reymond (1816–96), known for his electrophysiological instruments and methods, von Helmholtz, who showed that muscles were the seat of heat production and also discovered the opthalmoscope, and Brücke (1819–1892), who studied optics and acoustics.[7] In 1836 he commenced microscopic examination of tumours and in 1838 published the first part of his work, 'On the Nature and Structural Characteristics of Cancer and of those Morbid Growths which may be confounded with it'. His pupils included Schwann (1810–82) who was soon to propound his cellular theory with Schleiden, Kölliker (1817–1905), Henle (1809–95) and Virchow (1821–1902). With this list of important men it can easily be seen how German medicine obtained its leading role later in the century. Another famous school arose at Leipzig under Karl Ludwig, who founded a Physiological Institute there in 1869. He had previously taught physiology at Zürich (1849) and Vienna (1855). He studied a wide variety of aspects of Physiology including renal permeability, endosmosis, gases during muscular exertion, and capillary blood pressure. He attracted a number of foreign visitors including Pavlov from Russia and Horsley from England, for he was regarded by some as the greatest teacher of Physiology of all time.[7]

During the above period there was no parallel advance in Physiology in Great Britain, and this has been attributed by some to the traditionally conservative nature of the British mind. The clinicians pursued their anatomical approach and their study of gross pathological lesions. This went on throughout the century as can be seen in the reports of the Pathological Society of London which was dominated by physicians and surgeons during its existence from 1846–1907. There was even some resistance to the use of the microscope in pathology, and Hughes Bennett was deploring this attitude in 1845 when he gave a course of lectures on Histology and the use of the microscope.[9] Such physiological research as had been carried out was concentrated on nerve conduction and reflexes. In 1811 Charles Bell had distinguished sensory from motor roots in the spinal nerves, but was reluctant to carry out animal experiments. In 1833 Marshall Hall (1790–1857) established the existence of reflex action. William Stirling (1851–1932), a pupil of Ludwig's, described the summation of electrical stimuli and much later in 1876 Ferrier (1843–1928) discovered the motor areas of the cerebral cortex.

This remarkable delay in the study of physiology and experimental medicine can be traced to another cause. The British have always been closely attached to their domestic animals and were thus unwilling to perform experiments which would cause pain and suffering in a world that was still devoid of anaesthetics. It appears that this feeling existed particularly amongst the upper classes who ironically enough did not seem to recognise similar sufferings inflicted on animals in their blood-sports such as hunting. The early 19th century British physiologists included A. P. Wilson Philip (1770–1847), James Blundell (1790–1878) and Charles Bell.[10] Bell was not altogether certain of the ethical status of animal experiments and this viewpoint contrasted strongly with that of the French school and in particular with Magendie (1783–1855) whose work was essentially experimental. In 1822 the efforts of 'Humanity Dick' Martin (1754–1834) and Lord Erskine (1750–1823) resulted in the passage of Martin's Act which outlawed cruelty to the larger domestic animals such as horses and cattle, though excluding cats and dogs.[11] It should be realised that all this time 'cruelty' included bull-baiting, cock-fighting, blood sports and casual cruelty to beasts of burden as well as experimental procedures referred to as vivisection. The public concern was first aroused when in 1824 Magendie came to London to give a series of lecture demonstrations involving live animals.[12] The resulting outcry must have been considerable for in the same year the Society for Prevention of Cruelty to Animals was founded.[13] When it was known that Magendie intended to return in 1826 for further lecture-demonstrations, Martin made an attack on him in the House of Commons. A second society appeared named the Animals' Friend Society which offered a reward for anyone who would be able to procure a conviction and in 1835 Martin's Act was extended to cover all domestic animals.[13] With this climate of public opinion it can well be understood that doctors were reluctant to take up Physiology and to use the experimental method. Marshall Hall (1790–1857) in 1831 and again in 1847 suggested laying down guidelines for experiments and the formation of a society for physiological research but it came to nothing.[14] By mid-century and soon afterwards the antivivisection movement had gained momentum. In 1847 the Rev. David Davis, a dissenting minister, presented Queen Victoria with a petition drawing her attention to the fact that living animals were being dissected in England.[11] Further afield, in 1861, a delegation from England had an audience with the French Emperor protesting against the live dissection of old horses at the Veterinary Colleges at Alfort, Toulouse and Paris.[15] This protest naturally came from the English gentry whose favourite animal was the horse. The whole subject of vivisection received additional publicity when an international congress on the topic was held at the Crystal Palace in

August 1862. The medical press pointed out that (1) vivisection was only carried out on a small scale compared with the Continent where there were many workers in dozens of such laboratories in Germany, France, Austria, Switzerland, and Italy and (2) that while vivisection was permissible for scientific purposes its use for practising operative dexterity was not acceptable. With the discovery of anaesthesia the number of animal experiments increased. Amongst others a sometime physiologist, Sir Benjamin Ward Richardson (1828–96), maintained that with anaesthesia there could be no pain and therefore no cruelty. Far from reassuring the antivivisectionists it led them to press for the total abolition of all animal experiments.

By 1870 there were signs of development in British physiology. The Royal College of Surgeons had just revised its examinations and were demanding more physiological knowledge.[16] Medical schools had to respond to this and a number of posts in Physiology were created. In 1870 J. S. Burdon Sanderson (1828–1905) was appointed Professor of Practical Physiology and Histology at University College London; in 1871 E. A. Schäfer (1850–1935) became Assistant Professor of Physiology under Burdon Sanderson; in the same year Michael Foster (1836–1907) was made First Praelector of Physiology at Trinity College, Cambridge. Also in 1870 the General Committee of the British Association for the Advancement of Science appointed a ten-man committee of anatomists and physiologists (including Burdon Sanderson and Foster) to lay down guidelines for the performance of physiological experiments. In 1871 they issued a report in which anaesthesia was advocated if possible for all experiments and urged that painful experiments should only be carried out by skilled persons. It would be reasonable to conclude that this action might have reassured the antivivisectionists and possibly also the general public. But between 1870 and 1874 when Physiology was progressing in Cambridge, London and Edinburgh, two events occurred which stirred up the controversy afresh.

(1) the newspaper 'Scotsman' carried an advertisement for dogs and cats to be used in the Edinburgh Physiological Laboratory (1873).

(2) J. Burdon Sanderson published a two-volume handbook for use in the physiological laboratory (1873). The other contributors were Emanuel Klein, histologist and bacteriologist at the Brown Institute, Michael Foster, physiologist at Cambridge, and T. Lauder Brunton, pharmacologist to St. Bartholomew's Hospital. The cause of the trouble that followed was an indiscreet sentence in the book which ran as follows: 'This book is intended for beginners in physiological work'.[18]

As can be imagined the outcry which followed was given full publicity at the Sixth International Congress of Societies for the Prevention of Cruelty to Animals which was held in June 1874. Worse was to follow when the British Medical Association, rather unwisely, arranged for a French experimentalist, Eugene Magnan, to give a demonstration of the production of epilepsy in a dog by the intravenous injection of absinthe at their Annual Meeting in Norwich in August of the same year. Legal proceedings were taken against those arranging this demonstration by the Royal Society for the Prevention of Cruelty to Animals (the RSPCA) but they were unsuccessful.[19] The stage was now set for a confrontation between the antivivisectionists and the protagonists of experimental medicine. The former were supported by John Colam (secretary of the RSPCA from 1861–1905) and the powerful Richard Holt Hutton (1826–97) the editor of 'The Spectator', a member of the Senate of London University and one who later attempted to stop experimentation at the Brown Institute;[20] the supporters of the medical scientists included T. H. Huxley (1825–95) and his assistant Edwin Ray Lankester (1847–1929). Although this matter was becoming one of national concern, the Government was reluctant to act for at the time it was pre-occupied by European events in general and the Bulgarian atrocities in particular.

At last in 1875 the Government was forced to act and appointed a Royal Commission to investigate the matter.[21] It consisted of seven members who met between the 5th July and the 15th December 1875 and issued their report on 8th January 1876. Information was obtained by examining 53 witnesses, receiving some written submissions and asking over 6,000 questions. The enquiry seems to have been carried out admirably, but there is one part of it which merits our special attention, the testimony of Emanuel Klein, Burdon Sanderson's assistant at the Brown Institute. Klein (1844–1925) was an Austrian who had trained in Vienna, had come to London in 1871 on the invitation of Burdon Sanderson, and by 1875 was assistant Professor at the Brown Institute and Lecturer in Histology at St. Bartholomew's Hospital.[22] In his testimony he shocked the Commissioners by saying 'that his whole mind was absorbed in the experiment itself, and that he did not regard the pain inflicted on the animal'. Worse still, it was said that 'his manner of giving utterance to those views was even more cynical than their substance'. When his evidence was sent to him in proof he attempted to alter it but the Commission refused to accept his alterations.[23] Two years later when Burdon Sanderson left the Brown Institute he was succeeded by Prof. W. S. Greenfield, and Emanuel Klein to some people's surprise was passed over. This is perhaps less surprising when it is remembered that R. H. Hutton was a Commissioner and doubtless heard Klein's testimony, and was also a member of the Senate of London University which appointed Sanderson's successor.

If legislation was to follow the report of the Commission both sides were going to have plenty to say. However, for Burdon Sanderson the year 1876 started disastrously, for three weeks after the appearance of the Report he lost his brother, sister-in-law, and two nieces, all killed in the Abbott's Ripton railway disaster.

For the purpose of legislation a Bill had to be drawn up and the Government invited proposals from the Victoria Street Society. This Society had been founded in late 1875 by Frances Power Cobbe, and was officially known as The Society for the Protection of Animals Liable to Vivisection, though it was subsequently always referred to as the Victoria Street Society. At this time it was particularly vocal, and in this it was not alone as by midsummer 1876 ten new societies came into being in various parts of the country. After much discussion and lobbying by pressure groups on each side the Bill was amended and was given Royal Assent on 15th August 1876, thus becoming Act 39 and 40 Victoria. or the Cruelty to Animals Act. In future any individual wishing to perform experiments upon living vertebrate animals must submit an application to the Home Secretary, endorsed by both a President of one of the eleven leading scientific or medical bodies in Britain (such as the Royal Society of London, Royal College of Surgeons of Edinburgh, Royal College of Physicians of Dublin) and a professor of medicine or one of the medical sciences. In addition these experiments could only be performed at a place registered by the Home Secretary and subject to inspection at any time.[24]

When the Bill was passed neither side was really satisfied. The antivivisectionists felt that it had not gone nearly far enough and were disturbed at the inclusion of a clause permitting experiments on live cats and dogs. The medical scientists were shocked at the restrictions which were to be imposed on them.

The activity of the antivivisectionists soon revived, and developed further in the next 20 years. At the time of discussion of the Bill, the House of Commons received 805 petitions supported by 146,889 signatures demanding the total abolition of animal experiments.[25] The movement was a large one, but one in which there was a measure of disunity. After the passage of the Bill most of the societies favoured total abolition and between 1876 and 1884 petitions demanding this had been submitted, but without success. However, throughout this period the RSPCA had behaved with considerable restraint and, guided by Colam, their Secretary, they hoped to gain their ends by moderation and negotiation. Between these two extreme views lay the Victoria Street Society, which soon settled for total abolition, like the rest, and maintained this policy in 1898. The antivivisectionists adopted several methods of attack including examination of research reports in an attempt to detect violations of the Act. They called for a boycott of contributions to any institution which had a vivisector on the staff, and they launched a special campaign against the newly formed British Institute of Preventive Medicine. All these efforts brought little success, chiefly due to consolidation of opinion amongst medical scientists, disunity in their own ranks, and lastly a misjudgement of the reaction of the general public.

The medical scientists had become better organised but they still had not achieved unity. Many were not in favour of any legislation while the remainder felt that by the Act the advance of physiology and experimental medicine in Great Britain would be further hindered. They pursued their policy of avoiding confrontations with the antivivisectionists, and moved towards consolidation of their ranks by the formation of the Physiological Society in March, 1876. However, little was achieved until August 1991, when they fortunately obtained a platform for their views at the International Medical Congress held in London.[26] Experimental Medicine was supported by eminent men such as Rudolph Virchow, Sir John Simon and Thomas R. Fraser (Professor of Materia Medica in Edinburgh, who had had his application for a license refused!). The Congress ended by endorsing the value and necessity for experiments on living animals. At this time the medical scientists had voiced their displeasure at the administration of the Act, including delays and also refusals of applications for licenses from some very reputable workers. Indeed Rutherford, Professor of the Institutes of Medicine in Edinburgh, on being refused transferred his research work to France.[27] In examining the requests for licensure the Home Secretary obviously needed expert advice, and for this he turned to George Busk (1807–86) FRS, FRCS who was a Fellow of both the Linnaean and Zoological Societies. Further support followed the formation of the Association for the Advancement of Medicine by Research in March, 1882. By this time the medical scientists had realised that they needed support from the rest of the profession and also from the general public, which they now attempted to educate. The members of the new Society included some impressive names and was to be under the Chairmanship of the Presidents of the Royal Colleges of Physicians and Surgeons alternately.[28] The Home Secretary looked with increasing favour on this body and in 1885 gave all license applications to the Council of the Society for approval before examining them himself, a procedure which was followed until 1913. When it is noted that in that year the President was a professional physiologist and not a President of a Royal College it can be seen that Physiology had come a long way.[29] Thus by the mid-1890s the antivivisectionists realised the result of the gradual progress of its antagonists. Instead of being opposed by a small group of scientists they now faced a body which had not only a close link with the Government, but possessed also the support of the medical profession as a whole, to say nothing of a considerable portion of the general public. By now, as a result of the discoveries of bacteriology and immunology, the demand for animal experiments had become much greater. In the year 1896 the experiments performed under the Act increased from 4,679 to 7,500.

Thus, after a long struggle Physiology had become recognised as an independent discipline, and the British school was now in a position to make a considerable contribution.

REFERENCES

1   Singer, Charles, 'A History of Biology'. Henry Schuman, New York 1959 (Revised Ed.), p. 280.
2   Ibid pp. 224–5.
3   Ibid pp. 208–12.
4   Sigerist, Henry E., 'The Great Doctors'. Transl. by Eden and Ceder Paul. Doubleday Anchor Books, 1958, pp. 287–291.
5   Garrison, F. H., 'History of Medicine'. W. B. Saunders Company, 4th Ed., 1929, p. 428.
6   Singer, Charles, 'A History of Biology'. Henry Schuman, New York 1950 (Revised Ed.), pp. 218–20.
7   Taton, Rene, 'Science in the 19th Century'. Basic Books, Inc., New York 1961, pp. 410–21.
8   Singer, Charles, 'A History of Biology'. Henry Schuman, New York, 1950 (Revised Ed.), p. 388.
9   Bennett, J. Hughes, 'Lancet'. (1845) *i*, pp. 517–22.
10  French, Richard D., 'Antivivisection and Medical Science in Victorian Society'. Princeton Univ. Press (1975) p. 18.
11  Ibid p. 25
12  Ibid p. 20
13  Ibid pp. 29–30.
14  Ibid p. 21.
15  Ibid p. 32.
16  Cope, Zachary, 'The Royal College of Surgeons of England'. London 1959, p. 143.
17  French, Richard D., 'Antivivisection and Medical Science in Victorian Society'. Princeton Univ. Press 1975, p. 18.
18  Ibid pp. 47–8.
19  Ibid pp. 55–6.
20  'Lancet'. London (1883) *i*, p. 795.
21  French, Richard D., 'Antivivisection and Medical Science in Victorian Society'. Princeton Univ. Press 1975, p. 96.
22  J. Path. Bact (1925) *xxviii*, pp. 684–97 (Obituary notice).
23  French, Richard D., 'Antivivisection and Medical Science in Victorian Society'. Princeton Univ. Press 1975, pp. 103–6.
24  Ibid pp. 143–5.
25  Ibid p. 129.
26  Ibid pp. 199–200.
27  'British Medical Journal'. (1877) *i*, p. 79.
28  French, Richard D., 'Antivivisection and Medical Science in Victorian Society'. Princeton Univ. Press 1975, p. 204.
29  Ibid p. 216.

# THIRTEEN
# John Simon and Public Health 1848–71

A general outline of the early Public Health Reforms between 1830 and 1850 has already been given in chapter 5. These had been chiefly brought about by such persons as the Earl of Shaftesbury, Dr. Neil Arnott, Dr. Southwood Smith and others and had resulted in considerable improvement. But the dominating influence underlying it all belonged to Edwin Chadwick with his enormous energy and unquestionable administrative ability. This phase was now drawing to a close because of the many problems which threatened to engulf the Board of Health and also because of the growing opposition to the ever-unpopular Chadwick. By 1854 he had resigned from the Board and by 1858 he had retired from the public service for good, though he lived on in retirement till 1890. Southwood Smith continued working until his death in 1861. With the abolition of the Board of Health in 1858 health matters were brought under the Privy Council and a new phase began. At this time no one could have foreseen that John Simon would provide new leadership in Preventive Medicine, and would take over where Chadwick had left off. In order to see how this occurred, it will be necessary to study in some detail various aspects of his versatile career and how it stimulated advances in both Medicine and Pathology. This information has been drawn freely from the excellent biography of Simon written some years ago by Royston Lambert.[1]

John Simon was born in 1816 in London and his family lived in the fashionable suburb of Blackheath in that well known architectural gem, 'The Paragon'. He was educated locally, but also spent a year in Germany living in the home of a parson in 1832. On his return in 1833 he decided on a career as a surgeon, and was accordingly apprenticed for 6 years to Mr. J. H. Green, a surgeon at St. Thomas's Hospital who had just been appointed Professor of Surgery at King's College Hospital. Green was a cultured man and an expert lithotomist, and appeared to be on the threshold of a very successful career. He soon commanded the respect of his young pupil, and under his care Simon made a very auspicious start. In 1838 he obtained the Diploma of the Royal College of Surgeons, and in 1844 was made an Honorary Fellow. In 1840 he had been appointed Senior Assistant Surgeon to King's College Hospital and showed some research ability, possibly because of the influence of a colleague, William Bowman, then a physiologist and later to become a famous opthalmogist. In 1844 Simon was elected FRS for his paper on 'The Comparative Anatomy of the Thyroid Gland'. During these years in London he developed a wide variety of interests, made a good many friends, and broadened his outlook by holidays on the Continent where he met a number of eminent scientists. In Heidelberg he met and was probably much influenced by Jacob Henle, the well known anatomist and pathologist. By this time Simon's two great interests were Pathology and Surgery. In 1846 he served on the Council on the newly-formed Pathological Society of London, and by 1853 had published over 20 short papers in the Transactions of the Society.[2] In 1847 he had been appointed Lecturer in Pathology at St. Thomas's Hospital. This post was said to have been the first of its kind in the hospitals of this country,[3] though it should be remembered that Thomas Hodgkin was made Lecturer in Morbid Anatomy and Curator of the Museum at Guy's Hospital in 1825.[4] Simon had also been put in charge of a ward of surgical patients at St. Thomas's, and in 1853 on J. H. Green's retirement he was appointed Surgeon to the hospital.[5] He never missed an opportunity of witnessing a post-mortem examination, and when facing an operation of some difficulty he frequently practised it beforehand on corpses. He was held in great respect by such men as Sir William Fergusson and Sir Richard Owen, and was well known for his skill at lithotomy. In 1851 he performed a remarkable operation for the diversion of urine through the rectum in a case of extroversion of the bladder, and this had been preceded by intense experimental preparation.[6] In addition to these activities he had also gone into private practice. At this stage Simon appeared to be well on the way to a very successful career as an orthodox surgeon and no one could have imagined the change in his future, which had commenced in 1848 with his appointment as Medical Offer of Health to the City of London. This post was initially temporary, and also part-time, thus enabling him to continue his surgical, pathological, and experimental work. In 1850 he published his lectures as 'General Pathology' and in so doing became the first systematic writer on the subject in this country. He must have been well known for it is said that the great Virchow classed him as amongst 'the cleverest of all modern pathologists'.[7] It is of interest that although he gave up private surgical practice in 1855 he maintained his post as Surgeon to St. Thomas's until 1876 and his Lectureship in Pathology until 1870. With his new post the next phase of his career was to unfold. He had developed a sound academic basis in medicine, which decided the methods that he was to adopt in solving his future problems.

His appointment as Medical Officer of Health of the City of London had occasioned some surprise because, although academically he was far superior to his competitors,[8] he had been little involved in public health matters, presumably because of his other numerous activities. Since 1844 he had been a member of the central committee of a pressure group, namely the Health of Towns Association, but had taken no part in the legislative struggles over sanitation in 1847–8. His hospital work had probably given him a good idea of the state of the poor, and when travelling abroad it is known that he had examined the sanitary systems of towns which he had visited.[9]

In 1838 the Poor Law Commissioners had sent Arnott, Kay-Shuttleworth, and Southwood Smith to investigate the state of the

London poor. Their findings, together with Chadwick's report in 1842 on the sanitation of the labouring population, drew attention to the gravity of the situation.[10] By the time that the Commission on Health of Towns had made its report in 1844, improvement in hygiene and sanitation had become recognized as an urgent necessity. Compared with the health of other towns, that of the Metropolis did not seem too bad, though the health administration was chaotic.[11] Chadwick was anxious to remedy this by bringing the whole of it under one central administrative body, but at this stage the City of London, traditionally independent, became the centre of dispute. The population of this 'square mile' was still increasing and though this was nothing like the increase in the rest of the Metropolis it was sufficient to give rise to overcrowding in some areas. The Lord Mayor and City Corporation considered the City as the healthiest town in the world,[12] while the rest of the Metropolis and other English towns considered it one of the worst. Indeed, the Health of Towns Association had referred to it as a 'city of cesspools'.[13] There was something to be said on both sides, for while in many parts of the City the drainage, sanitation and living conditions were fairly good, there were also a few overcrowded areas and it was in these that the drainage and water supply were deficient. At this juncture the City Corporation became apprehensive of Chadwick's centralisation plan, for the last thing that they wanted was to be under his control. Many discussions were held, and as a result the City Sewers Act was passed in 1848, leaving the City independent of the rest of the Metropolis.[14] In 1847 the old Metropolitan Commission had been disbanded, and a new Crown-appointed Commission of 23 members came into existence.[15] As a result, with the passing of the Metropolitan Bill in 1848, Chadwick was able to centralise the sanitary arrangements of the Metropolis, exclusive of the City of London.

Amongst the provisions of the City Act was the appointment of a Medical Officer of Health, the event which was to change Simon's life. It should be realised that when Simon took over this new post in 1848 there was no example for him to follow. Although the Royal Commission of 1834 had recommended the appointment of Medical Officers of Health, nothing had been done, and the only city in the country with such an officer was Liverpool where Dr. W. H. Duncan had only been appointed as recently as 1847.

At this time, about a generation before the discovery of pathogenic bacteria, the prevailing theory of epidemic diseases was that of 'miasmas' or 'vapours' which pervaded the environment. The sanitary reformers believed that the remedy lay in an attack on the environment, rather than a study of the personal health of the individual. They advocated general cleansing of streets, disposal of organic material, and improvement of drainage and water supply. In this respect John Simon's views were remarkably similar to those of Edwin Chadwick. Nevertheless, there were fundamental differences between the two men. Chadwick, with his administrative zeal and ability, favoured centralisation in dealing with problems, while Simon believed in encouraging controls at a local level. Most important of all Chadwick, being non-medical, did not think doctors were very important in solving public health problems, which seemed to him to be more related to sanitary engineering than to medicine. Simon on the other hand, who had been trained as a doctor and therefore understood the basic importance of Pathology, believed that the solution to public health problems lay in a better knowledge of disease and therefore depended on the work of medical men. Lastly, although he was a determined man and on occasion could be very forthright and outspoken, he often displayed a tact and understanding of his fellow men which was simply non-existent in Chadwick. It was therefore likely that Simon would succeed where Chadwick had failed.

The duties of the new Medical Officer of Health included the following:

(1) to inspect and report on the City's sanitary condition in general.

(2) to take cognisance of epidemic diseases and to 'point out' their local causes and the best means of preventing their spread.[16]

He was concerned with the treatment of disease, this being the province of practitioners, Boards of Guardians, Charity hospitals, and Dispensaries. After the passing of the Act the City Corporation, in appointing the new Medical Officer of Health, acted with a haste which was activated by the fear of an epidemic of cholera. Simon had therefore his fair share of problems and the ultimate triumph of his first year of office made it a memorable one. The events were numerous and of some complexity, and are available elsewhere,[17] but their importance is such that brief reference to them must be made.

Simon's original plans were simple and based on common sense, the two key words being 'coordination' and 'subordination'. It was not possible to assess the health of the city, for the only statistics available to him were those of death which could be obtained from the Registrar General. Statistics of sickness were non-existent and to obtain them assistance from such sources as the City workhouses, the prisons, and the Poor Law Medical Officers were necessary, and this meant 'coordination'. Once areas had been identified where sickness was prevalent, sanitary measures would be proposed and then carried out by the staff of the City Commissioners – and this meant 'subordination'. In the early months Simon soon found that the co-operation which he needed in these two fields was not forthcoming, though he made some progress by his powers of persuasion. There were many other difficulties, as for instance the finding of areas where disposal of refuse was deficient and sanitation bad. The problem here was that the traditional 'domestic privacy' of the City dwellers made the inspection of private houses impossible. It was here that the 1848–9 outbreak of cholera proved of value as people came to regard inspectors as friends and not with suspicion as heretofore. Permission for house-to-house inspection had not been easy to obtain and was only given when the Lord Mayor himself fell victim of cholera.[18] As the epidemic grew worse Simon proposed a scheme to provide medical assistance for victims of the disease, although this was outside the jurisdiction of the commissioners. With the larger London hospitals overflowing with cholera cases, he proposed a Marquee Hospital on the site of the old Fleet prison, but to his dismay the plan was rejected. During this year his sanitary inspections had revealed innumerable areas with sanitary deficiencies, the so-called 'nuisances'. With cholera at its height he pleaded, cajoled, and argued with the various City authorities, but with limited success. With matters coming to a head in September when there was an upsurge in the number of cases, 'The Times' surprisingly hastened to Simon's support. This newspaper attacked the City Commissioners as well as several 'anti-sanitary' individuals in the strongest possible language. Henry Lowman Taylor, who had opposed Simon's attack on the disgraceful conditions in the slaughterhouses, was referred to as 'Defender of the Filth'. Between the 9th June and the 17th October 854 persons died in the City. Then, ironically, just as Simon was beginning to get his own way, the epidemic subsided.

Thus ended the first year which, one imagines, Simon could never have forgotten. Frustration and opposition he had received in plenty, but it was mingled with much success. The Committee of Health, originally opposed to him, now began to give him its respect, and the Poor Law Doctors who initially refused to co-operate now eagerly gave him their support. During the year he had issued weekly, monthly, and quarterly reports, and now that the year had ended, he prepared his first Annual Report to present to the Commissioners. This occurred on the 6th November, 1849 and its effect was like that of a bombshell.[19,20] The quality of the report was outstanding, and consisted of 71 pages which gave details of the cholera epidemic as well as a broad survey of the whole public health problem in the City. All the daily newspapers carried the report in full, and the comments of 'The Times' can only be described as rapturous. Indeed John Simon became a national figure overnight. He had not only outlined the existing public health problems, but had included recommendations for their improvement. It was a perfect model of what a Medical Officer of Health's report should be. It is sad to read that the reception of it by the City Commissioners was decidedly cool compared with that given to it by the general public. Two weeks later the Commissioners met to discuss it.[21] While some appreciation was expressed, there was a certain amount of opposition in which, needless to say, the 'Defender of the Filth' played his part. The recommendations submitted were only partly accepted. His appointment was renewed, but a proposal for an increase in salary was rejected. Accordingly Simon continued his struggle and at the end of 1850 produced another outstanding report. Amongst other things he drew attention to the high rate of infant mortality in some parts of the City. The report, like the previous one, was published in the newspapers and 'The Times', in giving a favourable comment, remarked that 'even the city Commissioners were mildly gratified'.[22] But during these two years Simon had learned a great deal and was getting his own way more often, because of a more conciliatory attitude which he had developed towards his employers.

Further progress was made in 1851 as Simon continued to fight for legislative measures to support his proposals. In addition to controls of disgraceful slaughter-house conditions, meat inspection was introduced for the first time. Inspection of the interior of certain housing, especially 'lodging houses', was extended and the urgent necessity of slum clearance began to be recognised. But the really important achievement during the year was in administrative reconstruction. Simon was now able to organise his group of inspectors and other sanitary activity around himself.[23] He arranged for systematic inspection of each area and recorded the findings of his inspectors in a series of weekly reports. All this was to feature in his 3rd Annual Report which he presented in November 1851, and which was received with an enthusiasm similar to that of the previous two years. There remained the problem of the water-supply and the opposition of the private water companies, whose supply was often substandard and who strongly resisted any proposals for improvement.

Simon was to continue to occupy his post as the City Medical Officer of Health until 1855. Each year his Annual Report appeared and was received with the usual acclamation. Although there were no great changes during this period, substantial advances were made on a number of smaller items. He had changed his technique and was showing great ingenuity in turning apparently unrelated events to the advantage of his cause. Simon continued to show the same persistence and perseverance and gave his Commissioners little peace. He was now adopting an essentially practical approach, so different from the unsuccessful theoretical approach of Chadwick. He had now become accepted as a sanitary authority, though the previous publication of his lectures in pathology in the early 1850's was a constant reminder of his eminence as a medical scientist. Relationships between him and the Commissioners had improved greatly and in 1853 even the 'Defender of the Filth' praised him for his work and for his annual reports. In March 1853 his tenure was no longer subject to annual renewal and his salary, initially £500, now became £800 per annum. After the cholera epidemic of 1848–9 interest in health matters seems to have waned in the Metropolis, but not so in the City, as Simon ploughed relentlessly on. When the 1854 epidemic arrived, its effect on the City was very much less and the death rate during the year was only 211 compared with 728 in 1849.

At this time two events occurred which indicated that the influence of

Simon on health matters had spread far beyond the City of London. In February 1853 he was consulted by the Croydon Local Board of Health following an outbreak of typhoid in the town. This was an unfortunate event, for it had followed the installation of a new system of drainage pipes by Chadwick, and consequently did much damage to his reputation.[24] Simon endorsed Chadwick's arterial drainage system, and dismissed the possibility of water propagation in favour of the theory of 'fog of faecal evaporation' from the sewage farms. In January 1854 after some agitation on the part of 'The Times', the government was pressured into appointing a three-man Royal Commission to investigate a severe outbreak of cholera in Newcastle, which had occurred in late 1853. The men chosen for this were J. B. Hume, John Simon, and J. F. Bateman, an engineer.[25] Their report castigated the local authorities for the appalling sanitary conditions of the town and attributed the cause to 'Atmospheric impurity', but blamed unfiltered water from the Tyne as the 'chief vehicle of transmission'. In these two instances we see less reluctance to believe in the water-borne theory, which at the time lacked experimental proof and was not generally accepted till much later. It seems certain that Simon was considering it for he would have known that John Snow had written the following in 1849, some five years before the famous Broad Street pump incident.

> 'There is often a way open for it to extend itself more widely, and that is by the mixture of cholera evacuations with the water used for drinking and culinary purposes, either by permeating the ground and getting into wells, or running along channels and sewers into rivers'.[26]

This had been written in the 'London Medical Gazette', and in the same issue of this journal William Budd had published a similar article saying that cholera spread 'principally in the drinking waters of infected places'.[27]

In retrospect, it is remarkable how long it was before cholera and typhoid were finally accepted as water-borne diseases, and in the meanwhile what a controversial subject it had become. Even when Koch isolated the 'comma bacillus' of cholera in 1883, it was not readily accepted as the cause of the disease. One of Koch's chief opponents was Max von Pettenkofer, who occupied the Chair of Hygiene at Munich. The following incident, which relates to his successor, Rudolf Emmerich, is so surprising that it may be mentioned briefly. In Gelsenkirchen in 1901 there had been a severe outbreak of typhoid which claimed 3,000 victims of whom 8% died. In 1904, a criminal prosecution was taken out against the local waterworks. The prosecution witnesses included Koch and some other experts, while Emmerich appeared for the defence. It is amazing that at that time, more than 50 years after John Snow's work, Emmerich was able to maintain that typhoid was not a water-borne disease, and cited in support the views of his old chief, Pettenkofer, who had committed suicide some three years earlier.[28]

Looking back to the 1850s there were some good pieces of evidence that cholera was water-borne, though lack of knowledge of the nature of the disease prevented its recognition. The experience of cholera outbreaks at the time showed that the peak period was in the summer months when flies were more numerous and decaying excrement at its worst. In 1849, however, following a decline in severity in August a fresh upsurge of cases occurred in September. It would seem that this may have been water-borne possibly aggravated by sanitary measures such as the frantic flushing of sewers into the Thames which provided the water supplies.[29] Clearer evidence was forthcoming in 1854 when the overall severity was less but had a peculiar distribution, being related to the two main sources of water supply. South of the Thames the Southwark Company provided unfiltered water from the river, and in this area the incidence was high; north of the Thames, water came from the New River Company, which now provided filtered water from further up the river at Thames Ditton, and in this area the incidence was much lower, the main mode of transmission being by flies or by contact.[31]

In spite of the lesser overall severity of the 1854 epidemic, Simon's scientific caution prevented him from jumping to the conclusion that the sanitary improvements which he had instituted between 1849 and 1854 were completely responsible. As he said, 'links of cause and effect may, in the particular instance, be beyond our means of demonstration'.[29] But by 1856, aided by the work of Snow and Budd, he was ready to accept that water was at least one method by which cholera was spread.[13]

In the midst of all this concern about cholera in England, there came news of the high mortality from cholera and other fevers in the Crimea, where war had broken out in 1854. So serious was it that the Government appointed and sent out a Sanitary Commission,[32] which included Sir Robert Rawlinson, a well-known sanitary engineer, Dr. Sutherland, and Dr. Gavin, the latter of whom was tragically killed, accidentally shot by his brother.[33] It seems ironical that at a time when the possibility of water-borne cholera had been considered, it seems to have been either overlooked or disbelieved as a method of spread in the Crimea. In fact it appears that everything except water was suspected! However, the sanitary measures instituted by the Commission did much to improve hospital care and its report was to be instrumental in the appointment of a Royal Commission to reorganise the Army Medical Services and to create an Army Medical School (see chapter 14).

By the summer of 1854 the first Board of Health was moribund, and following the resignations of Chadwick, Shaftesbury, and Southwood Smith it was completely reorganised. Sir Benjamin Hall was made President responsible to Parliament for the new Board's activity.[34] During his first year of office he showed remarkable energy and made two basic changes of policy. Firstly he decided to favour the principle of local self-government, so successful in the City under John Simon, rather than that of centralisation, so dear to Chadwick's heart. Secondly, he realised the importance of medical knowledge of disease in the pursuit of Hygiene and Public Health, and in the immediate future sanitary engineering was to give place to medicine. With the current cholera epidemic still uncontrolled, one of Hall's first actions was to appoint twelve doctors as cholera inspectors, and to form a Medical Council to investigate the present outbreak. This consisted of thirteen eminent practitioners or scientists nominated by the Royal Colleges and approved by himself, and included Farr, Owen Brodie, and Simon.[35] Once the epidemic had subsided and the Council had done its job, there was pressure from the Council members, the 'Lancet', the Epidemilogical Society, and the Board's officials for a permanent and prominent representation of medicine in central sanitary administration.[36] That Hall saw the importance of this, and acquiesced, is much to his credit for at that time there were many lay persons who believed that, in health matters, doctors were only needed in times of epidemics. Accordingly he insisted on the appointment of Medical Officers of Health in all the metropolitan districts. More important still, he decided to have a medical Officer on the new Board of Health[37] to advise the Government, and for this responsible post there was no one more suitable than John Simon, whom he had already consulted frequently. Thus Simon resigned from being Medical Officer of Health to the City, a post which he had held from 1848 till 1855. He was succeeded by Dr. Henry Letheby, who had been the City's Gas Analyst since 1848. The City Commissioners can hardly be accused of generosity for they offered him a salary of £400 per annum, £100 less than that originally paid to Simon. It is significant that, before accepting his new appointment to the Board of Health, Simon stipulated certain conditions. He was willing to give up his private practice, but he insisted on retaining his Lectureship in Pathology and his post as Surgeon to St. Thomas's Hospital. He was well aware of the value of his scientific standing, which had stood him in good stead in the recent years and would do so even more in the future.

Thus another phase in Simon's life began in which his influence in medicine became increasingly wider. His success in his previous job had been such that he had set a pattern for any future Medical Officer of Health. The Government had benefitted from his example and their decision for the compulsory appointment of a Medical Officer of Health for every Metropolitan district was a milestone in the history of public health. Many of these Medical Officers proved to be men of high quality and when in 1856 they formed a professional association, they showed their respect for John Simon by electing him to be their first President.

With wider responsibility Simon hoped to design a national policy for Public Health and to obtain the necessary legislation in much the same way as he had done in the city on a smaller scale. One very important step towards the recognition of his subject came when he persuaded St. Thomas's Hospital to appoint a Lecturer in Public Health.[38] This was the first of its kind in this country and, no doubt due to Simon's influence, E. H. Greenhow was elected.

The newly formed Board of Health was to enjoy a precarious existence and to come to an early end. By its terms of appointment it had been made renewable yearly and on one occasion survived by only 101 votes to 95.[39] Thus it was no surprise when the Board was finally disbanded in 1858, and its medical duties and public health functions transferred to the Privy Council. John Simon then became Medical Officer to that body, a post which he held until 1871.

Probably the most fruitful years of John Simon's life were those from 1855 until 1871. He had overcome much opposition in the early years and he had established the central position of the doctor in public health matters. But there was much research to be done, for improvements in health could only follow a better understanding of the prevalent diseases, and it was there that his academic background proved so useful. During these years, as will be seen, an enormous field was covered and it was a pity that circumstances changed in 1871. In that year it was decided to transfer public health matters to the newly-formed Local Government Board, and John Simon as Medical Officer to it was to have new masters again. This had been the recommendation of the Royal Commission of 1869–71 and it seemed that his position would be similar to his previous one with the Privy Council. The first President of the new Board was Mr. James Stansfeld M.P., the first Secretary Mr. Lambert, and the Medical Officer Dr. John Simon. Stansfeld and Lambert, imbued with the traditions of the old Poor Law Office, set out to make the Medical department of the Board subordinate to lay control and John Simon, whose advice had been disregarded, finally resigned the post in dissatisfaction in 1876. Thus, the medical control which Simon had so successfully instituted was at an end, at least for the time being.[40]

When in 1858 health matters had come under the Privy Council, the outlook could not have appeared very rosy, although one great advantage was that the controversial Board of Health was now out of the way. In the past there had been a tendency to load the Privy Council with a number of unrelated responsibilities and this of course did not make for unity. Nevertheless John Simon was to find that, if there was a lack of organisation, there was also a lack of interference. Owing to a shortage of accommodation, he was housed away from the main body of the council, and this made for some degree of independence. Lastly, he found that he was obtaining co-operation from the Lord President and also from the Clerk to the Council. The latter, although occupying a relatively subsidiary position, was very influential and Simon was delighted to hear that his old friend, Arthur Helps, the sanitary writer and reformer, had been appointed to this post in 1860.[41] From that time on, he was encouraged to act independently and to decide the lines along which he wished to develop his department.

As already mentioned Simon now realized that, before the health of the nation could be improved, a great deal more would have to be learned about disease in general and febrile complaints in particular. In tackling this problem, his background of Pathology naturally led him to attempt to unravel the pathogenesis and more widely the natural history of disease. With the existing state of knowledge this was not easy, for the cause of infectious diseases, his primary concern, had not yet been discovered and the prevalent views on their spread were often erroneous. The sanitary viewpoint that cholera was due to an 'atmospheric fog' resulting from decaying excrement and filth was still popular and, as previously emphasized, the concept of water-borne spread was only beginning to be accepted. There was also a lack of knowledge of the distribution of disease for, although the Statistical Society had been founded in 1833, the only available figures were those relating to death, and these had first been issued by the Registrar General in 1839. Research was therefore needed in plenty, though some information came from the newly appointed Medical Officers of Health amongst whom there were some outstanding men, who would naturally follow the example set by John Simon. These included Dr. John Burdon Sanderson, Dr. Odling, Dr. Parry, Dr. Robert Barnes, Dr. John Bristowe, and Dr. Thomas Stevenson.[42,43] When it came to his own research, Simon was severely limited as he had neither medical nor technical staff. The 1858 Act transferring public health matters to the Privy Council had made no provision for staff and stated that temporary assistance for problems as they arose would be the only form of help available, a rule which would certainly prevent any rapid expansion in the staff of the department! But discouraging as it may sound it worked out in the end to Simon's advantage. He was quick to see that he could not easily obtain the full-time services of outstanding men, if only because he could not afford to pay them. To employ them for a specific job on a temporary basis was quite possible, and a man with Simon's scientific reputation was able to command their cooperation and respect. Amongst those who provided him with reports were Dr. E. H. Greenhow, Dr. Burdon Sanderson, Dr. George Buchanan, Dr. Milroy, Dr. Edmund Parkes, Dr. E. C. Seaton, Dr. H. Stevens, Dr. John Bristowe, Dr. Augusus Guy, Dr. Thudicum, Dr. Edward Smith, Mr.Netten Radcliffe, and Dr. Thorne-Thorne.[44]

The research of this period was to prove exceedingly important, for the information which it yielded, when added to the discovery of bacteria, and the significance of wound sepsis did much to produce a rapid flowering of Bacteriology and its recognition as an independent discipline by the end of the century. At this stage it might be wondered how this piecemeal type of research could attain any degree of unity. The personality of John Simon did much to achieve this, but in addition the group of workers which he recruited were all very active in one or more of the following societies, namely the Pathological Society of London (1846), the Epidemiological Society (1850), and the Association of Medical Officers of Health (1856). At the meetings of these bodies there was ample opportunity for these men to discuss their work and their current problems.

The amount of work covered by this group in the succeeding years was very considerable, and a few examples may give some idea of what was achieved. One of the earliest subjects which attracted Simon's attention was vaccination. This is not surprising because at the time it was the only known preventive method against any infectious disease. Furthermore, although it was more than fifty years since Jenner's publication in 1798, vaccination was by no means universally applied, and the technique had not yet become standardised. In 1855 the Epidemiological Society (founded in 1850) had been pressing for the extension and improvement of vaccination, but had encountered some opposition. John Simon made a thorough study of the technique and in 1857 published his 'Papers relating to the History and Practice of Vaccination'. This outstanding document dispelled the opposition and paved the way for the passage of the Vaccination Acts of 1867.[59] But the immediate effect of Simon's activities was that vaccination and the provision of lymph came under the Privy council, and no longer under the Poor Law authorities.

In dealing with the existing deficiencies of vaccination, Simon went for assistance to Dr. Edward C. Seaton (1815–1880), who had been in practice first in Rochester and then in London from 1837 until 1862. Since 1840 he had been greatly interested in public health matters in general but especially in smallpox and vaccination. As a result, when the Vaccination Committee of the Epidemiological Society was formed, he became the first secretary.[45] Together with Simon, whom he had joined in 1858, he established fifteen vaccine-supplying centres to ensure adequate amounts of lymph of good quality. They used these centres for instruction in the technique of vaccination and empowered them to grant Privy Council Certificates of proficiency.[46] Boards of Guardians were forbidden to employ public vaccinators unless they possessed this certificate. These steps amounted to a system of central control, but while it was one thing to lay down regulations, it was quite another matter to see that they were carried out. Some form of inspection was necessary, and by 1861 Seaton, aided by George Buchanan, Henry Stevens, and John Burdon Sanderson, who acted as inspectors, had visited 125 Unions and 687 Vaccination Districts. Instructions for vaccination were made generally available and in 1867 Seaton published a very complete and detailed handbook on the subject.[47] All of this represented considerable progress, but smallpox had by no means disappeared for later in 1871 there was the worst epidemic on record, in which over 23,000 persons lost their lives.[48] The source of such outbreaks had been indicated when Simon found in 1861 that many children were not vaccinated at all and that 56% of all deaths from smallpox were in children under five years of age.[49] In 1876 Seaton succeeded Simon as Medical Officer to the Local Government Board, but by the end of 1879 was forced to retire on account of ill-health. He died in the following year, having devoted much of his life to smallpox and vaccination. As a final note it should be mentioned that it was not until 1867–8 that the University of London agreed that a Vaccination Certificate was essential for anyone entering the medical profession.[47]

Another good example of how these enquiries advanced medicine and pathology relates to diptheria. Until 1855 this disease was relatively unknown in England, but its growing prevalence prompted Simon to set about collecting what was known about the disease at the time. After the 1858–9 epidemic he employed E. H. Greenhow and Burdon Sanderson to visit 70 places in 17 countries to gain information about the disease.[50] Details recorded were the general features of the locality, the duration of the disease, symptamatology, and communicability. At the same time Simon himself made enquiries from practitioners, and with the assistance of J. S. Bristowe wrote some notes on the pathology of the condition. This material together with a special article by William Gull on 'Diptheria in the Metropolis' was published in his second Annual Report. The advantages of this information were limited, especially as the cause of the disease was not yet known, but it was a move in the right direction and provided a basis for further scientific study later.

It seems likely that the direction of Simon's activities was largely determined by the work of Edward Headlam Greenhow (1814–1888). Greenhow came from a Northumberland family whose members had been on the staff of the Newcastle Infirmary for over 100 years. He joined his father in practice in Tynemouth for a period of 18 years (1835–53). As a student in Edinburgh he won a Gold Medal from the Argyle Square School of Medicine for the class of Pathology and the Practice of Medicine.[51] He showed an interest in public health at an early stage and had experience of cholera in the epidemics of 1831 and 1849. It is likely that his sanitary activities during the epidemic of 1853 were responsible for the outbreak in Tynemouth being much less severe than the corresponding one in Newcastle. Whether this work attracted Simon's attention we do not know, but we find that they were friends some time in 1854 and that this friendship developed rapidly over the succeeding years. Between 1854 and 1858 Greenhow made a very extensive statistical study of the causes of death for the years 1848–54 in 105 out of 623 Registration Districts. It covered very many diseases such as smallpox, measles, whooping cough, typhus, etc. in addition to occupational pulmonary hazards and other aspects of industrial medicine.[52] The real importance of all this work was that it showed for the first time the great variation which existed in the death rates of the same disease in different districts. Obviously a number of local enquiries were needed to explain these discrepancies, and this was the line that Simon proposed to follow. Before giving a few examples of these investigations, it will be necessary to give a few more details of Greenhow. Simon had the greatest regard for him, for it will be remembered that he became (on Simon's recommendation) the first Lecturer in Public Health in the country at St. Thomas's Hospital. From 1859–62 he travelled widely in the country making epidemiological studies of such conditions as diptheria, diarrhoea, lung diseases and infant mortality. On coming to London in 1853 he had become physician to the Western Dispensary,[53] and in 1861 his attention turned to Clinical Medicine and Pathology. He became Lecturer in Public Health and Medical Jurisprudence at the Middlesex Hospital, where he was Assistant Physician in 1861, and full Physician in 1870. He was mainly responsible for the foundation of the Clinical Society in 1867 and was President from 1870 until 1880. His interest in Pathology is evidenced by his activity in, and his contributions to, the Pathological Society of London. In particular his papers on the 'Pathology of Pulmonary disease in Operatives' (1864–66) remind us that by his interest in industrial disease he was continuing the pioneer work started by Thackrah (1795–1833) a few years previously.

In his early years at the Privy Council Simon had relied chiefly on Seaton and Greenhow, though he had also received substantial help from Henry Stevens with whom he had been previously associated during the cholera enquiry in the City of London. For his future investigation he was to rely on a group of younger men. Some of these, such as Murchison, Orde, and Whitley were on the staff of large hospitals, whilst others such as Hillier, Conway Evans, Andrew Barclay, Buchanan, Bristowe, and Burdon Sanderson were Medical Officers of Health.

Greenhow had investigated pulmonary disease associated with industry and now several different trades were examined. Edward Smith reported malnutrition in cotton operatives in Lancashire,[54] and also found over-crowding in the tailoring trade with a high incidence of tuberculosis. Bristowe made a study of the health of workers with phosphorus and also the infections liable to occur in the rag trade. Dressmaking trades examined by Orde showed overcrowding similar to that found in the tailoring trade. Whitely surveyed the health of workers in mercury and lead, while Augustus Guy investigated arsenic poisoning in the paper-colouring industry.[55] Other workers for the Privy Council included Henry Julian Hunter (1823–1908) who reported on housing in both towns and rural areas; Thudicum on the nature of meat infestation, and Wagstaffe on the incidence of veneral disease. In addition many local surveys were made by various other Medical Officers of Health.

It has been pointed out that many of Simon's temporary workers were men of high academic standing, and held appointments at the large teaching hospitals. It is interesting to learn how many of these eminent men had a good background in natural history, which gave them a broader outlook on their work. In some cases it proved to be of great value. Sir William Henry Power (1842–1916) after extensive experience in public health, became Medical Officer to the Local Government Board in 1900. For some years prior to 1887, the year in which he had been made Assistant Medical Officer, the East London Water Company found that some of their service pipes were blocked with dead eels, which gave a putrid flavour to the water. The problem facing an enquiry was how the eels got into the system, because there appeared to be no fault in the filtering system. It was then that Power's knowledge of natural history came in useful, for he pointed out that eels were perfectly capable of wandering overland for considerable distances especially when grass was wet with dew in the autumn. Simple preventive measures were taken and no further trouble was experienced.[56]

Simon and his inspectors were men of broad outlook, and as such were concerned with the pathological basis of disease. Some of them including Simon himself had a special early interest in the subject, and among them was Edmund Alexander Parkes (1819–1876), one of the leaders in Hygiene who in his earlier days published a paper on 'Researches in the Pathology and Treatment of Asiatic and Algide cholera' (1847). Greenhow and his study of lung pathology in occupational disease has already been mentioned.[53] Charles Murchison (1830–79) became one of Simon's inspectors in 1861. He had been educated at Edinburgh University, had the outlook of a naturalist, and graduated in 1851 with a thesis entitled 'On the Pathology of Morbid Growths'. After a period abroad he returned to England in 1855 and was appointed Physician to the Westminster General Dispensary. He was also Demonstrator of Anatomy and later Lecturer in Botany at St. Mary's Hospital. It is likely that in this latter post he succeeded Burdon Sanderson, of whom more will be said later. In subsequent years he became Assistant and later Full Physician to the Middlesex Hospital. Although he was primarily a physician he was deeply interested in Pathology and gave several communications to the Pathological Society of London. When in 1877 he gave his inaugural address as President of the Society it was stated that 'it will always be remembered as a terse and methodic exposition of the lines on which pathological research should be pursued'.[57] His interest in public health resulted from the six years that he spent at the London Fever Hospital, and he is probably best remembered for his great work, 'Continued Fevers of Great Britain', which was published in 1862.

John Syer Bristowe (1827–1895) was a brilliant student at St. Thomas's Hospital and was eventually to spend 39 years of his life as a Medical Officer of Health. His interest in Public Health began when as house-surgeon in 1849 and Curator of the Museum and Pathologist in 1850, he came under the influence of John Simon. At that time the post of Museum Curator may have been an interim appointment for those hoping soon to be elected to the hospital staff. Other men, later to be engaged in Public Health and who held such a post, were Conway Evans, who was Curator of the Anatomical Museum and Pathological Registrar at King's College Hospital and J. Netter Radcliffe (1830–1884), who was Curator at Leeds. Such appointments would naturally stimulate an interest in Pathology as they did in the case of Thomas Hodgkin at Guy's in 1825. Bristowe was best known for his skill as a teacher and writer in Clinical Medicine. In addition to becoming a Full Physician at St. Thomas's (1860), he was Lecturer in Medicine (1876), Botany (1859), Materia Medica (1860), General Anatomy and Physiology (1865) and Pathology (1870).[58] He was Medical Officer of Health for Camberwell, and during his lifetime was President of several societies, including the Association of Medical Officers of Health and the Pathological Society of London (1885). His field work on the incidence of 'phossy jaw' in the match-making industry was memorable. In later years his background interest in Pathology may have been responsible for his visits to practically all the major hospitals in the country with the surgeon, Mr. Timothy Holmes. Stimulated by the current interest in wound infection they studied the sanitary circumstances of the hospital and the effect upon infections in surgical and puerperal cases.

The quality of many of the men who assisted Simon in his research has already been stressed. Of these the most outstanding was probably J. (later Sir John) Burdon Sanderson. His versatility would be hard to match and some idea of it is suggested by the fact that his first post, after graduating MD in Edinburgh, was Lecturer in Botany at St. Mary's Hospital, London, and his last one Regius Professor of Medicine at the University of Oxford. When he died his obituary notice and the several tributes from most of the leading medical scientists occupied twelve pages of the 'British Medical Journal'.[60] A natural observer, his original approach was that of a biologist, but early in his medical career he became interested in what is now called Forensic Medicine and Toxicology. This period was followed by one in which he was a physician, and one of the earlier Medical Officers of Health (1860). By 1870 he had turned to basic research and Physiology, and this interest dominated his thoughts until he became Regius Professor of Medicine at Oxford in 1894. Many regard him as a Physiologist at heart, though they point out that he was equally interested in Pathology, and it is significant that when towards the end of his career he was made Regius Professor of Medicine at Oxford, he gave the lectures in Pathology. But at that time the distinction between Experimental Physiology and Pathology was not at all clear, and it was not uncommon for posts in the two subjects to be combined. The early influence which determined his outlook probably came from John Hughes Bennett, a leading enthusiast for Pathology and the use of the microscope, to whom he became attached as a Demonstrator before he graduated MD. Not surprisingly, his thesis was related to a study of the blood for it was about the time when Bennett described leukaemia. He carried out much physiological research during his life, but that related to Pathology was done mostly between 1860 and 1880. As Medical Officer of Health for Paddington he became interested in infective conditions, and with Greenhow surveyed some epidemics of diptheria.[61] This disease had only recently appeared and was therefore of current concern. In 1865 he went to Northern Germany to study epidemics of cerebrospinal meningitis, a disease which was practically unknown in England at the time. This epidemiological study was the first of its kind and Sanderson doubted whether the disease was communicable. Later in the year when working for the Royal Commission on Cattle Plague, he was able to show that this disease could be transmitted by the blood of infected animals. He had shown that the agent did not diffuse through parchment paper, but his colleague Dr. Lionel Beale was unable to find any particles under the microscope. These observations led Sanderson to wonder about the possibility of some infective agents being ultra-microscopic.[62] Some years later Koch was to congratulate him on this piece of work.

About this time the question of communicability of disease was attracting great attention. Villemin, in France, claimed that the tubercle of tuberculosis could be transmitted in rabbits. This was received with frank disbelief by many including the great Virchow, for up to that time tuberculosis was thought to be a disease determined by 'diathesis' and not by an outside agent. In retrospect this is surprising, for there had been hints of its communicability. William Budd, who had some years previously established that typhoid could be water-borne, wrote a remarkable statement about tuberculosis in December 1866, which he gave in a sealed envelope to Dr. G. E. Paget. In October 1867 he gave permission for it to be opened and it was published in the 'Lancet' on the 12th.[63] It revealed Budd's views on tuberculosis and showed that in his thinking he was far ahead of his time. He regarded it as a specific disease, and of a type which could be transmitted because the 'specific morbid matter' is cast off in a liquid form and could therefore spread from one person to another. He indicated the tendency for it to occur in areas where people were crowded, and gave examples of how prevalent and severe tuberculosis could be when first introduced into a population in which the disease had previously been non-existent. David Livingstone, the famous missionary and explorer, had pointed out to him that in the interior of Africa tuberculosis was not seen, but that nearer the coast it was quite common because of contact of the natives with European traders.[64] Although Budd wrote this in 1866, he claimed to have thought of it first in August 1856 when he was convinced that there were many similarities between typhoid and tuberculosis. He seems to have feared that his views would not be readily received (as often happens!), for he emphasised that they were not conceived in a hurry and he added that he had 'considerably exceeded the ten years which the Roman poet prescribed as the time to be given to every composition intended by the writer to endure'.[63] It was therefore essential to repeat Villemin's work, and this was confirmed by an experimental animal study carried out by Simon and Burdon Sanderson.

Simon, as a surgeon, had been much concerned with wound infection, and was one of the few persons at the time in England to be interested in the techniques of Semmelweiss in Vienna to reduce the high mortality from infection in puerperal cases. This matter must have been one of discussion between Simon and Sanderson, for we find the latter embarking on a study of the transmission of pyaemia. On May 7th, 1872 Sanderson gave a paper on this work to the Pathological Society of London.[65] It described the effects of injecting 'pyaemic liquids' from a case of pyaemia into guinea pigs and a dog. The material injected was a purulent liquid from the ankle joint. The results were confusing for it appeared that there were two types of reaction, (1) a rapid one with formation of metastatic abscesses, i.e. pyaemia, and (2) a slower one with nodules resembling miliary tubercles, i.e. tuberculosis. He investigated the presence of bacteria in pyaemic liquids, and found them to be numerous in cases of pyaemia. At this stage Dr. Edward Emanuel Klein had come to England and started collaborating with Sanderson in his experiments which were performed at the recently opened Brown Institution (1871), of which Sanderson was now the director with the title of Professor Superintendent (see chapter 16). As a result of these experiments they concluded that 'pyaemia' and 'tuberculosis' were caused by a poison which was itself a product of inflammation. They tried to define pyaemia and stated that it resembled tuberculosis in its mode of origin, but differed from it in the rapidity of its progress.[65] It is here that we get an insight into the workings of Sanderson's mind. He placed the experimental results before his audience and posed the question, 'Do these experiments concern us as physicians or not?' In the same way that he recognised the necessity of a link between curative and preventive medicine, he also recognised the necessity of a link between work carried out in the laboratory and its practical application. He was also asking his audience whether these experimental animal results would be valid in man. He may well have been disappointed at the negative response which he received.

The subject of septicaemia and pyaemia continued to be discussed, but at this stage Sanderson ceased to pursue this line of research as he had been appointed Professor of Practical Physiology and Histology at University College, London. In many ways this was a pity for he and Klein had already made some important discoveries. They reported that the 'poison' in a pyaemic abscess could be greatly enhanced by injection into a suitable animal, i.e. by animal *passage*.[65] Sanderson had also shown that passage of anthrax through a guinea pig lessened its virulence for the ox.[66] These observations take us to the borders of immunology and it is interesting to speculate what might have been discovered had these lines of research been pursued.

During the succeeding years interest in inflammation was further pursued and the Pathological Society of London attached sufficient importance to the subject to appoint a committee to 'investigate the nature and causes of pyaemia, septicaemia, and purulent infection'. The Report appeared in 1880 and consisted of statistics collected from 1869–78 in the London Hospitals, and included 156 detailed reports of cases, arranged according to their clinical and pathological features. They were compared with diseases produced artificially in animals, and with observations on the blood, urine, and microscopical appearances of organs from typical cases. This report was published in the Transactions of the Pathological Society of London for the year, and summarised in the British Medical Journal.[67] From the findings it did not appear that there had been much clarification in the concepts of pyaemia and septicaemia since the paper given by Sanderson some eight years previously. The bacterial aetiology had still not become accepted. There was the old tendency to blame the environment, for when it was found that the highest incidence of pyaemia occurred during the months of February and March, meteorological data are given in an attempt to provide an explanation. The writers found difficulty in defining septicaemia and pyaemia, but they appeared to accept the experiments of Koch, in which he distinguished 'septic or putrid intoxication' from 'septic or putrid infection'. The former produced by injection of a large amount of putrid fluid caused rapid death in animals without inflammation and was therefore regarded as a chemical poisoning. The blood contained no bacteria and the condition could not be transmitted by injection of blood. In septic infection, which followed the injection of a small amount of putrid fluid, there were signs of inflammation around the injection site, and after a period of about '24 hours immunity', the animal rapidly developed acute blood poisoning. The blood contained many bacteria and became highly infective for other animals. But the writers were unable to explain the circumstances which produced one or other condition, and they found that the two states were by no means always clear cut. The Committee then decided to classify cases of pyaemia into groups according to the presence, association or absence of one or more of the well-known pathological features of the condition, such as visceral abscesses, thrombosis, embolism, etc. The blood was found to have an increased number of white cells, the examination having been done during life. Bacteria of about 6 varieties were found in the blood but it was shown that 'no one form of bacterium is peculiar to any one kind of disease'. Microscopic examination of the tissues showed micrococci in many organs, frequently in the blood vessels, but in some cases this may have been a post-mortem invasion. Thrombi were noted in the lung and there were a few cases with ulcerative endocarditis.

The contribution of Public Health to Medicine and Pathology during the years 1855 to 1871, the active part of Simon's life, was considerable. The difficulties encountered by Simon and Sanderson in their experimental work on basic or general pathology were great as had been seen in the case of pyaemia. A few years were to elapse before Cohnheim's masterly research clarified the process of inflammation,[68] and the studies of Metchnikoff explained the mechanism of phagocytosis.[69] In 1877 Cohnheim was to confirm Villemin's demonstration of the infectivity of the tubercle, by injecting it into the anterior chamber of a rabbit's eye. These great contributions by Cohnheim are all the more remarkable when it is remembered that he died at the early age of 45. But Simon, for all his work in Preventive Medicine, always seems to have been well abreast of new ideas. He was acquainted with the theories of Semmelweiss, and he also followed Pasteur's researches. Later he followed Lister's research on antisepsis and asepsis.

While studies in Sanitary Science had been progressing, there had been many advances in other fields of Medicine. The discovery of anaesthetics in the 1840s gave a new lease of life to Surgery, and of course more operations at this time inevitably meant more cases of wound infection. Pathological histology made enormous strides, thanks to a remarkable sequence of German pathologists, and to further improvements in microscopy. General Medicine had been handicapped by lack of knowledge in Physiology, and the need for experimental research was being realised. Use of animals for this work became widespread; this had existed far into the past, but opposition to it suddenly developed in the 19th century, when some antivivisection societies were founded.[70] Burdon Sanderson's appointment as Professor of Physiology in Oxford was opposed by many, who claimed that he was a vivisectionist. Yet in spite of this progress in Experimental Physiology continued. Then, with all these advances progressing side by side, Bacteriology burst upon the scene and showed that some organisms could be pathogenic to man. For so long, practically no one was able to conceive of a living organism causing disease, even though it was well-known that certain diseases could be transmitted from one person to another. Even when bacteria were discovered the idea of specific bacteria for specific diseases was not appreciated immediately. But once this fact was realised the advance in Bacteriology was phenomenal and most of the organisms pathogenic for man were identified in the 1880–1900 period. The effect on Pathology was dramatic, and for the time being attention was diverted away from Histopathology.

The general effect of this flood of new knowledge was to reinforce the need for more and wider research, and resulted in the development of many experimental laboratories (see chapter 16). The effect on Pathology was a great expansion of the subject leading to its becoming an independent discipline, recognised at last by the Universities.

The appreciation of Sir John Simon at the time is indicated in a book written by an American doctor Joseph Payne and entitled 'A Manual of General Pathology designed as an introduction to the practice of Medicine'. This work the author dedicated to Sir John Simon 'in recognition of the great services, which by his own researches, and by those carried out under his direction, he had rendered to the Science of Pathology.'[71]

REFERENCES

1  Lambert, Royston, 'Sir John Simon 1816–1904'. Macgibbon & Kee, London 1963.
2  Ibid p. 46.
3  Ibid p. 26.
4  Foxon, G. E. H., 'Thomas Hodgkin, a biographical note'. Guy's Hosp. Rep. (1966), p. 244.
5  Lambert, Royston, 'Sir John Simon 1816–1904'. Macgibbon & Kee, London 1963, pp. 17–26
6  'Lancet'. London (1852) ii, pp. 568–70.
7  Lambert, Royston, 'Sir John Simon 1816–1904'. Macgibbon & Kee, London 1963, pp. 17–26.
7  'Lancet'. London (1852) p. 47.
8  Ibid p. 105.
9  Ibid p. 64.
10  MacNalty, Sir Arthur Salusbury, 'The History of State Medicine in England'. The Fitzpatrick Lectures for 1946 & 1947. Royal Institute of Public Health and Hygiene, London 1948, p. 18.
11  Lambert, Royston, 'Sir John Simon, 1816–1904'. Macgibbon & Kee, London 1963, p. 65.
12  Ibid p. 79.
13  Ibid p. 83.
14  Ibid p. 70.
15  Ibid p. 68.
16  Ibid p. 113.
17  Ibid pp. 112–142.
18  Ibid p. 129.
19  Ibid p. 154.
20  'Lancet'. London (1849), ii, p. 511.
21  Lambert, Royston, 'Sir John Simon 1816–1904', Macgibbon & Kee, London 1963, pp. 157–8.
22  Ibid p. 165.
23  Ibid p. 180.
24  Ibid p. 199.
25  Ibid p. 200.
26  Snow, J., 'On the pathology and mode of communication of cholera'. 'Lond. Med. Gazette' (1849) *44*, pp. 730–2.
27  Budd, W., 'Malignant cholera; its mode of propagation, and its prevention'. 'London med. Gazette' (1849) *44*, pp. 724–5. References 26 & 27 quoted by Schönberg, B. S., and Ruth Mann Mayo Clin Proc. (1974) *49*, pp. 680–4.
28  Howard-Jones, N., 'British Medical Journal'. (1973) *i*, pp. 103–5.
29  Lambert, Royston, 'Sir John Simon 1816–1904'. Macgibbon & Kee, London 1963, p. 206.
30  Ibid pp. 206–7; 247.
31  Ibid p. 248.
32  MacNalty, Sir Arthur Salusbury, 'The History of State Medicine in England'. The Fitzpatrick Lectures for 1946 & 1947, The Royal Institute of Public Health and Hygiene, 1948, p. 26.
33  'Builder'. (1855) *xiii*, p. 226. Quoted by Lambert, Royston. p. 107. Ref. 34.

34  Lambert, Royston, 'Sir John Simon 1816–1904'. Macgibbon & Kee, London 1963, p. 223.
35  Ibid p. 227.
36  Ibid p. 228.
37  Ibid p. 208.
38  Ibid p. 261.
39  Ibid p. 278.
40  MacNalty, Sir Arthur Salusbury, 'The History of State Medicine in England'. The Fitzpatrick Lectures for 1946 & 1947, The Royal Institute of Public Health and Hygiene, 1948, pp. 42–3.
41  Lambert, Royston, 'Sir John Simon 1816–1904'. Macgibbon & Kee, London 1963, p. 312.
42  Ibid p. 316.
43  MacNalty, Sir Arthur Salusbury, 'The History of State Medicine in England'. The Fitzpatrick Lectures for 1946 & 1947, The Royal Institute of Public Health and Hygiene, 1948, p. 23.
44  Ibid p. 32.
45  'British Medical Journal'. (1880) i, p. 188.
46  Lambert, Royston, 'Sir John Simon 1816–1904'. Macgibbon & Kee, London 1963, p. 324.
47  Ibid p. 438.
48  Ibid p. 444.
49  Ibid p. 357.
50  Ibid p. 318.
51  Brockington, C. Fraser, 'Public Health in the 19th century'. E. & S. Livingstone Ltd. Edinburgh & London 1965, p. 241.
52  Ibid p. 195.
53  'British Medical Journal'. (1888) ii, pp. 1104–6.
54  Brockington, C. Fraser, 'Public Health in the 19th century'. E. & S. Livingstone Ltd. Edinburgh & London 1965, p. 251.
55  Lambert, Royston, 'Sir John Simon 1816–1904'. Macgibbon & Kee, London 1963, p. 334.
56  'British Medical Journal'. (1916) ii, p. 205.
57  'Lancet'. London (1879) i, pp. 645–6.
58  Brockington, C. Fraser, 'Public Health in the 19th century'. E. & S. Livingston Ltd. Edinburgh & London 1965, pp. 257–9.
59  MacNalty, Sir Arthur Salusbury, 'The History of State Medicine in England'. The Fitzpatrick Lectures for 1946 & 1947, Royal Institute of Public Health and Hygiene, London 1948, p. 32.
60  'British Medical Journal'. (1905) ii, pp. 1481–9.
61  MacNalty, Sir Arthur Salusbury, 'The History of State Medicine in England'. The Fitzpatrick Lectures for 1946 & 1947, Royal Institute of Public Health and Hygiene, London 1948, p. 33.
62  Ibid p. 38.
63  'Lancet'. London (1867), ii, p. 452.
64  Dubos, René & Jean, 'The White Plague'. V. Gollancz Ltd., London 1953, p. 97.
65  'British Medical Journal'. (1872), i, pp. 508–10.
66  MacNalty, Sir Arthur Salusbury, 'The History of State Medicine in England'. The Fitzpatrick Lectures for 1946 & 1947, Royal Institute of

Public Health and Hygiene, London 1948, p. 39.

67 'British Medical Journal'. (1880), i, pp. 134–6.

68 Garrison, Fielding H., 'History of Medicine'. W. B. Saunders Company, Philadelphia and London, 4th Ed. reprinted 1929, p. 573.

69 Ibid p. 584.

70 Goodrich, June E., 'The first 100 years of Antivivisection'. Mayo Clin Proc. (1977) *52*, pp. 257–9.

71 Payne, Joseph F., 'A Manual of General Pathology designed as an introduction to the practice of Medicine'. Lea Brothers & Company, Philadelphia 1888.

# FOURTEEN
# Army Medicine and Pathology 1742–1907

Two pioneers of military medicine came from Scotland. The first was John Pringle (later Sir John) who came to Edinburgh to become a medical student. He was destined to become the pioneer in Military Medicine as distinct from Military Surgery. He completed his education in Leyden and Paris before returning to Edinburgh where in 1734 he became Professor of Moral Philosophy. In spite of this appointment he continued to practise as a physician. Recommended in 1742 to be a physician to the Earl of Starr who was commanding the British forces in Flanders in the War of the Austrian Succession, he was present at the battle of Dettingen. It was due to his initiative that the French general agreed not to attack buildings occupied by casualties. He became Physician-general to the Duke of Cumberland and went with him in his campaign against Prince Charles Edward. He kept special records of sickness amongst soldiers during their long march from Perth to Edinburgh. He realised the importance of hygiene, both personal and in hospital, and the dangers of the spread of illness due to overcrowding. In 1752 he wrote a medical classic, 'Observations on the Diseases of the Army', and is always regarded as 'The Father of Military Medicine'.

The other Scottish pioneer was an 18th century graduate of Marischal College, Aberdeen, namely James McGrigor, (later Sir James). He is chiefly remembered for his contributions to Military Medicine generally. In most references to Military Medicine he is overshadowed by his predecessor, Sir John Pringle, but if Pringle is justly described as the 'Father of Military Medicine', then McGrigor deserves to be remembered as the 'Father of the Army Medical Corps'.

Born in the Highlands, he was brought up in Aberdeen where he graduated BA and then MA from Marischal College. He thought of becoming a surgeon, and in the absence of a Medical Faculty in Aberdeen he studied for a year at the University of Edinburgh. Returning to Aberdeen he and eleven friends founded the Medicochirurgical Society, which played an important role in stimulating medical education in the city.[1] McGrigor became apprenticed to a physician at the County Infirmary, but in 1793 went to London where he was apprenticed to a surgeon in Islington. In the same year his army career started when he obtained a commission in the Connaught Rangers.

In 1794 McGrigor's regiment joined the Flanders campaign in the War of the First Coalition, which proved disastrous, and the regiment had to be withdrawn. The experience, though short, was sufficient to show the young doctor that casualties from disease were about ten times as great as those resulting from battle wounds. In 1795–6 McGrigor participated

227

in the West Indies campaign, and soon realised the additional hazards in hot climates where a number of 'new fevers' were encountered. His tropical experience concluded with a period in India and Egypt, from which he returned in 1803. With this experience he had improved his medical services by better organisation of supplies, more attention to hygiene in hospital, and accurate records. In 1805 he wrote a thesis on 'Regimental Hospitals' for which Marischal College awarded him an MD degree. His ability was now generally realised and during the next four years he became Inspector of Hospitals.

His greatest period came when he was ordered to join the Duke of Wellington's Army and put in charge of the Medical Department for the Peninsular war where the casualties were very heavy. The Duke soon came to admire the organising power of McGrigor, though it took him somewhat longer to agree to his hospital policy. It is likely that McGrigor was somewhat frustrated by not being allowed to organise rapid evacuation of casualties as advocated by Napoleon's surgeon, Larrey. With the war won, McGrigor returned to London and enrolled for courses in Chemistry and Anatomy at the Windmill Street Academy. By now he had been made Director General of the Medical Board, and he held this authority until he retired in 1851. This appointment had taken place only five days before the battle of Waterloo. It appears that the casualties were very heavy and that the medical services left something to be desired. McGrigor came over to Waterloo and visited the greatly overcrowded hospitals in Brussels. Civilian surgeons offered their help, including Charles Bell, George James Guthrie, and John Thomson. Immediately after the war McGrigor visited the army hospitals in the south of France and subsequently in Paris. In the latter he met Napoleon's surgeon, Baron Larrey, who was captured by the Prussians at Waterloo and only narrowly escaped being shot.[2]

It has been said that McGrigor was not a major innovator for his ideas had been pre-dated by Sir John Pringle. McGrigor held high office during an unusual period of peace, and there was really no occasion when organisation of a wartime army was necessary. But he made many improvements, as for example the strict screening of candidates for the Army Medical Service. He encouraged the training of officers which was carried out at Fort Pitt Military Hospital, Chatham. He established a Science library there which by 1850 had collected 67,000 books, and he also started a museum of Pathology and Natural History. He helped to found Chairs of Military Surgery at Edinburgh and Dublin. One thing that is surprising is the fact that McGrigor never seems to have supported the suggestion made by army surgeons of the 1790's for a State College of Naval and Military Medicine. Such a step did not occur until after the Crimean War and ten years after McGrigor retired. The difficulties of the time should not be overlooked for the medical officer of the day had a very much lower status than his army counterpart and this was not to be rectified until many years later. McGrigor could look back on a very successful army career extending over 58 years and he received many honours. Aberdeen still reveres him and he is commemorated by a granite obelisk in Duthie Park. His later years must have been saddened when he heard the severe criticisms which were levelled at the army medical services in the Crimean War.

The hundred years between the battle of Waterloo in 1815 and the outbreak of World War I in 1914 has often been spoken of as an era of peace. The Congress of Vienna in 1814 which followed the conclusion of the Napoleonic wars, like some other post-war conferences, aimed at devising treaties which would preserve peace. In attempting this it faced two problems, namely what to do with France, and how to sort out the turmoil in other European countries caused by the conquests of Napoleon. To some extent it succeeded in that no major European war occurred for a century, but there were a number of minor wars and in some of these Britain was directly involved. The importance of sickness and outbreaks of infectious disease must have been well-known at the beginning of the 19th century, for there are figures for the Peninsular War which indicate that the average monthly sick rate between 1811 and 1813 was approximately 25 per cent.[3] However, some of the minor wars fought in tropical countries were to yield figures for sickness and death amongst soldiers which were literally startling. In the first Burma war in 1824 the campaign was conducted in the monsoon season and there were extensive outbreaks of cholera and malaria in addition to many cases of scurvy. Among the British troops numbering 2,716 there were 1311 deaths, 1215 of which were due to disease.[4] In the Ashanti war in Africa malaria, cholera, dysentery, and yellow fever took their toll. Over an 18 month period in 1825–26 out of 108 healthy young soldiers 48 died, 21 were invalided and only 10 remained fit for duty.[5] Similar figures are available for the Sikh wars, the Afghan wars, and for various other campaigns in India. The danger of epidemics was also realized in civilian life for cholera had appeared in England in 1831 and was to return several times as a reminder, especially in 1853. During these years, thanks to the activities of Edwin Chadwick and Southwood Smith, the public became more hygiene- and sanitation-minded and came to realize how epidemic disease could be limited, even though the discovery of bacteria and the concept of infection were to be delayed for another generation. The importance of hygiene and proper sanitation was realised by the Army and their benefits were well-illustrated by an example from the China Wars. The first of these was fought in 1839–42 under appallingly bad hygienic conditions. Fever (probably typhoid), dysentery, cholera, and malaria were the main causes and among 2,500 personnel there were 3,239 hospital admissions within 6 months.[6] By contrast, in the light of this experience the planning of the medical services in the second China War in 1857 and 1860 was carefully considered. As a result the medical services were more than adequate and the sickness rate was only 3–5 per cent.[7] But it was the Crimean War of 1854–1856 with all its disasters which aroused public opinion to the pressing need for improved medical services.

Apart from military disasters, there were serious shortcomings in the medical services. The causes of the latter are many and complex but a short summary may be of interest. Although France and England declared war on Russia on the 28th of March 1854 the actual invasion of the Crimea and the battles which followed did not commence until September.[8] But in the general state of tension which preceded the declaration of war the British Government decided to send an Army of Observation to Malta. Its departure on the 28th of February had something of the air of a weekend outing. Some soldiers took their wives while many officers took not only their wives but even their mothers.[19] Many of these women were to go as far as Bulgaria where they saw some of the horrors of the war. One officer's wife, Mrs. Duberly, an excellent horsewoman, went all the way to Balaclava, and was virtually an eyewitness of the whole campaign.[10] In 1855 she published her 'Journal during the Russian war'.

The Army of Observation which left on the 28th of February for Malta proceeded to Gallipoli which was reached early in April.[11] This army consisted of 10,000 men and it was only 18 days before they sailed that the Director General of the Army Medical Department had been asked to make arrangements for medical officers, medicines, and equipment to be provided.[12] This would have been difficult under ideal conditions of provision, but England had not been at war for 40 years and in some instances the mechanism for obtaining materials was not in existence. Drugs would normally be obtained through an apothecary, but this appointment in the Army had been discontinued as an economy measure. Thus the Army sailed with virtually no medical provisions. After the declaration of war the army proceeded on its way and was augmented until a force of 25,000 had reached the Black Sea and landed at Scutari and Varna. Medical supplies followed but they were always deficient. In the summer months and before the fighting had started a severe outbreak of cholera occurred amongst the troops in Bulgaria. Almost 1,000 cases were admitted to hospital with a mortality of 64 per cent.[13] Medical supplies ran out for no one had foreseen this disaster. When the time came for invasion of the Crimea the regimental hospitals had to be cleared and the sick transported to the base hospitals at Varna and Scutari. Transport which had always been a problem for the medical services was now totally inadequate. An additional disaster for this army related to the transport of cavalry horses. Horses travel badly by sea and with shortage of shipping they were crammed into the holds of sailing ships and endured tortures during rough seas. One ship which carried 100 horses lost 75 of them *en voyage*.[14] Equipment was also affected and in some cases had to be left behind for lack of transport space. The army which now prepared for battle had thus suffered grievous losses before the war had begun. The biggest irony relates to the cholera disaster. The medical staff, overwhelmed by the suddenness of the outbreak, attributed it to climate, unripe fruit, and unwholesome wine, in fact to everything except the water. Yet while the epidemic was at its height, unknown to them, John Snow in London had shown that the disease was water-borne in his famous investigation of the Broad Street pump.[15]

When the war proper started in September 1854 conditions grew worse. There was the same shortage of supplies accentuated by the failure to distribute them where they were most needed. Even when realized, this was not easy to rectify because of shortage of transport. With no hospital beds attached to the regiments, transport of wounded from the field and to the base hospitals became a major problem. In the absence of ambulance wagons the wounded were often left on the field to die or were transported to base in springless country carts, travelling in which was hazardous because of the state of the roads. Evacuation to the base hospital by ship was disastrous. The ships were poorly equipped for the purpose and grossly overloaded. The resulting mortality en route was thus very considerable. To all of this can be added the gruesome fact that cholera was still there together with many cases of dysentery and other fevers.[9]

At home Miss Florence Nightingale had heard of the terrible sufferings of soldiers at the battle of the Alma in September 1854. The medical supplies were totally inadequate, the surgeons were too few, and there were neither medical orderlies nor nurses. Accordingly, with permission from the Secretary for War, Mr. Sidney Herbert, she mobilized a small group of 38 nurses and sailed to the Crimea on the 21st of October. They arrived at Scutari on the 4th of November to witness the dreadful conditions at the hospitals there.[10]

The war dragged on for more than a year but by the close of 1855 the end was in sight and in March of 1856 the peace treaty was signed in Paris. By this time, the general public was fully aware of the deficiencies of the Army Medical Services and the reason is not far to seek. There were the eye-witness accounts of Miss Nightingale and her nurses, to say nothing of Mrs. Duberly's journal.[16] Moreover the Crimean war was the first one in which there were war correspondents of the press, and photographic records into the bargain.[17]

In the public outcry which followed, the influence of Florence Nightingale and of Sidney Herbert, the Secretary of War, was predominant.[18] As a result the government appointed a series of Royal Commissions to improve sanitation in the Army and to re-organize the medical services. One of the recommendations of the Sanitary Commission was the formation of an Army Medical School at Fort Pitt, Chatham. It is significant that in addition to professors of Surgery, Military Medicine and Pathology there was also a Professor of Hygiene. The areas of investigation of the Royal Commission were wide and are very fully dealt with in Cantlie's History of the Army Medical Department.[19] The conditions in the Chief Army Hospital at Fort Pitt were found to be appalling and considerably inferior to those at the corresponding naval hospital at Hasler. Approval was given in 1856 to build a new hospital at Netley near Southampton to replace the old one at Fort Pitt though it was not opened by Queen Victoria until 1863. But in addition to poor accommodation the Army suffered from the poor quality of its medical personnel. The terms of employment and the financial remuneration were not such as would attract high quality, if they attracted any at all. The fact that they were not given authority equal to combatant officers led to difficulties, for the latter made the decisions about medical problems on which they had neither knowledge nor interest. The Commission made recommendations to rectify these anomalies, and their implementation, though not welcomed at the time, greatly improved the quality of the medical services. In addition, another great advance was the setting up of a branch of medical statistics and there were plans for an improved nomenclature of diseases to replace Cullen's nosology of 1780 which was still in use.

In the new Army School, hygiene emerged for the first time as an independent subject, and soon this department won an international reputation, thanks to the activities of the new professor, E. F. Parkes. Parkes had been superintendent of the Renkioi Civil Hospital in the Crimea and became Professor of Clinical Medicine at University College. Unfortunately, his career was cut short in 1876 when he died of pulmonary tuberculosis, but the basic work had by then been completed.

The first Professor of Pathology was a civilian doctor called William Aitken who like the other professors was given a life-appointment. He retired in 1892 and died later in the same year. He was probably chosen because he had acted as assistant during the Crimean War to another civilian doctor, namely R. D. Lyons of the Catholic University in Dublin. Lyons was a pathologist who was employed by the Army to investigate the causes of disease in the Crimea and his chief task was to perform post-mortem examinations in which Aitken assisted him. In 1856 Lyons and Aitken published a Blue Book of 120 pages 'On the pathology of the diseases of the Army in the East'.

When the School opened in 1860 it was planned to run a four month course for 42 officers. The first group, selected by examination, consisted of 29 officers from the British and 14 from the Indian Army. In 1863 the School moved from Fort Pitt to Netley. Aitken must have been fully occupied with his training courses for although he published a few papers during his earlier days he published little after his appointment as professor. However, his work entitled 'Science and Practice of Medicine', which reached seven editions and was very popular amongst students, must have taken up much of his time.[20] He is chiefly remembered for his excellent post-mortem demonstrations and for his ability at clinicopathological correlation. Prior to his death he was writing a descriptive catalogue of the specimens in the Pathological Museum of the Army Medical Department at Netley which was published soon after his death. He died respected by all as a man of fine character who had received many honours including the FRS in 1873 and a knighthood in 1887.

The army professors, apart from the unfortunate Parkes who died in 1876, held their positions for a long time. Appointed in 1860, Maclean (Miliary Medicine) retired in 1885, Longmore (Surgery) in 1891, and Aitken (Pathology) in 1892. It was decided that their successors should be appointed for seven years only, but this was renewable. It should be mentioned that during their tenure the original professors had felt the need of assistants and so Assistant Professors were appointed, the tenure being for five years, and to some of these we shall return later.

At the time of Aitken's retirement, his assistant was David Bruce and he was a candidate for the Chair. In this he was unsuccessful for Almroth Wright, strongly supported by German Sims Woodhead (see chapters 6, & 16 part 2), received the appointment. Wright seems to have thought highly of Bruce for he asked that he might be able to stay as his assistant. But Bruce's term of office as assistant had expired, and the Secretary did not agree. As a result the new assistant was Surgeon Captain Semple.

The choice of Wright was not surprising for he had already shown signs of amazing versatility. He had graduated with 1st Class Honours in modern languages and literature at Trinity College Dublin, and in medicine a year or so later. Deciding to devote himself to research in physiology and pathology he visited several continental laboratories before changing his mind and becoming a law student at the Middle Temple. But this latter intention he did not pursue and we next hear of him working at the Admiralty for two years in the Higher Civil Service. But once more he changed his mind and reverted to medical research, working in Cambridge on diabetes before becoming a demonstrator in physiology at the University of Sydney, Australia. Two years later he was back in London, working on diabetes and blood coagulation at the Laboratories of the combined Royal Colleges on the Embankment where his chief was German Sims Woodhead. In his new post Wright lectured on a variety of subjects and carried out research on diabetes, blood coagulation, hemophilia and acidosis. His interests at this stage underwent a sudden change after the visit to Netley in 1893 of the Russian bacteriologist, Haffkine, who had recently made a vaccine against cholera. The typhoid bacillus had been identified by Eberth in 1880 and cultured by Gaffky in 1884, and Wright now determined to see if a vaccine could be made against it.[21] Wright made the vaccine and was well pleased with the results of his preliminary trials, so much so that he wanted to make its administration compulsory for soldiers. To this the War Office was reluctant to agree but Wright continued to offer his vaccine on a voluntary basis. Statistics became available at the time of the South African War and a Medical Advisory Board was appointed to assess them. The Chairman of the Board was Lieutenant Colonel David

Bruce, the assistant professor who had been passed over for the professorship of the Army Medical College in favour of Wright. When Bruce's committee gave an unfavourable report, Wright was furious and considered that Bruce was biased against him. This is unlikely but after all the controversy which followed and which involved civilian doctors, Wright resigned his professorship and subsequently became Director of the Institute of Pathology at St. Mary's Hospital, Paddington. While at Netley, Wright had worked with great energy, had produced diptheria antitoxin for both the Army and the Navy, and worked on a vaccine for Malta fever, a disease which he contracted during his work. In his new post he was to pursue his work on vaccines and to be particularly interested in opsonins.

But Netley's days as a centre of Army education were numbered, for it was felt that such a centre should be in London. Thus it came about that in 1902 classes in Hygiene, Pathology, and Hospital Administration were given in the Examination Hall of the English Conjoint Board on the Victoria Embankment. Further classes were transferred from Netley which was finally closed in 1905. In 1907 the Royal Army Medical College was opened on its present site in Millbank.

Almroth Wright was succeeded by Major W. B. Leishman (1865–1926) who has been described as one of the greatest Army Medical Officers. He joined the Army at the age of 21 and was Professor of Pathology from 1900 till 1918 when he became Expert in Tropical Diseases to the Army Medical Advisory Board at the War Office. He was at that time one of the original members of the Medical Research Council. In 1918 he became Army Director of Pathology and in 1923 Director-General of the Army Medical Service. He was extremely talented and quite exceptional in being a first-class teacher, research worker and administrator. He owed a good deal to Wright during his earlier years and he is best known for his work in developing Leishman's stain for blood parasites, for his quantitative study on phagocytosis and for his observations on Leishman-Donovan bodies.[22,23]

Since that time there have been other distinguished pathologists holding the Army Chair, including J. S. K. Boyd who made valuable contributions in the field of dysentery and did much to ensure the high standard of pathological services in World War II.

Mention must be made of a few other Army Pathologists who made significant contributions. With the posting of army pathologists to various parts of the Empire it is not surprising that many of the advances made were in tropical pathology.

David Bruce (1855–1931), who has been already mentioned, was a logical thinker and research worker, and was greatly aided by his wife who had much technical ability. In 1886, when serving in Egypt and Malta, he identified the Micrococcus melitensis as the cause of Malta fever. In Africa he showed that the tsetse fly, Glossina morsitans, was responsible for transmitting trypanosomes to man. He also found an animal reservoir for the disease called 'Nagana' in Zululand, and the causative organism was named Trypanosoma brucei. Both he and his devoted wife died during the same week in 1931.[24]

Timothy Lewis (1841–1886) first worked as a dispenser before graduating in Medicine at Aberdeen University. He was one of the top students of the Army Medical School which he entered in the following year (1868). In 1883 he became Assistant Professor of Pathology to William Aitken at Netley. In his early days he studied on the continent and published some papers on cholera, the cause of which was in doubt. He is best known for making the first description of a trypanosome in the blood of a mammal, namely a rat. The organism was named Trypanosoma lewisi.[25] He later described chylemia in filariasis and eventually discovered the organism in the lymphatics. However it had been described the year before by Bancroft and was therefore named Filaria bancrofti.[26]

Ronald Ross (1857–1932) was born in India a few days before the outbreak of the Indian Mutiny. Soon after qualifying in Medicine he joined the Madras Medical Service and almost his whole military life was spent as a regimental medical officer. In his early days he displayed some literary talent and wrote several novels and plays. In 1892 he became interested in malaria and the probability of transmission by mosquitoes was suggested to him by Dr. (later Sir Patrick) Manson. In 1897–98 he succeeded in showing this to be true.[27] In 1902 he resigned from the service and became Professor of Tropical Disease at the Liverpool School of Tropical Medicine (see chapter 10). He was rewarded with a knighthood for his work and subsequently directed many expeditions attempting to eradicate malaria.

There were other distinguished Army pathologists, but the above examples will suffice. The Army Medical College, started in 1860, had made tremendous advances during its first 40 years and had laid sound foundations for its future. First of all it had established Hygiene as an independent subject and now the same had been done for Pathology. Yet in civilian life recognition of Pathology was delayed, for even at St. Bartholomew's Hospital which had the first full-time Chair in Pathology in London it was only established 52 years after the one at the Army College. But it would be wrong to assume that because there were no Chairs there was no pathology. Indeed many men not described as pathologists had been carrying out research in the subject as described in chapter 4.

REFERENCES

1  Hist. Scot. Med. Vol. II, pp. 545–6.
2  Dible, J. H., 'Napoleon's Surgeon'. William Heineman Medical Books, 1970, pp. 239–40.

3  Cantlie, Lieut. General Sir Neil, 'A history of the Army Medical Department'. Churchill, Livingstone, Edinburgh and London 1974, Vol 2, p. 373.
4  Ibid Vol 1, p. 459.
5  Ibid Vol 1, p. 462.
6  Ibid Vol 1, p. 78.
7  Ibid Vol 2, pp. 251–3.
8  Ibid Vol 2, p. 9.
9  Ibid Vol 2, pp. 46–86.
10  Ibid Vol 2, p. 91.
11  Ibid Vol 2, p. 15.
12  Ibid Vol 2, pp. 9–20.
13  Ibid Vol 2, p. 28.
14  Woodham-Smith, Cecil, 'The reason why'. McGraw-Hill Book Company, New York 2nd ed. 1971, p. 165.
15  Cantlie, Lieut. General Sir Neil, 'A History of the Army Medical Department'. Churchill, Livingstone, Edinburgh and London 1974, Vol 2, p. 30.
16  Woodham-Smith, Cecil, 'The reason why'. McGraw-Hill Book Company, New York 2nd ed. 1971, p. 138.
17  Barker, A. J., 'The war against Russia'. Holt, Rinehart, and Winston, New York 1970, p. 32.
18  Cantlie, Lieut. General Sir Neil, 'A history of the Army Medical Department'. Churchill, Livingstone Edinburgh and London 1974, Vol 2, p. 196.
19  Ibid Vol 2, pp. 196–237.
20  'British Medical Journal'. (1892) ii, p. 54.
21  Cantlie, Lieut. General Sir Neil, 'A history of the Army Medical Department'. Churchill, Livingstone, Edinburgh and London 1974, Vol. 2, pp. 229–230.
22  J. Path. Bact. (1926) 29, p. 515.
23  'British Medical Journal'. (1926) i, p. 1013.
24  Ibid (1931) ii, pp. 1067–9.
25  Singer, C. and Underwood, E. A., 'A short history of Medicine', Clarendon Press, Oxford 1962, p. 481.
26  Ibid p. 492.
27  'British Medical Journal'. (1932) ii, p. 609.

# FIFTEEN
# Growth of Physiology in France, Germany and Britain 1813–78

The birth of Physiology has been described in Chapter 12. Here further details are given of developments in the principal countries involved.

## French Physiology

When the Revolution was over, three new Schools of Health at Paris, Montpelier, and Strasbourg were approved and the first-named opened in 1795.[1] They were received with enthusiasm for they provided medical education for able students lacking the necessary finance. Without such assistance men such as Bichat, Laennec, and Claude Bernard would have been lost to Medicine.

The founder of what might be called 'the new physiology' was François Magendie (1783–1855). Born in Bordeaux, his early education was neglected for his mother had died when he was aged nine and his father, a surgeon, seems to have been largely occupied in activities of Revolutionary Committees. When he did start his education, his progress was rapid and at the age of sixteen he became apprenticed in Paris to the surgeon, Alexis Boyer. His work at this stage consisted in making anatomical dissections. He became a medical student in 1803 and in 1807 was appointed an assistant in anatomy at the Ecole de Medicine. There he gave courses in Anatomy and Physiology, and finally obtained his medical degree in 1808. In the next year he reported the results of his first experimental work. It related to the toxic effects of vegetable material containing strychnine and this was followed by the discovery with Pelletier of emetine, the active principle of ipecachuana. This work might well qualify him to be the pioneer of experimental Pharmacology. Although not regarded as a genius, he made a surprising number of worthy observations over the succeeding years. He was a firm believer in the experimental method supported by accurate observations and in 1813 decided to devote his life to a study of experimental physiology. He gave private courses which included experiments based on vivisection. They soon proved so successful that he published a two-volume work, 'Précis elementaire de physiologie', in 1816–1817. It was a new type of text-book of Physiology, designed to show how vital phenomena could be investigated by the experimental method. By 1821 he was becoming well known and was elected to both the Academie des Sciences and the Academie Royale de Médicine. In the same year he founded the 'Journal de Physiologie', the first periodical consisting exclusively of physiological matters.

Probably his most important discovery was in 1822, when he confirmed and extended Bell's work on the spinal nerves and showed that the anterior nerves controlled movement and the posterior nerves, sensation, the so-called Bell-Magendie law. In 1823 he described the production of decerebrate rigidity by experimental methods. In the following year he visited England at the invitation of William Hyde Wollaston (1766–1828) and gave a number of public demonstrations on living dogs of section of the cranial nerves. It will be recalled that they provoked an outburst on the part of the anti-vivisectionists (see chapter 12). Over the years he had not abandoned Clinical Medicine and in 1831 had succeeded Recamier in the Chair of Medicine at the Collège de France. In this capacity he gave his famous lectures on the physical phenomena of life in which he aimed at a physical explanation of vital phenomena and the building up of Clinical Medicine on a basis of pathological physiology. It should be added that at this period he described the production of anaphylaxis by injections of egg-white.[2]

Magendie's contributions to Physiology had been considerable but most of all he had encouraged a young assistant, Claude Bernard (1813–1878), who will be seen to have been one of the greatest physiologists of all time.

One cannot fail to notice the amount of research at this time which was directed at the nervous system. We have seen it in the case of Magendie, and there are two others who should be mentioned. Julien Jean Cesar Legallois (1770–1814), who took part in the Revolution, was one of the first experimental physiologists and the first to localise the respiratory centre (1812). Further work by Marie Jean Pierre Flourens (1794–1867) resulted in its more precise location and he named it the 'noeud vital' – the vital node (1824). Flourens was Professor of Comparative Anatomy at the University of Paris and one of the greatest physiologists before Claude Bernard. He investigated the effects of removal of the cerebrum and cerebellum in a wide variety of animals. He described cerebellar ataxia and the function of the semicircular canals in the maintenance of equilibrium. Garrison[3] succinctly summarises Flouren's work in the following way:

'He had thus distinguished three centres in the nervous system:

(1) the cerebral hemispheres received and controlled sensation.
(2) the cerebellum coordinated bodily movements.
(3) the medulla was the vital point of existence itself.

The greatest moment in the history of French physiology occurred when in 1841 Magendie offered the post of assistant in his laboratory to Claude Bernard. Born near Villefranche, the latter was apprenticed to an apothecary in Lyons but he soon moved to Paris where he hoped to pursue a literary career. But he could not find a publisher for his five-act tragedy and was persuaded to study Medicine. We next hear of him holding the post of House Surgeon to the Paris Hospitals. Whilst in

Magendie's laboratory, he received encouragement from a physician, Alexis Rayer, and he obtained his Doctorate of Medicine in 1843. He continued to work with Magendie and took charge of the laboratory in later years.[4]

Although it was some time before he definitely decided on a career of Experimental Physiology, his outstanding ability soon became recognised. In 1854 he was appointed Professor of General Physiology in the Faculty of Sciences and on the death of Magendie in 1855 succeeded him as Professor of Experimental Medicine at the Collège de France. Finally, in 1868 he followed Flourens as Professor of General Physiology at the Museum of Natural History and succeeded him also at the Académie Francaise.[5] He benefitted much from his training under Magendie from whom he learned the value of experiments and accurate observations. It is tempting to suggest that his work on curare as a muscle poison stemmed from his master's earlier work on strychnine. Magendie was a pure experimentalist but Bernard was a genius who went farther and wider. He made an observation, proposed a theory, and carried out a carefully designed experiment to test its validity. His contributions to Physiology involved whole fields of the subject, and the applications of his results to disease made him a pioneer of Experimental Medicine. Written near the end of his life, his 'Introduction to the study of Experimental Medicine' became a classic.

When Bernard commenced his research there was a belief in France that plants alone could build up complex chemical compounds and that animals could only break them down. Anxious to find out what happened to food materials after digestion, he started with carbohydrates and demonstrated that glycogen could be either built up or broken down in the liver, and in some other tissues as well. At the same time, this surprising discovery also dispelled the idea that the sole function of the liver was to produce bile. He next turned his attention to the pancreatic enzymes and showed the great part that they played in intestinal digestion. Prior to this it had been believed that all digestion took place in the stomach. The third great advance concerned the demonstration of vasoconstrictor and vasodilator nerves and opened up the whole field of vasomotor physiology. It remains to mention a concept always associated with the name of Claude Bernard. One refers to the 'milieu interieur' or internal environment for the proper regulation of the parts of the body in relation to one another, and depending on the constancy of the composition of the blood and lymph, which bathe all the cells of the body.

There are two final physiologists to whom brief reference must be made even though they lie outside the period at present under consideration. The first of these is Charles Edouard Brown-Sequard (1817–1894). Born in Mauritius and therefore a British citizen, he was of Franco-American parentage. When he finally succeeded Claude Bernard as Professor of Experimental Medicine at the College de France in 1878, he became a French citizen. As a young man he, like Bernard, favoured a literary career and had some initial success. But he decided to study medicine and obtained his MD degree in 1846 in Paris. His thesis was entitled 'Researches and Experiments on the Physiology of the spinal cord'. He pursued this line and in 1849 described the syndrome for which he is best remembered, and one which follows experimental hemisection of the spinal cord. In 1852 he demonstrated the presence of vasoconstrictor nerves, and in 1856 that removal of the adrenals in animals always proved fatal.

Brown-Sequard was a restless and impulsive character and the story of his travels backwards and forwards between France, the United States, and England is one of bewildering complexity.[6] In these countries he held academic appointments and gave many courses in Physiology and Pathology. But like the French physiologists of earlier years, he retained a lifelong interest in the nervous system. Thus between 1860 and 1863 we find him practising as a Physician at the newly-formed National Hospital for paralysed and epileptics at Queen Square, London. In his later years, when appointed to the Collège de France in 1878, he divided his time between Paris and Nice. But the greatest surprise that he ever created was on the 1st of June, 1889. He had previously been showing unmistakable signs of advancing age but on this day he addressed the Societe de Biologie looking twenty years younger. He claimed to have 'rejuvenated' himself by subcutaneous injections of a liquid obtained from the testicles of freshly-killed guinea-pigs and dogs.[7]

Lastly, we turn to Paul Bert (1833–1884), the favourite pupil of Claude Bernard, and one who succeeded him as Permanent President of the Society of Biology. It says much for his quality that he obtained this appointment in the face of competition from scientists such as Brown-Sequard. Bert's education had been very diverse. He commenced with Engineering, changed to Law at his father's request (1853–1857), and finally decided on Medicine. Stimulated by the Parisian Comparative Anatomist Gratiolet,[8] he had graduated MD in 1863 with a thesis on grafting of animal tissues. From 1866–67 he was Professor of Zoology at Bordeaux and became Professor of Physiology from 1872–1885. But during this last period he had become involved in politics, being particularly interested in educational problems in the Colonies. As a result of this, he was sent out in 1886 to be Resident General in French Indochina. Here he survived only six months and died from dysentery in Hanoi.[9]

But in his relatively short lifetime he had carried out a remarkable amount of scientific work. He performed grafting experiments and attempted transfusion. His real interest lay in the physiology of respiration and in 1874 he published a large book 'Leçons sur la Physiologie comparée de la Respiration'. This was followed in 1878 by his 'Pression barométrique', his most famous work. In it he described his investigations on blood gases, the toxic effects of oxygen at high pressures, and caisson disease, the pathogenesis of which he discovered.[10] Interested always in education, he played a prominent part in the foundation of the universities of Lille and Lyons, at a time when Strasbourg had been lost to the Germans.

## German Physiology

The 18th century had seen advances in Physics which had indicated the nature of heat, and in Chemistry the discovery of the elementary gases had paved the way for an understanding of respiration. The phlogiston theory had been disproved but the belief in 'vitalism' still prevailed. The ensuing century revealed many applications of Electricity and Organic Chemistry to physiological problems, and the need for experimental work became realised. In the space of five years, four men were born who in this field would make a substantial contribution. They were Carl Friedrich Wilhelm Ludwig (1816–1895), Emil Du Bois Reymond (1818–1896), Ernst Wilhelm von Brücke (1819–1892), and Hermann Ludwig Ferdinand von Helmholtz (1821–1894).

Carl Ludwig graduated at the University of Marburg in 1839 and became Professor of Comparative Anatomy in 1846. In 1849 he moved to Zürich and in 1855 to the Josephinum in Vienna, in both places he was Professor of Anatomy and Physiology. The year 1865 was the culmination of his distinguished career when he accepted an invitation to the new Chair of Physiology at Leipzig. There, he established his famous Physiological Institute of which he was Director for the remaining 30 years of his life. He was a magnificent teacher with an extensive knowledge of his subject, comparable with that of the great Johannes Müller. As such, he attracted an enormous number of pupils to his Institute.

As early as 1842, interested in physiochemical processes probably as a result of contact with R. W. Bunsen (1811–1899), the Professor of Chemistry and Physics, he proposed a physical theory to explain renal secretion. In 1847, on a visit to Berlin, he met by chance three young pupils of Johannes Müller, with whom he established lifelong friendship. They were Brücke, Du Bois Reymond, and Helmholtz, and though all four pursued divergent paths they all had one common aim, namely to interpret vital processes in terms of physics and chemistry. Their future work was to contribute to the downfall of 'vitalism'. Ludwig's most important contribution was the introduction of self-recording instruments into physiology. It should be remembered that in the experimental investigation of the problems of physiology he was badly handicapped. At the time, there were no laboratories, no instruments for experiments, and no mechanical experts to advise a young experimentalist. Knowledge of Physiology was essential but a much more important quality was ingenuity and this was possessed by Ludwig. For his early

241

work, he designed two pieces of apparatus which became of paramount importance. His kymograph was used by him for recording blood pressure; the stromuhr or mercurial blood pump was used for the estimation of blood gases. He covered a large field of research in his long life, and is always depicted as a generous man who published little independently, because he readily combined his work with the names of his many pupils. He wrote one book, a 'Text Book of Physiology' the first volume being published in 1852 and the second in 1856. Characteristically he dedicated it to his three great friends.[11]

Du Bois Reymond carried out his medical studies in Berlin and graduated in 1843. His early interest in Anatomy was fostered when he was Instructor in the subject at the Berlin Academy of Art. This changed with an invitation from Johannes Müller to lecture in Physiology in 1854 at a time when his interest in it was stimulated by his friendship with Ludwig, Brücke and Helmholtz. In 1855 he became Associate Professor and in 1858, when Müller's Chair became divided, he was appointed Professor of Physiology. He held this post for nearly 40 years and during this time attracted a number of excellent pupils. In 1877 he opened his Institute of Physiology which was said to be the best-equipped of its kind in the world.[12] He is always remembered as the founder of modern electrophysiology. This interest in electricity appears to have originated at the time of his graduation when Müller suggested that he write a paper on 'electric fishes'. This he did and throughout his lifetime maintained an interest in the nature and origin of the shock given by these fishes.[13] Most of his studies were performed with muscle-nerve preparations, and he showed that a nervous impulse was always accompanied by a change of electrical state and that chemical changes accompany contraction of muscle.[14] Although he lacked the ingenuity of Ludwig, he developed many useful aids for electrophysiology such as the mercury switch.

Brücke graduated MD in Berlin in 1842 and became Professor of Physiology at Königsberg in 1848. In the following year he became Professor in Vienna where he spent the rest of his scientific life. During his career he was greatly respected as a teacher and became regarded as one of the most versatile of physiologists. In 1847 he carried out a number of researches related to ophthalmology and this led to the publication of a book, 'Anatomical description of the human eye'. For many years it was the standard work for oculists. He also studied the physiology of digestion, and described the 'Peyer's glands' as the site of development of the lymphocytes. In 1867–8 he changed his research interest to the field of general nerve and muscle physiology, thus following the pathway of his friend, Du Bois Reymond. He resigned his Chair in Vienna in 1890 after a period of just over 40 years.[15]

Of this impressive group of Müller's pupils, Helmholtz was by far the most outstanding. Justice to his achievements cannot be done in this brief outline. He showed an early interest in Physics, but became a medical student in Berlin because as such he was able to obtain financial support. With Schönlein and Müller as his teachers, he graduated MD in 1842. His mind was still on physics for in 1845 with J. R. Mayer (1814–1878), he formulated the law of Conservation of Energy.[16] In 1848 he was appointed Associate Professor of Physiology at Königsberg. Here he measured the velocity of a nerve impulse, worked on physiological optics and acoustics, and in 1851 invented the opthalmo-scope. Of his many contributions to medicine, this was the greatest. By now he was regarded as the most brilliant young scientist in Germany and in 1855 became Professor of Anatomy and Physiology at the University of Bonn. But his stay there was not happy and in 1858 he moved to Heidelberg where he was provided with a new Physiological Institute. It was here that he spent his most productive years. Finally he returned to his first love and became Professor of Physics in 1871 at Berlin. He said that he had changed to Physics because Physiology had become too complex.[17]

The value of specialised institutes such as those of Müller and Ludwig in developing competent research workers has already been seen. At about the same time a similar institute came into being and proved to be the foundation stone of Chemistry in Germany. Born in Darmstadt, the young Justus von Liebig (1803–1873) had shown an interest in Chemistry and had been apprenticed to an apothecary for about a year. In 1820 he went to study at the University of Bonn with the chemist Kästner, accompanied him when he went to Erlanger, and obtained his Doctor of Philosophy degree in 1822. There being no practical instruction at either of these universities, he decided to go to Paris and fortunately obtained a study grant for two years from the Grand Duke Louis I of Hesse. There he attended lectures by Gay Lussac, Thenard, and Dulong, and carried out some research of his own on the fulminate compounds. It appears that this interest originated some years previously when he had observed an itinerant trader making the explosive silver fulminate. In 1823 he reported his work at the Académie des Sciences and greatly impressed the well-known explorer and scientist Alexander von Humboldt, who arranged for him to become an assistant to Gay Lussac, who was Professor at the Sorbonne. Here he learned the techniques of chemical analysis and the meticulous methods of his master which later proved to be so important in his career. Humboldt, impressed with Liebig's progress, now persuaded the Grand Duke of Hesse to establish a Chair of Chemistry in Giessen in 1824 and Liebig was appointed. From the outset he organised a school of training in the methods of basic chemistry and by 1827 had already attracted twenty students.[18] The laboratory at Giessen was almost the first to provide practical instruction though there had been similar teaching laboratories in Edinburgh in 1807 and in Glasgow in 1819. During the years 1824 till 1839, Liebig concentrated on pure chemistry and he and his pupils carried out a large amount of experimental work. One of his students had become well known, namely August Wilhelm von Hofmann (1818–1892). Born in Giessen, he had become Liebig's assistant before going to Bonn for a short period. In 1845 there had been founded in London a College of Chemistry and the Prince Consort, ever interested in scientific progress, invited Hofmann to take charge of it. This he accepted and stayed for 18 years during which time he did much for English chemistry, and returned to be Professor of Chemistry at Berlin in 1863.[19] There he was instrumental in stimulating the German dyestuffs industry.

In the meanwhile, Liebig had changed his research to applied Chemistry. He was now well known in Europe and had been invited to the Chair at Heidelberg. This he refused but in 1852 went to Munich where he spent the rest of his life. His new line of research commenced in 1846 and involved methods which he had invented for analysing plant and animal tissues. It consisted of a study of Organic Chemistry which could be said to have started in Giessen. The chemistry of living organisms and their products quickly led to the recognition of proteins and carbohydrates and the new subject of Biochemistry. Liebig soon perceived a kind of chemical life cycle. Plants absorbed certain salts from the soil which then passed into the animal which fed on the plants. He realised that these salts might be essential for life, and they were found in large amounts in Chile. They were nitrates formed from desiccated droppings from sea-birds and Liebig's suggestion led to their being used as artificial fertilisers.[20] He investigated some substances produced in animal metabolism such as urea and uric acid. He could not be called a 'Vitalist' for although he believed in vital processes he was sure that they could be explained on either a chemical or physical basis. Like many investigators with positive views he ran into some controversy, as in the case of fermentation, which he thought was a general chemical process. Pasteur by contrast believed that there was a specific ferment which controlled each type of fermentation.

He published several books and papers but for present purposes one on the application of his subject is particularly relevant. It is entitled, 'On the mutual relations existing between Physiology and Pathology, Chemistry, and Physics and the methods of research pursued in these sciences'.[21] Amongst his many eminent pupils the following three should be mentioned: Max Pettenkofer (1818–1901), Felix Hoppe Seyler (1825–95), who had been Virchow's assistant, and Ludwig Thudichum (1829–1901).

In 1842, Liebig had published his book on the chemistry of metabolism and had introduced the term 'stoffwechsel' or metabolism. In 1852 there were two main events. Friedrich Heinrich Bidder (1810–1894), a pupil of Johannes Müller and Carl Schmidt (1822–1894), who was a chemist trained by Liebig, published a brilliant work giving the idea of a balance sheet of metabolism.[22] Both these men occupied Chairs at the University of Dorpat. The other event in 1852 was that Liebig moved to Munich; two years later Pettenkofer had been promoted to ordinary Professor of Medical Chemistry and Theodor Ludwig Wilhelm Bischoff was appointed to the Chair of Anatomy and Physiology. In this period of activity Carl von Voit (1831–1908) returned to complete his medical studies after a period of absence at the University of Würzburg. At this time he studied chemistry under Liebig and Pettenkofer. A new Institute of Physiological Research was opened with Emil Harless (1820–1862) as Director. He died prematurely and von Voit, who was an assistant to Bischoff at the time, was appointed Professor of Physiology and Director of the Institute. He held this post for the next 44 years and it has been said that all modern research on metabolism stems directly from Voit.[23]

Some idea may now have been gained of the diverse origins which had led to the growth of Physiology. By 1860 the German schools had become predominant, and they maintained this position for at least the remainder of the century.

## British Physiology

There had been greater advances in German than in French physiology. The main difference between the two lay in the fact that in France there was no great university growth and no schools turning out several well-trained workers. A similar state of affairs existed in Great Britain where there were few physiologists. The earliest of these, like the Continental workers, seem to have been attracted by the nervous system. In 1811 Charles Bell (1774–1842) distinguished sensory from motor nerve roots and in 1833 Marshall Hall (1790–1857) established the existence of reflex action. But the most outstanding of all was John Hughes Bennett (1812–1875). A student of Edinburgh University, he had graduated MD in 1837 and had presented a thesis on 'Inaugural Dissertation on the Physiology and Pathology of the Brain; being an attempt to ascertain what portions of that organ are more immediately connected with motion, sensation, and intelligence'.[24] After graduating he spent two years visiting medical centres in the principal Continental cities. In Paris he studied clinical instruction in the hospitals and while there wrote a number of articles on central nervous system topics, which still claimed his attention. Amongst other subjects, he became very attracted by the use of the microscope (see chapter 5) and on his return to Edinburgh in 1841 he gave a course on the use of this instrument. He emphasised that diseased tissues should be studied by it, and this was probably the first attempt in this country to give practical instruction in Physiology and Pathology. In 1842 he was an unsuccessful applicant for the Chair of Pathology in Edinburgh when Henderson was appointed. But at this time his horizon was a wide one. He was Physician to the Royal Dispensary as well as Pathologist to the Royal Infirmary where he made a museum of Morbid Anatomy. With his background of Physiology and his current experience of Clinical

Medicine and Pathology, he was the ideal candidate for the Chair of the Institutes which became vacant in 1848. In his new post his teaching courses were brilliantly successful and he was almost certainly responsible for directing John Burdon Sanderson to an outstanding career in Physiology, Pathology, and Medicine. These practical courses which he gave were a far cry from the theoretical dissertations given by the earlier holders of the Chair of the Institutes.

If the North could claim Hughes Bennett as their champion of microscopy, it was not long before one would be also possessed by the South. Lionel Smith Beale (1828–1906), the son of a doctor, graduated in Medicine in London in 1851. He was destined to spend the whole of his life in this city. His interest in microscopy was stimulated when he was a student by John Quekett, the leading microscopist of the day. It led to his setting up a private laboratory in 1852 for original research, and he also used it for giving courses to students in Normal and Morbid Histology, and also in Physiological Chemistry. His success was rapid for when aged 25 he was appointed Professor of Physiology, a post which he held until 1869, when he was elected to the Chair of Pathological Anatomy, and Physician to King's College Hospital.[25] He carried out much microscopical research, published many papers, and also two books. These latter were completed in his younger days and were entitled 'How to work with the Microscope' and 'The Microscope in Medicine'. He appears to have had few close friends and he got involved in controversy on more than one occasion. The most famous was with T. H. Huxley when Beale stated his belief that a vital force was necessary for life. He made no great discovery and was nothing like as inspiring a teacher as was Hughes Bennett. It may be for these reasons that he has often been underrated. But there is no doubt that he made a significant contribution to Physiology, Pathology, and Pathological Chemistry. He greatly improved the quality of tissue preparation including especially vital staining which had just been introduced.[26]

One other worker of this period deserves mention, namely Henry Bence Jones (1814–1873), who commands our attention because of his interests in Chemistry. Graduating BA at Cambridge in 1836, he proceeded to St. George's Hospital, London where in 1844 he passed his examination for graduation in Medicine. In 1841 he had attended a course in Chemistry given by Baron Liebig in his laboratory at Giessen.[27] His advance was rapid for in 1845 he was appointed Physician to St. George's Hospital; in 1846 he became a Fellow of the Royal Society and in 1849 obtained his MD degree. It is not surprising that the first paper which he published was on 'Cystine calculus'. He studied urinary contents and wrote articles on 'Animal Chemistry', 'Animal Electricity', and 'Pathology' for which he advocated the use of the microscope. His name is preserved by its attachment to a urinary protein found in cases of myelomatosis. The story of this discovery is of some interest.[28] It concerns a 45 year old man who consulted his doctor because of what we now realise was a pathological rib fracture. He was referred to a consultant physician, William Macintyre, who tested the urine and found a substance which although like albumen, displayed some unusual features. Specimens of it were sent to Bence Jones, who was described as 'an able pathologist'. He was at the time 31 years of age and a physician on the staff of St. George's Hospital. At this stage bone disease was not suspected (1845) and was only established just over a year later at post-mortem examination. It is strange to read that this was carried out by John Dalrymple (1803–1852), a well-known ophthalmic surgeon on the staff of Moorfields Hospital, who became famous for a beautiful atlas on the 'Pathology of the Eye'. He was interested in general pathology, had given several papers on this subject to the Medicochirurgical Society, and of course examined the bony lesions of this case under the microscope. He published his findings in 1846. In the meanwhile, Bence Jones had confirmed Macintyre's urinary findings, regarded the substance as an oxide of albumen, and reported the case as one of 'mollities ossium'.[29] It has at times been contended that Macintyre should have been given credit for the discovery, and not Bence Jones. This may be so, but it should be remembered that Bence Jones carried out a very extensive study of the protein and certainly did not wish to deprive Macintyre of any credit, for in reporting the case he said, 'a peculiar state of urine was discovered through the carefulness of Dr. Macintyre'.[30] It was only in the next century that this interesting condition came to be understood.

Such was the limited progress made in Physiology in England in the early years of the century. Workers on the Continent realised the value of experiments carried out in the living animal in advancing Physiology and England lagged behind because of the general opposition to the method. The public demonstrations given in England on live animals in 1825 aroused a violent anti-vivisection movement in a general populace already appalled by the 'body-snatching' of the time (see chapter 12). It was to be many years before this could be overcome. Thus in England at the middle of the 19th century there were no pure physiologists and in many medical schools teaching of the subject was deputed to a junior member of the clinical staff. The one exception was at the recently founded University of London (or University College as it was later called) and Physiology was kept alive in those dark days by the efforts of one man, William Sharpey (1802–1880). In 1836 a new Chair of General (or physiological) Anatomy and Physiology had been founded and Sharpey was its first occupant. At the time he was an extramural lecturer in Edinburgh where he was also engaged in anatomical and microscopical research. He was destined to hold the London University post for 38 years by which time his two outstanding pupils, Michael Foster (1836–1907) and John Burdon Sanderson (1828–1905), were ready to continue his good work.

William Sharpey's appointment to London University occasioned some surprise for he was not well-known in London and had carried out little research work apart from a description of ciliary action. In Anatomy he had been well-trained by Barclay as a student, but appeared to have had little experience in Physiology. Graduating from Edinburgh University at the age of 21, he spent a few years on the Continent working with some outstanding men, including Dupuytren in Paris, and Rudolphi and Kölliker in Berlin. Rudolphi was an inspiring teacher who had produced a large work on Helminthology (1808–19).[31] Under him Sharpey spent nine months dissecting in his department. Kölliker, commencing as a physiologist, had become the leading histologist of his day. Sharpey's extensive travel accounts for the wide knowledge for which he became famous. His broad experience of Anatomy explains why, when appointed to London University, he gave the first complete course on Physiology and minute Anatomy. At this time he gave up investigative work and concentrated on administration and teaching. He soon became well known and influential, holding such offices as membership of the Council of the Royal Society, the General Medical Council, and the Senate of the University of London. He was thus well-placed to watch and to guide the growth and development of his subject. He proved to be a magnificent teacher who maintained a close relationship with his students whose names he knew because of a remarkable memory. Although limited in experimental experience, he had an excellent knowledge of the problems of Physiology. Because of this, he was able to guide his students in research, but it must be admitted that a few more years had to elapse before adequate laboratory accommodation became available for practical work. The years 1869–1882 were to witness some very important developments. In 1869 Sharpey persuaded his favourite pupil, Michael Foster, to give up general practice in Huntingdon and become Professor of Practical Physiology at the University. His stay was short, for in 1870, he became the first Praelector in Physiology at Trinity College, Cambridge. But before he left he had greatly developed the practical aspects of his subject. In 1874, with his health failing, Sharpey resigned and was succeeded by his other favourite pupil, John Burdon Sanderson. He stayed in London till 1882 when he was appointed Waynflete Professor of Physiology at Oxford. As indicated elsewhere (see chapter 8), two of Sharpey's best students were to direct the future development of Physiology in the two older English Universities.

In the meanwhile there were other developments such as the appointment of a Royal Commission on Vivisection. In spite of advancing years, Sharpey still had sufficient energy to watch and to influence the deliberations of this body which issued its recommendations in 1876 (see chapter 12). The findings were encouraging up to a point, but Foster realised that there was still much to be done. The small group of Physiologists needed the sympathy of the general public and the support of the rest of the medical profession. But first of all, they must achieve unity amongst themselves. The first step was taken in 1876 when, largely due to Foster, it was decided to found the Physiological Society at a meeting held in Burdon Sanderson's house. This was followed on the 26th May by an Inaugural Meeting in the Criterion Restaurant, London when 22 members and 14 guests attended.[32] It might be mentioned that one of the founder Members was George Henry Lewes, the author and journalist well-known for his association with the novelist Mary Ann Evans (George Eliot). Although he did not study Medicine, he always showed great interest in Physiology. After his death in 1878, George Eliot founded the George Henry Lewes Scholarship at Cambridge, the first holder being Charles S. Roy, who in 1883 became the first Professor of Pathology in the University of Cambridge.

The new society flourished. When founded, there was a limit of forty members, which was increased to fifty in 1878 and abolished in 1884. A number of Pathologists became members and it is interesting to find that Dr. C. S. Roy demonstrated on one occasion a microtome for cutting frozen sections, and on another two cardiographs recording the motions of the mammalian heart chambers.[33] There was still one more thing lacking, namely a journal in the English language entirely devoted to Physiology. Once more Foster came to the rescue. As a result the Journal of Physiology appeared in 1878, the initial expenses having been met by a rich man who was a close friend of Foster's. His name was A. G. Dew-Smith and he was an original member of the Physiological Society. The story of the Journal is a complex one which has been well recorded in Sir Edward Sharpey-Schafer's 'History of the Physiological Society during its first fifty years'. Suffice it to say that the journal was ultimately acquired by the Society, but not until 1926.

By the end of the century the leeway in British Physiology had been made up. It was a remarkable achievement brought about by a relatively small number of outstanding men. The new century now commenced with such famous names behind it as Bayliss, Gaskell, Gotch, Horsley, Langley, Sherrington, and Starling.

REFERENCES

1 Booth, C. C., 'British Medical Journal'. (1979) i, p. 1471.
2 Dict. Scient. Biog. (1974) Vol ix, pp. 6–11.
3 Garrison, 'History of Neurology'. Revised by McHenry, L. C. Chartes, C. Thomas, Springfield, Illinois 1967, p. 193.
4 'Lancet'. (1878) i, pp. 256–7.
5 Foster, M., 'Claude Bernard', 'British Medical Journal'. (1878) ii, pp. 519–21.
6 Dict. Scient. Biography (1970) Vol. II, pp. 524–5.
7 Robinson, V., 'Pathfinders in Medicine'. Medical Life Press, New York 1929, pp. 585–6.
8 Bull. Hosp. Med. (1944) Supp. 3. pp. 16–31.
9 Ibid Supp. 31. pp. 16–31.

10 Castiglioni, A., 'A History of Medicine'. Translator Krumbhaar E.B. Alfred A. Knopf, 2nd. Ed. 1947, pp. 794–5.
11 Dict. Scient. Biog. (1973) Vol viii, pp. 540–1.
12 Garrison, 'History of Neurology'. Revised by McHenry, L. C. Chartes, C. Thomas, Springfield, Illinois 1967, pp. 534–5.
13 Dict. Scient. Biog. (1971) Vol. iv, pp. 200–205.
14 Surges, C., 'History of Biology'. Henry Schuman, New York Revised Ed. 1959, p. 411.
15 Dict. Scient. Biog. (1970) Vol II, pp. 530–2.
16 Singer, C., 'History of Biology'. Henry Schuman, New York Revised Ed. 1950, p. 396.
17 Dict. Scient. Biog. (1972) Vol vi, pp. 241–3.
18 Idem (1973) Vol viii, p. 330.
19 Partington, J. R., 'A short History of Chemistry'. MacMillan & Co., London 2nd Ed. 1948, p. 250.
20 Crowther, J. G., 'A short History of Science'. Methuan Educational Ltd., London 1969, pp. 139–40.
21 'Lancet'. (1846) ii, pp. 549–52.
22 Castiglioni, A., 'A History of Medicine'. Translator Krumbhaar, E. B. Alfred A. Kopf. 2nd Ed. 1947, p. 788.
23 Singer,C. & Underwood, E. A., 'A short History of Medicine 1962'. Clarendon Press, Oxford pp. 581–3.
24 'British Medical Journal'. (1875) ii, pp. 473–6.
25 Idem (1906) i, p. 836.
26 Dict. Scient. Biog. (1970) Vol I, pp. 539–40.
27 'Lancet'. (1873) i, p. 614.
28 Snapper, I. & Kohn, A., 'Myelomatosis'. University Park Press, Baltimore, London 1971, pp. 1–9.
29 Phil. Trans. Royal Society London. 1848, p. 55.
30 'Lancet' (1847) ii, p. 91.
31 Sharpey-Schafer, Sir Edward, 'History of the Physiological Society during its first fifty years, 1876–1926'. Cambridge University Press, London 1927, p. 17.
32 Ibid p. 15.
33 Ibid pp. 55, 64.

# SIXTEEN
# The Research Establishments 1871–98

The growth of experimental physiology and laboratory medicine led to an increased demand for laboratory space which was not adequately met by the Universities. In the latter part of the 19th century it was partly supplied by research institutes, the best known being the Brown Institute, the Conjoint Laboratories of the Royal Colleges of Physicians and of Surgeons, and the Lister Institute. They are described below.

## The Brown Institute

The Brown Institute was opened at the end of 1871 and continued to function until 1944 when the buildings were destroyed by bombing. It is of importance because it must have been one of the first, if not the first, Research Institute in this country. Information concerning it has been hard to find and consists of fragmentary details from journals such as the 'Lancet' and 'British Medical Journal'. It does not seem to have issued any reports though there are occasional references to the work in the above journals. Fortunately a very complete and detailed description of the Institute was given in a series of articles by Sir Graham Wilson in recent issues of the Journal of Hygiene (vols 82, 83). For the brief outline that follows the author has drawn freely on this excellent account.

The bequest which gave rise to the Institute was a peculiar one. Thomas Brown, a citizen of London and Dublin, made a bequest of £15,000 in 1852. One account says that the fund was intended for 'the establishment of an Animal Sanatory Institution for the study of Comparative Pathology, and the treatment of the maladies and injuries of quadrupeds and birds useful to man'.[1] The monies were to be allowed to accumulate for 15 years so that by 1867 they amounted to about £30,000. Unless this was made use of in terms of the will within 4 years, it would pass into the hands of the University of Dublin for the establishment of professorships in Welsh and Oriental languages, such as Persian, Chinese, Coptic, and Sanskrit.[2] One writer with a whimsical turn of mind said that it would be used to teach Welsh to the Irish![3] A further condition was that the site of the Institute must be within a mile of Southwark, Westminster, or Dublin, and by the laws of Mortmain the money could not be used for purchasing a site or for erecting buildings.[1] In 1867, a bill was promoted by the Charity Commissioners to enable the University of London to utilise Mr. Brown's bequest by substituting the foundation of scholarships in Veterinary Medicine for that of a hospital for the treatment of diseased animals. This was, however, thrown out in the House of Lords owing to opposition from the University of Dublin.[2]

With time running out, for the 4 year period alluded to above would expire in 1871, the University of London took action and thanks to some 'great energy and liberality' by medical members of the Senate and a gift of £2,000 obtained by Dr. Burdon Sanderson from a city merchant, Mr. John Curliffe, a site was purchased in the Wandsworth Road and some buildings erected. The staff of the Institute was to consist of a Professor Superintendent, his Assistant, a Veterinary Surgeon, and three Servants. The Chamber of Agriculture made a handsome grant and the staff was appointed. The Professor Superintendent was Dr. J. Burdon Sanderson, who up to this time had been Medical Officer of Health for Paddington and had shown considerable enthusiasm and ability for research. His assistant was Dr. E. E. Klein, an able pathologist from Vienna, whom Burdon Sanderson had invited to come to London in May 1871. Klein was employed on a voluntary basis though it seems that some finance was obtained for him in return for carrying out work for the local Government Board. The Veterinary Surgeon was engaged later and was a Mr. Duguid.[4] The first work of this promising team was to 'study treatment and comparative pathology of pleuropneumonia, an epizootic which commits the most costly ravages amongst our herds'.

The new centre was to have several different functions and at the time it must have been difficult to see how it would evolve. To conform with the terms of the will it had to provide care for sick animals, that is to say to be an animal hospital. This was certainly fulfilled, for a review of the first sixteen years claimed that 'over 45,000 animals had been admitted, and of these 34,650 had been completely cured'. That these animals were mostly 'pets' is suggested by a later report which stated that, during 1920, 6,040 were treated, including 2,383 dogs, 2,660 cats and 221 horses.[5] Each year the Professor Superintendent gave the Brown lectures, which formed a series of five and were given towards the end of the year. These lectures gave him the opportunity of reporting the research work of the Institute. Obviously the nature of the research would depend on the interests of the Professor Superintendent. At that time when animal experiments were becoming more essential because of the growth of Physiology and its demand for research, the antivivisectionists were extremely active. Every effort was made to publicize the fact that physiological investigations formed no part of the work at the Institute, which was devoted entirely to Pathology.[6] Again, at a meeting of the Pathological Society of London the retiring President, Dr. Richard Quain, mentioned the newly-formed Institute and added, 'So pathology will more and more completely fulfil its mission of throwing light upon the genesis of disease and will afford a more solid foundation for therapeutic practice'.[3]

The outcry by the antivivisectionists was so great that the Government appointed a Royal Commission to report on the subject (see chapter 12). The report was issued in early 1876 and later in the year a Cruelty to

Animals Act based on the findings was passed. Under its terms a worker had to obtain a licence for animal experiments, and in addition the Institute in which he carried out his research had to be registered. In the same year Burdon Sanderson's assistant, Emanuel Klein, made application for registration of the Brown Institute.[7] An unsuccessful attempt was made to refuse this by Hutton, a prominent antivivisectionist and a member of the Senate of London University. The Secretary of State had granted a license to Klein, and it was therefore ruled that the Institute should be registered. It was some years before opposition died down and again in 1883 the antivivisectionists tried to have experiments at the Institute prohibited, but again they were unsuccessful.[8]

One can only hazard a guess as to how the Institute functioned in its earlier years. We are told that there was a laboratory where the origin and progress of disease were investigated, and a hospital for sick animals. But although the Institute was primarily intended for the prevention and treatment of animal diseases, apart from Horsley's work on rabies and Greenfield's preparation of an anthrax vaccine human diseases were studied using animal models. This was inevitable as all the superintendents were medical men, and for many years research workers in the veterinary profession were virtually non-existent. The only one to study animal disease in a research animal was J. (later Sir John) McFadyean who had both medical and veterinary qualifications. But he founded no school of animal research, and veterinary research was only promoted by the activity of the Agricultural Research Council as late as the 1930s.[9] In its earlier years, the Institute had financial difficulties and was very short of equipment. The shortage was such that a microscope was not purchased till 1900.[10] An appeal to the public was made in 1890 when a new operating room was needed in addition to wards for after-care, equipment and extra staff.[11] Such appeals generally yielded little, for the Institute was unpopular as a result of repeated attacks on it by the antivivisectionists.

Presumably the Veterinary Surgeon ran the hospital and if so he must have been busy! The Assistant probably carried out most of the research work and Dr. Klein must have been sadly missed when he left after failing to become the successor to Burdon Sanderson in 1878. The Professor Superintendent organised the programme of research which was related to his own particular interest. During its existence the Institute had eight Professor Superintendents who held office as below:

| 1871–78 | John Burdon Sanderson | (1828–1905) |
| 1878–81 | William Smith Greenfield | (1846–1919) |
| 1881–84 | Charles Smart Roy | (1854–1897) |
| 1884–90 | Victor Horsley | (1857–1916) |
| 1890–95 | Charles Scott Sherrington | (1857–1952) |
| 1895–1902 | John Rose Bradford | (1863–1935) |
| 1903–08 | Thomas Gregor Brodie | (1866–1916) |
| 1909–44 | Frederick William Twort | (1877–1950) |

Looking over this list of names one is very impressed with the quality of these men. Apart from the last-named, they all held other posts while working at the Brown Institution, as for instance Victor Horsley, who was made Professor of Pathology at University College in 1887; they were mostly clinicians or pathologists with clinical orientation, and stayed at the Institution for a relatively short time, the longest being eight years and the shortest three years. It may well be that appointment to the Brown Institution was regarded as an interim one and especially attractive to young men because of the research facilities which were available. The outstanding ability of these men is indicated by the posts which they ultimately held. Dr. J. (later Sir John) Burdon Sanderson stayed seven years and after becoming Professor of Physiology at University College, London, ultimately held Professorships at the Universities of Edinburgh and Oxford. Dr. C. S. Roy became the first Professor of Pathology at the University of Cambridge; unfortunately he suffered from ill-health and died at the early age of 43. Mr. (later Sir Victor) Horsley had a most distinguished career becoming Professor of Pathology and later Surgeon to University College, London. C. S. (later Sir Charles) Sherrington became the leading neurophysiologist of the day and held the Holt Chair in Physiology at Liverpool and subsequently the Waynflete Chair of Physiology at Oxford. Dr. (later Sir John) Rose Bradford became Professor of Materia Medica and later of Clinical Medicine, in addition to being Full Physician at University College Hospital, London. Thomas G. Brodie became Professor of Physiology at the University of Toronto, and organised a department which became internationally known. Some idea of the work carried out by the Professor Superintendents may be obtained from the topics of the annual lectures. This is fully dealt with in the articles by Wilson previously referred to. Only a few brief comments need be made here.

With his public health background and experience of infective diseases, Burdon Sanderson naturally spoke on more than one occasion on pyeaemia which he had been studying experimentally since 1867.[12] Soon after his appointment he lectured in 1879 on 'Researches on the Infective processes carried out in the Institution during the present year'.[13] The extent of Greenfield's contribution has only been realised recently. Two months before Toussaint and a year before Pasteur, Chamberland and Roux, Greenfield reported the success of a vaccine against anthrax made with organisms attenuated in aqueous humor.[14] His breadth of interest must have been considerable for at about the same time he had given one of the earliest descriptions of the histology of Hodgkin's disease.[15] When it is noted that Greenfield was the only Professor Superintendent of the Brown Institute who did not become F.R.S. it seems quite certain that he was underestimated at the time. Dr. C. S. Roy, no doubt influenced by a year's study in Professor Goltz's Physiological Institute in Strasbourg, and a further period with Cohnheim in Leipzig, made the action of the mammalian heart his major study at the Brown Institute.

On one occasion he was given three months' leave of absence to investigate an epidemic of cattle disease in the Argentine which turned out to be anthrax. In 1890 Victor Horsley chose as his lecture topic 'The arrangement of the Central Nervous System and the Pathological conditions produced by Compression'.[16] His main subjects of study while at the Brown Institute were the functions of the cerebral cortex with localisation of the motor impulses, the functions of the thyroid gland, and the diagnosis and prevention of rabies.[17] From a practical point of view the last-named study was the most important for it led to the Dogs Muzzling Order of 1885 which eradicated rabies from London and subsequently from the rest of the country. The level of activity at the Institute was probably at its highest during the periods when Horsley and Sherrington were in charge. Certainly there was a large number of outside workers who were given laboratory space. In Horsley's term of office, namely 1884–90, several special investigations were carried out for the Medical Department of the Local Government Board.[18] Also we read that Dr. L. C. Wooldridge, a most promising physician and physiologist from Guy's carried out research on blood at the Institute where he became friendly with Professor Horsley and Dr. Lingard.[19] It is sad to relate that this friendship was interrupted by the death of Wooldridge at the age of 31 from an intestinal disorder. Lastly, Horsley's interest in idiopathic epilepsy should be mentioned. Working with Hughlings Jackson he produced epilepsy in animals by the injection of absinthe,[20] a technique similar to that of Magnan, which was demonstrated in England in 1874 at a B.M.A. meeting in Norwich and which aroused the anger of the antivivisectionists (see chapter 12). It was during his time at the Brown Institute that Sherrington developed his interest in neurophysiology. His studies included reflex actions and he continued his work on secondary degeneration in the spinal cord which he had commenced with Mott. Sir Graham Wilson in an intriguing story suggests that Sherrington may have been the first person to adminster diphtheria antitoxin successfully to a patient, the young son of his brother-in-law. The antitoxin was obtained from a horse in process of being immunised by Dr. Armand Ruffer, but on which trials had not yet been made.[21] In 1896 Dr.J. Rose Bradford selected two subjects and gave two lectures on 'The work of the Brown Institution with special reference to rabies' and three on 'Observations on the Pathology of the kidneys'.[22] He also reported his research work at the Institute in his Gulstonian lectures in 1897. Although he maintained his interest in renal disease he does not appear to have done further research after leaving the Institute. Dr. T. F. Brodie published papers on a wide variety of subjects, though his outstanding work was on the kidney and the functions of the glomerulus. He is particularly remembered for his student handbook, 'Essentials of Experimental Physiology'.[23] He seems to have had a delightful personality with the ability to attract good workers and inspire them by his great enthusiasm.

The last superintendent, Dr. F. W. Twort, stands apart from the other seven. He was a full-time research worker who held no other appointments and he remained as Superintendent for 35 years, more than four times longer than any of his predecessors. He came to the Institute with a good reputation as a bacteriologist having trained under Dr. Louis Jenner at St. Thomas's and Dr. William Bullock at the London Hospital. Within six years he had performed some preliminary studies which led to the discovery of bacteriophage, probably the most outstanding contribution to come from the Institution. This work was interrupted by a period of war service, and strangely he did not pursue his original observations. In the meanwhile, d'Herelle had published some more detailed observations and so this feature of bacterial lysis became known as the Twort-d'Herelle phenomenon. The future was to hold little happiness in store for Twort for as early as 1914 the Medical Research Committee refused a request for a research grant. It is perhaps significant that in 1921[24] his appointment was still on a yearly basis even though he had been Head of the Institute for 12 years. In 1930 the finances of the Institute were in better shape and he was able to purchase apparatus for his work. At this time he was working on many aspects of virology, but in the succeeding years the Medical Research Council grew anxious at the paucity of his results. From then onwards it became a battle between the Council and Twort which resulted in some unwise and fruitless litigation on his part; he also voiced his grievances in the press. The bombing of the Second World War made work increasingly difficult and after five attacks the Institute was completely destroyed. Twort expected that the Institute would be rebuilt and that he would be restored to his position as Superintendent, but it was decided not to rebuild and in 1949 the London County Council made an order for the compulsory purchase of the whole area. It had been a very sad story, for Twort had been credited with an attractive personality, and certainly had scientific ability. But he had suffered from being an isolated worker, though he attributed his lack of results to the obstruction of his arch enemy, the Medical Research Council, which nevertheless seems to have gone a long way in attempting to resolve the impasse. In any case he could not expect to be re-engaged after the war for he was then two years over the normal retiring age. He did not live to enjoy a long retirement as he died in 1950 at the age of 72.[25]

After receiving the purchase money from the London County Council, the Trust Fund accumulated a considerable sum during subsequent years. Many suggestions were made for its use, but the legal complexities were such that it was not until the end of 1969 that it was agreed to divide the £96,000 equally between the University of London and Trinity College, Dublin. London University established a Fellowship at the Royal Veterinary College and in Dublin the University established a lectureship in Welsh, Slavonic, Russian, Persian, Chinese, Coptic or Sanskrit, or in a near Eastern language.[26]

## The Conjoint Laboratories of the Royal Colleges of Physicians and of Surgeons

These laboratories were opened in 1890 for general research and although they functioned for this purpose for only about fifteen years, they were of great importance at a time when laboratory accommodation was hard to find.

The Medical Act of 1858 did much to promote unity within the medical profession. For many years the usual qualification for the general practitioner was the MRCS and the LSA. The Act took this function of the Apothecaries away, and thus indirectly led to discussions between the two English Royal Colleges and other bodies and which ultimately led to the establishment of a Conjoint Diploma given by the RCP and RCS. Such a plain statement might give the impression that it was a straightforward affair. On the contrary, the discussions extended over a period of 25 years and the various stages are outlined in the excellent 'History of the Royal College of Surgeons' by Zachary Cope.[27] The matter was one of great complexity for in 1880 it was stated that there were 'nineteen licensing bodies in Great Britain, including Universities and Corporations, conferring amongst them between fifty and sixty different qualifications or licenses to practise'.[28] As far back as 1868 a Bill had been passed in the Lords and debated in the Commons which would abrogate 'the licensing powers of all the medical authorities, and substitute for their diverse proceedings a single licensing or examining board in each division of the United Kingdom'.[29] But nothing happened and when in 1880 a new government had been elected, the Council of the Royal College of Surgeons threatened to withdraw from the discussions as they appeared to have lost all confidence in legislative measures for the amendment of qualifying examinations. Happily the Council did not proceed further with this threat, and in 1884 the 'British Medical Journal' published the following in two successive issues, namely: 'At an ordinary meeting of the Royal College of Physicians it was said that the Medical Bill had been withdrawn and the President advised that the College should at once proceed with the scheme for conjoint examinations with the Royal College of Surgeons, which only awaited the sanction of the Medical Council'.[30] In October 1884 full sanction was given for the Conjoint Diploma of the two Royal Colleges. It might be thought that all would now be plain sailing but in 1885, there was a movement to obtain permission for the Royal Colleges to grant an MD degree to holders of the Conjoint Diploma. This had been under discussion many years before and in 1862 a correspondent claimed that the Diploma given by the King and Queen's College of Physicians in Ireland contained the following wording: 'Licentiates are entitled to the Degree Title and qualification of Doctor of Medicine'.[31] A second letter contested the above and quoted a case in the Queen's Bench Division in Dublin. The Registrar of the Branch Council for Ireland stated that 'no such degree was recognized by the Medical Act and that it was not a registerable qualification'.[32] Later and towards the end of 1863 there appeared a leading article in the BMJ in which Trinity College Dublin questioned the right of King and Queen's College to confer the MD degree. The College had assumed this right since 1860 and was now challenged to make good this right in Chancery.[33] The whole matter turned out to be both complex and protracted and at one time there was even proposed the formation of a second university in London. But in spite of the fact that discussions went on from 1885 till 1903 no agreement was ever reached.[34]

It has been said that the first Conjoint examination was to be held in January 1885,[35] but the 'British Medical Journal' mentions that one was held in October 1884.[36] A really striking feature was the number of candidates who presented themselves. In this case it amounted to 400, of whom 200 presented for the first examination alone. The Pall Mall buildings were totally inadequate and in August 1885 the 'Lancet' reported that there were 520 candidates at a recent examination, and that accommodation had to be obtained in distant localities. It was felt that accommodation for 650 students would be required and the Building Committee was asked to proceed with plans for the erection of a new Examination Hall.[37]

A suitable site was found on the Embankment and on March 24th, 1886 Queen Victoria laid the foundation stone for the Examination Hall in the presence of a distinguished gathering.[38] There was some vacant land adjacent to the new Hall and in May 1887 it was decided to erect a new building with classrooms, laboratories, and a lecture theatre fully equipped for 'research and exposition'.[39] It is possible that this decision may have been influenced by a petition from British proponents of experimental medicine (including J. E. Erichsen, then an inspector under the Vivisection Act of 1876). In this, they appealed to the Royal College of Surgeons to use a large benefaction recently received to set up a Physiological and Pathological laboratory at the College. As can be imagined the Antivivisectionists immediately counter-petitioned the College and succeeded in receiving from the Council assurances that vivisectional research would not be permitted.[40] This incident seems to confirm the suggestion that experimental laboratory space was hard to find. The final design of this extension consisted of a wing on each end of the main building. These wings were connected by two galleries of rooms, and the building was ready for use in early 1890. The laboratory committee included John Marshall, Sir William Roberts, Dr. P. H. Pye-Smith, Dr. J. F. Payne, J. W. Hulke and Anthony Bowlby, and met on the 1st January, 1890.[39]

The first duty was the appointment of a Director of the Laboratories and there were fifteen applicants. Dr. G. Sims Woodhead was unanimously elected and he was well-suited for his new post as he was at the time superintendent of the Laboratory of the Royal College of

Physicians in Edinburgh.[41] The appointment was for a year but was renewable for up to six years and carried with it a salary of not more than £500 per annum.[42] About £2000 had been spent on laboratory equipment and it was anticipated that a further £2500 might be needed.[43]

Although the laboratories functioned for only twelve years it was said that 189 different persons made use of them during that period.[44] The following details give some idea of the variety of study that was being pursued a year after its opening:

(1) Dr. Parry FRS and Mr. Rowntree on glycogen and sugar metabolism.
(2) Mr. d'Arcy Power on cancer.
(3) Mr. C. A. Ballance and Mr. S. G. Shattock on tissue culture experiments with malignant tumours.
(4) Dr. Howard H. Tooth on paths of sensation in the brain.
(5) Dr. A. W. Macfarlance on anaesthetics and hypnotics.
(6) Mr. Watson Cheyne and Mr. Cheatle on tuberculous disease.
(7) Mr. Douglas Stanley on cancer.
(8) Dr. M. A. Ruffer on immunity against infectious diseases.
(9) Mr. James Galloway on malignant diseases affecting the peritoneum.
(10) Dr. A. E. (later Sir Almroth) Wright on coagulation of the blood.
(11) Mr. R. Cozens Bailey on surgical treatment of wounds of the intestine.
(12) Dr. Vincent Harris and Dr. W. Gow on the structure and function of the pancreas.
(13) Dr. W. P. Herringham and Mr. E. Groves on the excretion of uric acid and urea.
(14) Dr. Sidney Martin on the chemical products of infective micro-organisms.[45]

These research workers were relatively young and out of seventeen of the above only four were over 35 in 1890, and of the younger group four were still in their twenties. The research on breast carcinoma by Mr. C. A. Ballance and Mr. S. G. Shattock is of interest in that at that early stage they used a tissue culture technique. The work had been started in 1888 when malignant breast tissue was incubated at 100°F under sterile conditions. The epithelial tissues died but a number of dark-staining bodies appeared and underwent budding. There was no mention of any culture medium.[46] By 1893 they reported further experiments in which a culture medium of sterile milk and glycogen was used and incubation was at room temperature. Again after six weeks the epithelial cells had disappeared and been overgrown by the darker elements, which presumably were fibroblasts. When reporting their findings to the Pathological

Society of London they suggested that the elements might be leucocytes, some form of connective tissue cell, or even parasites.[47]

The enthusiasm must have been great for reports of the research at the Laboratories were soon being given at a number of societies. There was however an early misfortune when in 1892 Dr. Tylden, then only 35, was working on typhoid and with one of his young assistants succumbed to the disease.[48] At the Annual Meeting of the Royal College of Surgeons a very favourable report was given of the Research Laboratories and their Director.[49] During this short period the activity of Sims Woodhead seems to have been prodigious. Interested in the transmission of tuber-culosis from animals to man, he spoke on this subject at the Seventh International Congress of Hygiene and Demography in London[50] and also opened a discussion on it at the annual Meeting of the British Medical Association in Bournemouth[51] – both in the summer of 1891. In 1892 he addressed the Pathological Society of London on 'Phagocytosis and immunity',[52] and later in the year gave the Morton Lecture on 'Cancer and cancerous disease'.[53] In late 1892 he produced the 3rd edition of his book, 'Practical Pathology', which now consisted of 652 pages as compared with the 484 of the First Edition in 1883.[54] In the same year he founded the 'Journal of Pathology and Bacteriology', so the extent of his influence on the growing subject of Pathology is evident.

At this time the subject of Bacteriology was progressing by leaps and bounds. Some idea of the state of affairs in 1880, the year in which the typhoid bacillus was discovered, is obtained by reference to an address on Micro-organisms and Disease given at the Health Department of the Social Science Congress by its President, Dr. Charles Cameron.[55] At that time there was little knowledge of bacteria pathogenic to man, and much of this address relates to pathogens for animals. He dealt exten-sively with Pasteur's work and discussed at length the organisms of anthrax, fowl-cholera and other infections. It is small wonder that he advocated study of animal diseases and the institution of a Chair of Comparative Medicine and Pathology. At a time when relatively few pathogenic bacteria were known, there was yet a considerable under-standing of attenuation and enhancement of virulence and some remarkable studies on the effect of the portal of entry on the type of disease produced.

By 1894 at least a dozen human pathogens had been isolated including the diptheria bacillus, and bacteriological diagnosis was becoming a prac-tical reality. In 1891 the Society of Medical Officers of Health had urged the General Medical Council to insist that the clinical instruction in infec-tious diseases should be compulsory for students. In the same year the Conjoint Board laid down that all medical students should attend a certificated course at a fever hospital as part of their medical curriculum. With this enormous expansion of bacteriology the shortage of laboratory space can well be imagined. This was felt particularly by the

Metropolitan Asylums Board in London in their dealings with diptheria. In the absence of a central laboratory of their own it was agreed that space could be provided at the Conjoint Laboratories of the Royal Colleges on the Embankment. Cases of suspected diptheria were to have diagnostic tests performed both on admission and discharge, and these were to be carried out by bacteriologists paid by the Metropolitan Asylums Board, and under the direction of Sims Woodhead.[56] The work commenced on the 1st January, 1895, by which time further help was already required. In 1892 von Behring had produced diptheria antitoxin from horses for treatment, so the Metropolitan Asylums Board required antitoxin as well. Fortunately they were aided by a generous gift from the Goldsmiths' Company which enabled serum to be provided for those who could not afford to buy it. The Colleges agreed to this work being done by the bacteriologists in the Conjoint Laboratories provided that the Board would be responsible for the housing of the horses. The volume of work is indicated by the fact that during the year 1896 4,870 specimens were examined.[57] On the basis of his experience Sims Woodhead was able to give the Harben Lectures for 1897 to the Royal Institute of Public Health on 'Bacteriological Diagnosis'.[58] This phase of Woodhead's life was not to last much longer for in 1899 he was appointed to the Chair of Pathology at the University of Cambridge following the premature death of Kanthack. He was succeeded at the Conjoint Laboratories by Dr. T. G. Brodie.

By about 1901–02 the co-operation between the Board and the Royal Colleges started to come to an end as the Board was providing its own laboratory space and by 1904 the scheme was ended. By that time many other laboratories had been opened and the Royal Colleges felt that their facilities were no longer required. The ending was rather abrupt because Brodie, who had already had his space curtailed, was informed that he would have to vacate the rooms by Christmas 1902.[59] Early in 1903 Brodie became Professor Superintendent of the Brown Institute, a post which he held until 1908 when he left to become Professor of Physiology at the University of Toronto.[60]

The sudden change of policy on the part of the Royal Colleges may have been related to an important event in 1902. Sir Henry Morris announced the promise of a gift of £100,000 for Cancer Research which the donor wished to be administered by a conjoint committee of the two Royal Colleges. As a result in July 1902 a scheme was proposed whereby the rooms of the Research Department of the Examination Hall on the Embankment would be leased to the Cancer Research Committee. In this way the organisation of what is now the Imperial Cancer Research Fund commenced.

The examination Hall on the Embankment lasted till July 1908 when it was sold to the Institute of Electrical Engineers for £50,000, though the Colleges were permitted to use the buildings until a new site had been found. It is a strange coincidence that fifty years later in 1958, when a possible site was being considered for a College of Pathologists, a member of the Committee made enquiries about the building of the Institute of Electrical Engineers which was at the time up for sale. However it seems unlikely that the building was the one put up by the Royal Colleges for their Examination Hall.

In March 1909 three houses in Queen Square were purchased for £21,000 and a new building put up and occupied in May 1912 at a cost of £27,644.[61] The Examination Hall has remained on this site until the present day. The developments of the Imperial Cancer Research Fund were more complex. Its accommodation started on the Embankment as previously stated and it moved to Queen Square in 1912 with the Examination Hall. As the work expanded new buildings were taken over at Mill Hill. After World War II some work was also carried out at No. 48 Lincoln's Inn Fields. More recently, when Nos. 44, 45, and 46 Lincoln's Inn Fields were demolished, a large building was put up on the site which now houses the Imperial Cancer Research Fund.[61]

## The Lister Institute

The culmination of Louis Pasteur's remarkable experiments with rabies occurred in July 1885 when a boy called Joseph Meister was successfully protected against the disease after being bitten by a rabid dog.[62] On the 26th October of the same year Pasteur communicated his discovery to the Paris Academie des Sciences.[63] It was an outstanding date in the history of Medicine, but has also particular interest for our present purpose as it was indirectly responsible for the foundation of the British Institute of Preventive Medicine some six years later.[64] Paris became the centre for rabies treatment and during the next three years 5,384 patients passed through Pasteur's laboratories. Most striking of all was the fact that the mortality amongst these patients was only about 1 per cent. They came from many different countries and before long donations of money were forthcoming to finance this work and later to build a new centre. Thus on 14th November 1888, in the presence of a large body of scientists, President Carnot opened the new Pasteur Institute.[65] The rapid acceptance of the method was remarkable when one compares it with the resistance which vaccination had encountered 100 years previously. By the end of 1885 there were already twenty laboratories for rabies prophylaxis. These included seven in Russia (where rabies from wolf bites was common), five in Italy, and one each in Roumania, Austria, Brazil, and the Argentine Republic. Soon there was one in Chicago, and one in Malta which was the only one on British soil.[66] Cases from England were sent to Pasteur in Paris, where like others they were treated free of charge. Sir Henry Roscoe pointed out that 178 British subjects had been gratuitously treated during a matter of two years and asked the Government if it did not feel that it should provide some financial assistance for this service. The Chancellor of the Exchequer thought that this was a matter for individual patients as many of them had ample means. This of course was simply not true, and Sir Henry was quick to reply that very many were poor, and that shabbiness in appearances of patients was no excuse for shabbiness of behaviour by the Government.[67] Others such as the Lord Mayor of London agreed with Sir Henry, and this must have become widely known for on May 31st 1889 Pasteur wrote to the Lord Mayor and the letter was published in the 'British Medical Journal'.[63] It contained a number of observations, including the following:

(1) that Belgium and England were the only two countries in Europe without antirabic laboratories, presumably because cases could easily be sent to Paris.

(2) that they are in no way forbidden to contribute by subscription to defray the expenses of the Pasteur Institute.

(3) That if the British chose to set up an antirabic laboratory, he and his assistants would give them any help they could.

Lastly, he reminded the Lord Mayor that on his visit to the Pasteur Institute, he had presented to him a young English scientist from the University of Oxford named Dr. Armand Ruffer, who had worked in the Pasteur Institute for some months, was ideally suited for setting up a new laboratory for prophylaxis, and had expressed his willingness to help if required.

As a result, the Lord Mayor called a meeting of prominent scientists including Sir James Paget, Sir Henry Roscoe, Professor Huxley, and Professor Ray Lankester to discuss the matter. This led to a large meeting which was held at the Mansion House on July 1st 1889, when a public appeal for money was launched by a 'Mansion House Pasteur Institute Committee'. At a meeting in November 1889 this Committee asked the Lord Mayor to send 40,000 francs to Pasteur as a gesture of the country's gratitude,[68] and Pasteur hastened to express his appreciation. The question of building a British Institute had been raised at a meeting of the Committee in December. During the subsequent months a sub-committee had been considering the matter and it now issued a report recommending the establishment of a Bacteriological Institute of Preventive Medicine. The Mansion House Committee accepted this report and at the same time transformed itself into an Executive Committee for the purpose. London had not been favoured as a location and it was now proposed to set up the new Institute in Cambridge, preferably in connection with the University.[69]

By now there was much national enthusiasm for the project for it had been publicly stated that it was quite wrong that poor people bitten by mad dogs should have to go for treatment to Paris, and that 'our tuberculous patients should be inoculated with lymph prepared in Germany'. Also, at this time rabies in Great Britain was increasing. In addition to the human cases there was a severe outbreak amongst cattle and sheep in Galway;[70] some cases occurred in the deer in Richmond Park in the Spring of 1888,[71] and in the summer of 1889 an epidemic broke out amongst deer on the Marquis of Bristol's estate of Ickworth Park near Bury St. Edmunds, which ultimately resulted in the death of about 450 animals. An unusual event makes this epidemic of some interest. The disease had originally been diagnosed as anthrax by the Privy Council and the Park had been declared an infected area under the Contagious Diseases Act for animals. At this stage a promising young pathologist named Dr. J. G. Adami (later to become Professor of Pathology at McGill University, Montreal) working with Professor Roy at the University of Cambridge, was consulted by Dr. C. Scott Kilner, the Medical Officer of Health for the district. Adami did a post-mortem on one animal but was unable to find any trace of anthrax. Also, a careful enquiry into the symptoms of the disease led Adami and Roy to suspect that the condition might be rabies. Animal inoculation proved that they were right. There was however an unfortunate incident, for while carrying out post-mortem examinations on two further animals, Adami cut his finger. The wound was not large and was well-washed and treated with 20% carbolic acid. But healing was slow and in the meanwhile the diagnosis of rabies had been confirmed. Strongly persuaded by Professor Roy and his other colleagues, Adami finally consented to go to Paris for prophylactic treatment. Fortunately he never developed the disease, but about 26 days after the accident he experienced some peculiar nervous symptoms which might possibly have been evidence of a very mild rabies infection. Adam subsequently wrote an excellent account of this experience and ended by saying that he was possibly indebted to Louis Pasteur for the continuance of his days.[72]

The new Institute came into being at the end of 1891. Between 1889 and 1891 the whole matter of prophylaxis had been given much publicity. Victor Horsley gave a paper to the Epidemiological Society on Pasteur's treatment of rabies.[73] Pasteur was invited to give a Croonian Lecture at the Royal Society on preventive inoculation of anthrax and rabies, but he was indisposed, and the lecture was given by his assistant Dr. M. Roux.[74] Later in 1889 Dr. M. Armand Ruffer gave a summary of the whole subject of rabies, its treatment and its prevention, at the Society of Arts. This young man, who had worked at the Pasteur Institute, then became Honorary Secretary of the Council of the new British Institute. Other meetings were held all over the country and at a meeting in Birmingham in 1893 the objectives of the Institute were said to be 'The promotion of the study of experimental physiology and pathology, as these subjects are universally recognised throughout the world as vital to the progress of Medicine and the welfare of the people'.[75] The meeting appeared to favour the Government being the main contributor to the cost of the Institute. However, Victor Horsley thought it should be funded by public subscription. He also stressed the great use it would be

to the medical schools throughout the country for supporting Bacteriology and for teaching Public Health. Subscriptions had started to pour
in following the foundation of the Institute in 1891, and by the end of
1892 a sum of £32,000 had been accumulated. In 1894 Mr. Berridge
promised £20,000,if £40,000 could be raised from other sources and this
target was easily reached.[76] Later in the year the Grocers' Company, as
ever generous to medical endeavours, gave £10,000. There was a further
£25,000 from the Berridge Bequest and this was given to endow a
laboratory for the chemical and bacteriological examination of water
supplies. Lastly, with the amalgamation of the old College of State
Medicine and the new Institute, there was the transfer of about £4,000
in cash, securities, and plant.[77]

By this time the idea of having the Institute at Cambridge seems to
have been dropped, probably because of the offer of a suitable site in
London by the Duke of Westminster. It consisted of about an acre of
land on the Chelsea Embankment, which was purchased from the Duke
for £6,000. Plans for the Institute were drawn up, though it was to be
some four years before it was opened. There was some opposition to the
project, and this came from two sources. First of all there were the
antivivisectionists, but their activities soon died down. The other criticism
came from the local residents, who considered that the new Institute
would constitute a health hazard.[78] There was much urgent work to be
done, and 1894 was a year of considerable activity. Dr. Armand Ruffer
was appointed to be Director of the Institute for a period of three years,
and Professor Allan MacFadyean to be Lecturer in Bacteriology.
MacFadyean had previously been a Research Scholar of the Grocers
Company from 1889 till 1892, and at the time was also Lecturer in
Bacteriology at the old College of State Medicine.[79] For temporary
accommodation the Institute had offices in Great Russell Street, and a
laboratory was set up on these premises.[80] But at this time the great
need was for antisera, and for their manufacture accommodation for
large animals was necessary. Therefore the Institute at the beginning of
1895 acquired a farm, namely 'The Poplars' at Sudbury near Harrow,
where 21 horses were kept, 18 of which were ready to yield diptheria
antitoxin.[81] In addition tetanus antitoxin[82] and tuberculin could be
supplied.[83] It is interesting to find that three doses of the latter were
sold for a shilling. The enthusiasm of the early workers is much to be
admired when we read that in August 1894 they staged an exhibition of
bacteria at the meeting of the British Medical Association at Bristol. This
was said to have been the most comprehensive and complete display
which had ever been brought together in this country. It included over
1,000 cultures and about 50 microscopic preparations, all made by Dr.
H. G. Plimmer, a Fellow of the Linnaeian Society and Pathologist to the
Cancer Hospital, assisted by Dr. F. Blaxall, Lecturer in Bacteriology at
the Westminster Hospital. Even at this early stage both of these men
were carrying out research at the temporary Institute. In 1895 a large

party of British Medical Association members were entertained at Sudbury by Dr. Dean and his assistant Dr. Salter, and they commented very favourably on the excellent condition of the animals.[84]

The part played in these early days by Dr. Allan MacFadyean must have been considerable. In March 1896 he had been appointed Honorary Secretary of the Institute[85] and later in the year he succeeded Dr. Armand Ruffer as Director, when the latter left to accept a post in Egypt. By 1897 the Institute's work justified the publication of Transactions, and these were produced under the editorship of MacFadyean.[86]

Meanwhile the building of the new Institute was proceeding and was ready for occupation in 1898. Before dealing with its scientific developments it will be necessary to relate the events which led to a change in the name of the Institute. In 1896 a movement had started at St. George's Hospital to commemorate the centenary of Jenner's vaccination, which fell in that year. The form of the memorial depended on the sum of money which could be collected. It might even be an institute, or something less such as a Scholarship or Lectureship. In the event the sum of money was insufficient to finance the foundation of an institute. The cost of building the British Institute had been greater than anticipated, with the result that the original plans could not be completed. It was therefore agreed that the money collected for the Jenner Memorial should be transferred to the British Institute on condition that its name was changed to the Jenner Institute. This was brought about in 1898 and the new name used for the next few years. But it then became known that there was in existence a commercial firm known as the 'Jenner Institute for Calf Lymph' which had prior claim to the name 'Jenner Institute'. There was therefore likely to be some confusion, compounded by the fact that the British Institute had rented some of its laboratory space to the Local Government Board in order to prepare calf lymph for the public vaccinators. In 1903 it was decided that the Institute should once more change its name to that of the 'Lister Institute' and this it has kept until the present day. It should perhaps be added that Lord Lister himself was strongly opposed to this choice of name.[87] The Jenner Memorial Committee, naturally disappointed, agreed that their contribution should be used to finance a Jenner Memorial Studentship at the Institute.

The scientific development of the Institute was rapid and was greatly assisted by a generous gift in 1898 of a quarter of a million pounds by Lord Iveagh. In 1896 it had embarked on educational activities and ran a course of instruction, which was recognised by the various examining bodies, for the Diploma in Public Health.[88] By the time that the new building was occupied, the staff had expanded. In addition to the Director, Dr. Allan MacFadyean, there were two Bacteriologists, Dr. R. T. Hewlett, and Mr. Foulerton FRCS, and a chemist Mr. Arthur Harden. The production of antisera was still carried out at Sudbury where Dr. Dean was in charge, assisted by Dr. Salter.[89] As already mentioned, laboratory space had been rented to the Local Government Board for the production of calf lymph for public vaccinators. By 1901 further staff had been added. These included Dr. S. G. Hedin of the University of Lund, Sweden as Head of the Department of Pathological Chemistry; Mr. Beresford Leathes of St. Thomas's Hospital as Lecturer in Physiology; and Mr. W. J. Young of Owen's College, Manchester as Assistant in the Department of Chemistry. In addition there were three students, namely Drs. Moore, Petrie, and Mackenzie, the last-named holding the Grocers' Research Studentship.[90]

In 1903, when the Great Central Railway encroached on the farm at Sudbury, it was decided to look for a new site. This was found at Aldenham, near Elstree, and was called Queensberry Lodge. It consisted of some buildings and 28 acres of land. Dr. Dean was in charge and was assisted by two Bacteriologists, Drs. Todd and Petrie. Since the foundation of this section in 1895 many well-known men had carried out research work in it, including Ruffer, Washbourn, Hunt, Bullock, Symmers, Nolan and Salter.[91] It can be seen that the Institute was of great importance, even in its early days, in stimulating research, chiefly in Bacteriology, and also in providing laboratory space which at the time was hard to obtain. It would be far beyond the scope of this work to do justice to the outstanding contribution of the Lister Institute in recent years, but one or two examples of its lines of development may not be out of place.

As early as 1902 there were laboratories devoted to Cancer Research conducted by Dr. H. G. Plimmer, who resigned his post as Pathologist to the Cancer Hospital to devote himself to this work at the Institute.[92] In 1919 there was research work on the transmission of typhus by lice, the nature of accessory food factors in animal health, and some aspects of dietary deficiency diseases.[92] In 1926 the Annual Report stated that the annual expenditure of the Institute was £36,500. Research work on nutritional factors was still in progress, as well as on bacterial variation, the efficacy of plague vaccine, and many other subjects.[94] In 1929 a similar research programme was still in progress, but included work on preventive vaccination against implanted animal tumours. Its status as a research institute can be gauged by the fact that its workers were being supported by such bodies as the Medical Research Council, the Government Department for Scientific and Industrial Research, the British Empire Cancer Campaign, and the International Committee for the study of Infantile Paralysis.[95]

For its success during this period much credit must go to Charles J. Martin who was the Director at the time, having been appointed in 1903[96] and whose services were later recognised by the award of a Knighthood.

REFERENCES

1   'Lancet'. (1870) ii, p. 686.
2   Ibid (1867) i, p. 802.
3   'British Medical Journal'. (1871) i, pp. 16, 17.
4   Ibid (1872) i, p. 132.
5   Ibid (1921) i, p. 918.
6   'Lancet'. (1871) ii, p. 654.
7   Ibid (1876) ii, p. 871.
8   Ibid (1883) i, p. 795.
9   J. Hygiene, *82*, p. 507.
10  Ibid p. 158.
11  'Lancet'. (1890) ii, p. 190.
12  'British Medical Journal'. (1872) i, p. 508.
13  Ibid (1879) ii, p. 996.
14  J. Hygiene, *82*, p. 346.
15  Trans. Path. Soc, London, *29*, p. 272.
16  'British Medical Journal'. (1890) ii, p. 1077.
17  J. Hygiene, *83*, p. 176.
18  MacNalty, A. S., Fitzpatrick Lectures 1946-7, p. 54. Royal Institute of Public Health & Hygiene, London.
19  Guy's Hosp. Rep. 1889, *46*, xxxvii.
20  J. Hygiene, *82*, p. 502.
21  Ibid *82*, p. 342.
22  'Lancet'. (1896) ii, p. 1327.
23  J. Hygiene, *83*, p. 183.
24  'British Medical Journal'. (1921) i, p. 918.
25  J. Hygiene, *83*, p. 185.
26  Ibid *83*, pp. 193-7.
27  Cope, Z., 'History of the Royal College of Surgeons of England'. Anthony Blond, London 1959, Chap. 17. pp. 146–56.
28  'British Medical Journal'. (1880) i, p. 930.
29  Ibid (1862) i, p. 296.
30  Ibid (1862) i, p. 320.
31  Ibid (1863) ii, p. 674.
32  Ibid (1880) i, p. 818.
33  Ibid (1884) ii, p. 250.
34  Cope, Z., 'History of the Royal College of Surgeons of England'. Anthony Blond, London 1959, pp. 159–64.
35  Ibid p. 154.
36  'British Medical Journal'. (1884) ii, p. 1202.
37  Ibid (1885) ii, p. 273.
38  'Lancet'. (1886) i, pp. 563; 596–7.
39  Cope, Z., 'History of the Royal College of Surgeons of England'. Anthony Blond, London 1959, p. 167.
40  French, R. D., 'Antivivisection in Victorian Society'. Princeton Univ. Press 1875, p. 274.
41  'British Medical Journal'. (1890) i, p. 251.
42  Ibid (1890) i, p. 143.
43  Ibid (1890) ii, p. 1219.

44 Cope, Z., 'History of the Royal College of Surgeons of England'. Anthony Blond, London 1959, p. 158.
45 'Lancet'. (1891) i, p. 10000.
46 'British Medical Journal'. (1888) i, pp. 1058–9.
47 Ibid (1893) i, pp. 522–3.
48 Ibid (1892) ii, p. 696.
49 Ibid (1893) ii, pp. 1018–20.
50 Ibid (1891) ii, pp. 403–31.
51 Ibid (1891) ii, pp. 627–40.
52 Ibid (1892) i, pp. 373–80.
53 Ibid (1892) i, pp. 954–60.
54 Ibid (1892) ii, p. 947.
55 Ibid (1881) ii, pp. 583–6.
56 Ayres, G. H., 'England's first state hospitals and the Metropolitan Asylums Board 1867–1930'. Wellcome Institute of the History of Medicine, 1971, p. 186.
57 Wilson, G. S., 'History of the Public Health Laboratory Service'. 'British Medical Journal'. (1948) i, pp. 630–1.
58 Woodhead, G. Sims, 'The bearing of recent Bacteriological Investigations on Public Health'. Harben Lectures, J. State Med. London 1897, V, pp. 289–302.
59 Cope, Z., 'History of the Royal College of Surgeons of England'. Anthony Blond, London 1959, pp. 168–9.
60 'British Medical Journal'. (1908) ii, p. 1309.
61 Cope, Z., 'History of the Royal College of Surgeons of England'. Anthony Blond, London 1959, p. 253.
62 Taton, R., 'Science in the 19th century'. Basic Books Inc., New York 1965, pp. 395–6.
63 'British Medical Journal'. (1889) i, pp. 1313–14.
64 Ibid (1891) ii, p. 279.
65 Fleming, Sir Alexander, 'British Medical Journal'. (1947) i, p. 520.
66 'British Medical Journal'. (1888) ii, pp. 1122–3.
67 Ibid (1888) ii, p. 1406.
68 Ibid (1889) ii, p. 1050.
69 Ibid (1889) ii, p. 1363.
70 Ibid (1888) ii, p. 897.
71 'Lancet'. (1888) i, p. 542.
72 'British Medical Journal'. (1889) ii, pp. 808–10; 826.
73 Ibid (1889) i, pp. 342–4.
74 Ibid (1889) i, pp. 1269–74.
75 Ibid (1893) i, pp. 313; 317.
76 Ibid (1894) i, p. 483.
77 Ibid (1894) ii, p. 35.
78 Ibid (1894) i, pp. 926–7.
79 Ibid (1907) i, p. 601.
80 Ibid (1894) ii, p. 507.
81 Ibid (1895) i, pp. 262–3.
82 Ibid (1895) i, p. 268.
83 Ibid (1895) i, p. 997.
84 Ibid (1895) ii, p. 377.

85   Ibid (1896) i, p. 653.
86   Ibid (1897) ii, p. 1871.
87   Ibid (1903) ii, p. 156.
88   Ibid (1896) ii, p. 589.
89   Ibid (1898) i, p. 1675.
90   Ibid (1901) i, p. 350.
91   Ibid (1903) i, pp. 1513–15.
92   J. Roy. Microscopical Soc. (1918) pp. 349–57.
93   'British Medical Journal'. (1919) i, p. 717.
94   Ibid (1926) i, p. 1051.
95   Ibid (1929) i, p. 1051.
96   Ibid (1903) ii, p. 38.

# SEVENTEEN
# Parasitology 1835–1900

Throughout the 19th century Pathology had been steadily advancing and its impact on Medicine became greater and greater; in its contribution to the knowledge of pathogenesis of disease by the end of the century it was recognised as an essential part of a medical student's education. New branches of the subject were appearing and there were prospects of clinical laboratory tests which would assist in clinical diagnosis.

The discovery of fungal and parasite diseases preceeded the advent of bacteriology, as it did not depend on advanced microscopy or special laboratories. In 1835 the first living agent to cause disease was described by Agostino Bassi, an Italian trained for the law who subsequently studied natural science at Pavia.[1] He showed that a disease of silkworms called muscardine was caused by a fungus. This was followed in 1839 by Schonlein's studies, in which he had confirmed Bassi's findings, and also identified a fungus as the cause of a rare human skin disease, namely favus.[2] This stimulated further work on fungi and the characteristic pleomorphism of these organisms was soon recognised. Otherwise, little of note seems to have occurred, though the lesser known work of a very eccentric physician is of interest. David Gruby (1810–1898) was born in Hungary, educated in Vienna and practiced in Paris. Between 1839 and 1844 he described three fungi which were associated with ringworm. This work passed unnoticed for about 50 years when it was rediscovered by Sabouraud who very generously gave full credit to Gruby.[3]

Other pathogenic agents were Protozoa and parasitic worms or Helminths. Many of the latter are large enough to be seen with the naked eye or a simple hand lens. They are a heterogenous group and a number that occur in the tropics are usually listed under Tropical Diseases. Even though because of their size they were recognised early, a full understanding of their pathogenesis was often delayed because of the complexity of their life cycle. We shall confine ourselves to a few interesting events in their history.

Parasitic diseases do not always kill the host. In some cases there may be little effect whilst in others there may be considerable disability. Glancing through a table of their incidence, published in 1947, one is amazed at the prevalence of some of them.[4] Five different diseases each accounted for more than 100 millions of cases, namely, Roundworm (644 millions), Hookworm (359), Whipworm (227), Threadworm (208), and Filariasis (189). Schistosomiasis, of which there were 88 millions at the time, has probably advanced since then in areas where irrigation schemes have been installed.

No better introduction to the History of Parasitology can be made than reference to the Italian zoologist, Francisco Redi (1626–1698). His investigations of the tapeworms of cats and dogs earned him the title of 'The Father of Heliminthology'[5] (article by Shipley). Apart from this he showed great versatility and was many years ahead of his time. Interested in poisons, he showed that viper venom could be swallowed without any ill-effect. When he demonstrated that maggots were derived from flies' eggs it was the first attack on the theory of spontaneous generation.

By the middle of the 17th century, Parasitiology included only external parasites such as lice and fleas and a number of large internal parasites such as tapeworms and roundworms. For about a century there was little progress, until a great pioneer, K. A. Rudolphi (1771–1832), made a striking contribution.

Born in Stockholm, he spent most of his scientific life in Germany where he had graduated at Griefswald in Philosophy in 1793 and in Medicine in 1794. He showed an early interest in Parasitology, and 'Intestinal worms' was the subject of his MD dissertation. In 1808–10 he published his book on Entozoa. He described a number of new species of worms and seems to have been the first to have seen Taenia echinococcus. In 1810 he was invited to the Chair of Anatomy and Physiology at the newly-founded University of Berlin. There he attracted and influenced a number of foreign students including Richard Bright of Guy's Hospital, London.

Following Rudolphi's work on 'Entozoa' in 1808–10, there was a marked growth of interest in parasitic diseases resulting in the appearance of a number of treatises on the subject viz:

1853 'On Cestodes' by G. F. Kuchenmeister
1855 'Parasites in Man' by G. F. Kuchenmeister
1854 'On Taenia and Hydatids' by Carl Theodor von Siebold
1864 'On Entozoa' by Thomas Spencer Cobbold
1867 'Human Parasites' by Rudolf Leuckart

These were some of the leading names in Parasitology at the time and we single out for special mention Leuckart (1822–1898). After passing the State Medical Examination he became Associate Professor at Giessen where he was influenced by other staff members such as Justus von Liebig, the famous Chemist, and Theodor Bischoff, a well-known Anatomist and Embryologist. But Leuckart, although a Zoologist, was a Parasitologist at heart and known throughout the world for his expertise in this subject. It was therefore not surprising that when Wucherer (1820–1873) found a parasite (which turned out to be a microfilaria) in some blood clot in the bladder, he sent his preparations to Leuckart for confirmation. His contributions to his subject included some fundamental work on Onchocerciasis and a demonstration for the first time that in tapeworm disease T. Saginata occurred only in cattle and T. Solium only amongst pigs. But we must return to the discovery of a microfilaria by Wucherer, as the background of this is of interest and not generally well-known.

Otto Edward Henry Wucherer (1820–73), the son of a German merchant and a Flemish mother, was born in Portugal. He graduated in Medicine at Tübingen, and emigrated to Bahia in Brazil where he practised Medicine for the rest of his life. Wilhelm Griesinger, a Professor of Tübingen, went as Director of the Medical College of Cairo in 1850. He was described as 'a champion of German Physiological Medicine' and was also well known for his forensic work. He took with him as his assistant a young man called Theodor Bilharz. Bilharz had studied Natural History at Freiburg-in-Breisgau under Friedrich Arnold. In 1845 when Arnold went to Tübingen, Bilharz went with him and in this way met Griesinger. In Cairo Bilharz performed many dissections and found bladder lesions in which he discovered ova from the Nematode worm, Schistosoma. He observed the two different types of ova, later called 'haematobium' and 'mansoni', but did not associate them with two different diseases.[6] After two years work in Cairo, Griesinger returned to Tübingen and in 1852 was succeeded by Bilharz who later became Professor of Descriptive Anatomy. In this post he carried out some research on the electric organ of the thunderfish. It was sad that he lost his life at the early age of 37 from typhoid fever which he contracted on an expedition to Ethiopia with the German explorer Ernst von Coburg-Gotha.

While in Cairo with Bilharz, Griesinger had ample opportunity to see the parasitic ova of Schistosoma in the many cases of haematuria in Egypt. When Griesinger heard that his old pupil at Tübingen, namely Wucherer, was in practice in Brazil, he wrote and asked him to look out for these ova of Schistosoma in cases of haematuria in African slaves. The findings were negative until one day when he found the microfilaria in some blood clot in the urine. Some years later (1876) the adult female worm was found by Bancroft in an abscess of the arm.[7] This was the beginning of our knowledge of filariasis, a disease greatly advanced by Sir Patrick Manson (see later in this chapter).

Hook-worm disease or ankylostomiasis is historically interesting and illustrates the difficulties in putting together the pathogenesis of some parasitic conditions. The anaemia of the disease may have been observed in early times but was probably confused with the anaemia of chronic malaria, and the worm was not discovered until 1838 by an Italian named Angelo Dubini. But the lady possessing the parasite died of pneumonia and there was no indication of ill effects from the worm. In spite of this Dubini and others instituted a systematic search for worms at autopsy and obtained a number of positive results. In 1846 Pruner found the hook-worm in Egypt in association with 'Egyptian chlorosis', and in 1853 Bilharz pointed out the association of this worm which lived in the duodenum or jejunum with the presence of 'chlorosis'. In 1854 both Bilharz and Griesinger were emphasizing the worm and the anaemia as cause and effect. By 1866 Wucherer and other physicians in Brazil had found many similar cases.[8]

It was realised that hook-worm disease was one of the most prevalent in the world and by 1947 almost 400 million cases had been recognised.[9] It was generally considered to be a disease of the tropics though in temperate latitudes it occurred in the hot, damp atmosphere of mines and gave rise to what was called 'miners' anaemia'. Workers were exposed to high temperatures as ventilation was sadly lacking and hygiene and sanitation were non-existent. The importance of this disease in mines became obvious in the 1880s.

In 1872 the first railway in Switzerland was constructed, and it was a time when tunnelling was coming into vogue. It was therefore felt that the construction of a tunnel by boring through the Alps would greatly improve communications between Italy and Switzerland. As a result four such tunnels came into being, as follows, giving their time of commencement followed by their date of completion:[10]

| (1) | Mount Cenis | 1857–1871 |
| (2) | St. Gotthard | 1872–1882 |
| (3) | The Simplon | 1889–1905 |
| (4) | The Great St. Bernard | 1958–1962 |

From the time when the Thames Tunnel had been commenced in 1825 by Brunel, a number of hazards had been encountered. The Swiss tunnels proved to be no exception and a sharp lesson awaited the builders of the St. Gotthard. The construction of the tunnel by boring a single track resulted in very poor ventilation and made working conditions very difficult because of the dusty atmosphere. When the Simplon was bored with two tracks no such problem arose. The problems with the St. Gotthard continued for sudden large volumes of cold water on the Swiss side, and warm water on the Italian side, impeded the work of the men. Hygiene and sanitation were almost non-existent. In 1880 there was a sudden outbreak of anaemia, and investigation showed many cases to be infested with hook-worms. This infection was almost certainly brought in by Italian miners who had been recruited for the job. When the tunnel was completed in 1882 the miners dispersed and there were outbreaks of anaemia in the sulphur mines in Sicily, the lead mines of Spain, the coal mines in Germany, Belgium and France, and the tin mines of England.[11]

Studies of the hook-worm throughout the world have shown that there are two types of worm, similar but yet distinct and known as Ankylostoma duodenale and Necator americanus. For some time it was thought that these two worms existed in distinct areas, namely A. duodenale in the Old World in Europe and the Middle East and N. americanus in the New World in America and tropical Africa. This sharp distinction is no longer tenable.[12] The last episode in the story of ankylostomiasis unfolded in 1898. Up to this time it had been concluded that man became infected by mouth and that this was the only route. In 1866 Leuckart had shown that this could occur and Lichtenstein in 1887 had confirmed it experimentally.[13] But in 1898 the Professor of Parasitology in Cairo, Arthur Loos, accidentally let fall a drop of hookworm culture containing ankylostoma larvae onto his hand. He experienced some local irritation but gave it no treatment. When he subsequently examined his faeces he was able to find the tell-tale ova thus showing him that the larvae of ankylostoma were capable of infecting man by penetration of the skin. This is just one example of the difficulty in finding the mode of transmission of one of these parasitic diseases and brings to mind the pioneer work of Manson which came about in the later part of his life and in rather a fortuitous way. This work on the transmission of disease by insects has earned him the title of 'Father of Tropical Medicine' but Carmichael Low is careful to point out that there were many contributors to this subject as for example Martin, Annesley, Morehead, Chevers, Lewis, Cunningham and Fayrer in India; David Livingstone in Africa; and Finlay in Havana.[14]

Patrick Manson had graduated MB at the University of Aberdeen in 1865 and MD in 1866. In this latter year, on the advice of his brother in Shanghai, he went to Formosa as a medical officer, but in 1871 went to Amoy on the Chinese mainland. As a Customs Officer, with an appointment at the Baptists' Missionary Hospital and a certain amount of private practice, he saw much clinical material. It was at Amoy that he became interested in elephantiasis and found filariae in human blood for the first time. He devised a number of operative procedures for the disease and by the time he returned to London in 1874 was said to have removed a ton of tissue over a period of three years.[15] Over the next 15 years he made several journeys to London where he still pursued his interest in filariasis, and discovered the peculiar nocturnal appearance of Filaria bancrofti. Between the years 1885–9 he was in general practice in Hong Kong and founded the Medical School there for Chinese students.[16]

By now he had spent 23 years in China and had become an expert on tropical diseases. He returned to Scotland in 1890 to retire from active practice at the age of 45. But fate would have it otherwise for at this time the Chinese dollar depreciated sharply in value. As a result Manson was forced to return to London where he set up in practice once more and in 1892 was appointed Physician to the Seamen's Hospital Society. Two years later he was giving lectures on Tropical Diseases at Livingstone College, and at Charing Cross and at St. George's Hospitals. With filariasis there was the old problem, 'How did the larva get back from the mosquito to man?' For years Manson had always believed that mosquitoes died in water and man got infected by the larvae which had been liberated. He instituted a line of research in 1900 with Carmichael Low who was able to find larvae in the proboscis of the mosquito.[17] This new idea of transmission by the bite of an insect immediately led Manson also to consider its possibility in the case of malaria. As is well known Ross followed up Manson's suggestion successfully. As already mentioned, Manson was regarded as the Father of Tropical Medicine because of this concept of insect transmission of disease, which would not have been discovered at that time if he had not been forced to come out of retirement.

There are many points of interest in this world of parasites, not least the guinea worm. One wonders which should be more greatly admired – the skill of the witch doctor in removing the worm by means of his stick or the remarkable way in which the female locates an area of wet skin where she can deposit her larvae.

REFERENCES

1　Bullock, W., 'History of Bacteriology'. Oxford University Press 1938, p. 350.
2　Ibid p. 165.
3　'British Medical Journal'. (1898) ii, pp. 1705–6.
4　Stoll, N. R., 'This wormy World'. J. Parasitology, (1947) *33*, p. 16.
5　Shipley, A. E., 'Some ancient Worthies in Parasitology'. (1924–5) Vol. 10–11, pp. 182–3.
6　Dict. Scient. Biography, Vol II, p. 127. Charles Scribner's Sons, New York.
7　Friedheim, E., Schweiz. med. Wschr. (1966) *96*, No 34, pp. 1107–10.
8　Scott, W. H., 'A History of Tropical Medicine' 1939, Vol 2, pp. 840–53. Wilkins & Wilkins Co. Baltimore.
9　Stoll, N. R., 'This wormy World'. J. Parasitology, (1947) *33*, p. 16.
10　Beaver, P., 'A History of Tunnels'. Citadel Press, Secaucus, N. Jersey 1973 pp. 73–7.
11　Scott, W. H., 'A History of Tropical Medicine', 1939, Vol II p. 842. Wilkins & Wilkins Co. Baltimore.
12　Adams & MacGraith, 'Clinical Tropical Diseases'. Blackwell Scientific Publications, Oxford, 7th Ed. p. 163.
13　Scott, W. H., 'A History of Tropical Medicine' 1939, Vol II, p. 843.
14　Low, J. Carmichael, Trans. Roy. Soc. Trop. Med & Hygiene. 1929–30, *23*, p. 214.
15　Dict. Scient. Biography, Vol IX, (1974) pp. 81–3. Oxford University Press.
16　'Lancet'. (1922) i, pp. 767–9. Obituary.
17　Low, C. Trans. Roy. Soc. Trop. Medi & Hygiene 1929–30, *23*, pp. 220–1.

# EIGHTEEN
# The development of Bacteriology 1850–90

The advent of Bacteriology has been briefly mentioned and it was emphasised that it could only develop once the light microscope was sufficiently improved in order to visualise those small organisms, the bacteria. Their discovery revolutionised the knowledge of infectious disease and the progress can only be described as astonishing. In the short space of 20 years (1880–1900), the majority of bacteria pathogenic to man were discovered. In retrospect one is tempted to think of this period as one of the most exciting in the history of Medicine. Yet Frederick Andrews (later to become the first Professor of Pathology at Bart's), in writing of the early days of Bacteriology at Bart's, stated that there was not a great deal of enthusiasm, but rather more scepticism and doubt. Bacteriology developed along two main lines, namely Academic or pure bacteriology and Public Health or applied bacteriology. The latter became particularly important in the large English industrial towns where overcrowding was rife and strict public health measures became a necessity. It is interesting to note that in such towns as Birmingham, Leeds, Liverpool, and Manchester, the Chairs of Pathology when founded were designated 'Pathology and Bacteriology', a title not previously employed. Such was the progress of the new subject that in the early years of the 20th century independent Chairs of Bacteriology were being founded as for example in Manchester in 1905. It was not long before independent Chairs of Virology and Immunology were demanded. Concurrent with these advances were the needs for larger laboratory accommodation for experimental work and for practical instruction. Up to this time medical student education was almost purely theoretical. There were few laboratories, and it will be remembered that Beale with his enthusiasm for the microscope had his own private laboratory in 1851 as did Burdon Sanderson in 1868 for his experimental work on tuberculosis and pyaemia. But as mentioned earlier (chapter 16), laboratory space became more easily available with the foundation of the Brown Institute, the Institute of Preventive Medicine (later the Lister Institute), and the laboratories of the Conjoint Board.

Epidemics of infectious disease such as smallpox, typhoid, and typhus still occurred in the early 1800s though they were as yet not distinguished and were lumped together as 'fevers'. The gravity of such disease was accentuated when cholera made its first appearance in England in 1831. The theory of 'miasmas' was still in vogue, and as mentioned earlier in connection with Public Health, Chadwick regarded 'smell' and 'disease' as synonymous. Better sanitation led to improvement, though it should be emphasised that the measures adopted were those of simple hygiene and were instigated largely by a man (Chadwick) who had no medical qualifications. The cause of these fevers was not found for about another 50 years. Under the influence of medical men such as Sir John Simon and Dr. Southwood Smith hygiene was further improved, though when the next great development occurred it was related to the transmission of disease and not directly to its aetiology. John Snow, one of the earliest anaesthetists, was interested in Public Health as a hobby and the story of the Broad Street pump has been told many times. As a result, it now became realised that cholera could be transmitted by contaminated water, and Budd was soon to demonstrate the same for typhoid, though as yet nothing was known of the aetiology of these two diseases. John Simon, trained as a surgeon and a pathologist, realised that no further progress was likely until more was known of the natural history of disease. He therefore called for research to be carried out by his Medical Officers of Health including such outstanding workers as John Burdon Sanderson, who had been one of John Hughes Bennett's pupils in Edinburgh.

This was the state of affairs about 1868 when Sanderson had just confirmed the transmissibility of tuberculosis which Villemin had described in 1865.[1] Now the discovery of bacteria resulted in some startling progress when between 1880 and 1900 the majority of microorganisms pathogenic to man was discovered. As often happens progress is rapid once the first vital step has been taken, but in the case of bacteria this had been about 45 years in coming, and during these years there had been no lack of experimental work and certainly no lack of controversy.

There were, however, some other important discoveries, one of the most striking being the 'cell theory' of Schleiden and Schwann. This was to have far-reaching effects when it became taken up by Henle, and ultimately led to Virchow's great work on cellular pathology in 1858. Schleiden and Schwann had also believed that cells could arise *de novo* from 'a primordial fluid' but Virchow disproved it and maintained that a cell can only arise from another cell.

For some time past there had been other controversial matters including 'fermentation' and 'putrefaction'. Fermentation had been recognised for many centuries and was of importance because of its economic value. The formation of bubbles in the process bore some resemblance to effervescence and boiling, so that the chemists of the time regarded it as just another chemical reaction. It therefore came as a surprise when about 1836 three separate workers, namely, Cagniard-Latour, Theodor Schwann, and Friedrich Kützing, independently discovered yeast as the cause, thus establishing the 'germ theory of fermentation'.[2] Later Kützing was to recognise that different types of fermentation were brought about by different living microorganisms. Opposition from the chemists was not long in coming, for at the time great advances in chemistry had been made. Fermentation was firmly believed by notable chemists such as Liebig, Berzelius, and Wöhler to be a chemical process, and so the resentment at this sudden biological intrusion can perhaps be understood. The chemists' first response was to ridicule the whole idea, but they later maintained that yeast was a by-product of fermentation and therefore only secondary. Liebig accused the biologists of trying to explain everything on an anatomical basis in spite of their scanty knowledge, and raised once more the old problem of the 'Vital Force', which he thought would in the future be explained on a purely chemical basis.[3] But in 1838 Quevenna and Turpin had confirmed the results of the biologists[4] and so the controversy went on with the biologists steadily gaining ground. In 1857–60 Pasteur entered the field and in 1860 in his paper on alcoholic fermentation he showed himself to be diametrically opposed to Liebig and established the 'Germ theory of Fermentation'.

At this stage Pasteur also became involved in the dispute over 'spontaneous generation'. In the previous century it had been accepted that spontaneous generation did not occur in higher and more complicated animals, but the question whether it applied to 'animalcules' and hence to microorganisms was in doubt. The main argument ranged round 'putrefaction' and many experiments on this phenomenon were conducted. Redi (1626–97) had shown that maggots seen on decaying flesh did not arise de novo, but were produced from deposition of ova from flies. Spallanzani (1729–99) then showed that putrefaction did not occur if meat infusion was previously heated. An Irish priest named Needham (1713–81) entered the fray, disputed his findings and long arguments followed. Spallanzani refuted Needham's criticisms and his findings were subsequently confirmed by a number of workers including Schylze, Schwann, Schröder, and van Dusch and Tyndall.[5] It was established and accepted by most that microorganisms were carried in the air, and by the end of the 18th century it was generally agreed that spontaneous generation did not occur. There the whole matter might have rested, but about the middle of the 19th century the whole dispute erupted once more when an eminent French chemist named Pouchet (1800–72) claimed to have disproved Spallanzani's work. Pasteur took up the matter and conducted a series of complex experiments. Reading a summary of these,[6] one cannot but be impressed at the variety of places where Pasteur conducted his experiments and also the dusts examined by Pouchet from such places as the roof of the cathedral at Rouen, the Egyptian temple at Karnak, the banks of the Nile, the tomb of Rameses II, and the central chamber of the Great Pyramid at Gizeh.

The result of 20 years of controversy was that Pasteur's germ theory of fermentation and putrefaction was accepted by most scientists and that 'spontaneous generation' or 'heterogenesis' as it was more often called, was rejected. There were still some opponents, including Pouchet and Dr. Charlton Bastian, though their views differed somewhat. The terms 'homogenia' and 'heterogenia' indicated the two principal differences in the mode of origin of living things, i.e., in homogenia, an individual results from a pre-existing living thing similar to itself in organisation; heterogenia implied that living things came from matter of pre-existing organisms belonging to a totally different species.[7] Pouchet was therefore a heterogenist and was also a confirmed 'vitalist', who held that a pre-existing 'vital force' of some kind was necessary before a new individual could make its appearance. Charlton Bastian (1837–1915) was a physician at University College, London, who in 1887, when Assistant Physician, had also occupied the Chair of Pathology. He was later to become a Neurologist of some repute. In 1870 at the age of 33 he became embroiled in the dispute over 'heterogenesis'[8] and coined the word 'archebiosis' for his belief, namely that 'a living unit may originate from a non-living fluid, i.e., life begins *de novo* owing to the occurrence of new molecular combinations'.[9] He maintained this belief throughout his long life and in 1903 published a monumental work entitled 'Studies in Heterogenesis'.[8] In general, the contest had been between biologists and chemists and was fought on the battlegrounds of fermentation and putrefaction. Pasteur had observed different bacteria in different types of fermentation, but the application of his observations to medicine was still a few years in the future, during which the Germ Theory was to be disputed with heat and at some length. The concept of one living organism arising from a similar one, known as biogenesis, was a great biological milestone and was to find application in fermentation, putrefaction, and infectious diseases. For the moment, the opposite process, i.e., the derivation of a living organism from non-living material (abiogenesis) was shelved. It was therefore interesting to read in a recent symposium that abiogenesis might conceivably play a part in evolution. This conclusion, which would have delighted Bastian had he lived a further 40 years, runs as follows: 'Our concept of evolution and particularly the biochemical evidence seems to require that at some time in the distant past, life did emerge from a non-living milieu'.[10]

In the meantime there were some workers occupied in the study of bacteria related to disease in animals and man. About 1850 a French physician and pathologist, Pierre Rayer (1793–1867) described filiform rods in the blood of cattle dying from splenic fever, and a pathologist and parasitologist called Casimer-Joseph Davaine (1812–82) claimed to have made a similar observation independently. In 1855 a German worker, Franz Pollender (1800–1879) claimed to have seen these organisms back in 1849. The question was now raised as to whether these filiform rods could be the cause of the disease or only a by-product of putrefaction. But in the next 15 years Davaine and Rayer each showed that the disease could be transmitted to healthy animals by subcutaneous inoculation of blood from infected animals, and in 1864 Davaine and Raimbert found the same organism in malignant pustules in man.[11] They naturally maintained that this organism, which Davaine had called 'bacteridium', was the cause of splenic fever or anthrax, as it is now called. These experiments aroused a great deal of interest but some workers, notably Leplat and Jaillard at the Val de Grace military hospital in Paris, were unable to confirm them.[12] They claimed to have injected anthrax bacilli into animals but had been unable to recover them from the blood of dead animals. Davaine thought that his organisms were the same as those seen in the butyric fermentation by Pasteur, but Pasteur said that they were different. Davaine, Rayer and Pollender all found their filiform organisms non-motile, whilst Brauell in 1857 claimed that the organisms in his experiments were motile.[13] The dispute boiled down to whether Davaine's critics were really producing anthrax and Davaine maintained that they were not. It was not until 1876 that the whole problem became solved by Pasteur and Koch who, in a paper in 1876, confirmed that the organism was non-motile, that spore formation occurred under adverse conditions, and that germination could occur when favourable conditions returned. Lastly, they found that septicaemia appeared only very late in the experimental disease in mice.

The discovery of the cause of anthrax illustrates well the difficulties in correlating experimental results with clinical disease. Also the full picture of the disease had not been realised, because of the different forms that it may take.[11] The clinical features of the malignant pustule had been recognised in the 18th century and resulted from contact infection. The splenic fever observed in sheep and cattle was a septicaemic type of illness, this pattern being related to the mode of infection which is by ingestion of spores. The third type or 'wool-sorter's disease' was only recognised later and in a very interesting way. In 1878 in England a Bradford newspaper drew attention to three fatal cases of a disease amongst nine workers who were employed in the same shed in a wool factory. Further cases of this severe illness, which caused death in about 24 hours, were reported in the woollen industry in the West Riding district of Yorkshire. It transpired that about 1840 it had been decided to import mohair (from Asia Minor) and alpaca (from Peru), and in 1847 a similar case to the above had been noted. Subsequent examination of the wool showed it to be infected with anthrax spores, chiefly where blood had been spilled from the carcass.[14] Spores entered via the pulmonary route and spread throughout the body, chiefly by embolism from thrombosed vessels at the site of the primary infection. Again, the route of infection determined the clinical picture of the disease.

It was about this time that a striking application of Pasteur's discoveries became recognised. As far back as 1847 Semmelweiss in Vienna had reported his cases of puerperal sepsis which he had attempted to avoid by hygienic measures prior to maternal delivery. These observations had been rejected by other workers and 20 years later had been completely forgotten. Now was the time for surgery to be transformed into a modern art. Joseph Lister, born in 1827, was the son of a manager of a wine business, who had a remarkable interest in optics and had been elected FRS in 1832 for his researches on glass and the production of achromatic microscopic lenses. Young Lister had decided at an early age that he wanted to become a surgeon and having obtained a BA degree in 1847 at University College, London he commenced his medical studies in the following year. At the time University College and its hospital were noted for the quality of their work, and Lister as a student was fortunate in having amongst his teachers such men as Wharton Jones, William Sharpey, William Jenner, and W. H. Walshe. As a House Surgeon he later worked for Eric Erichsen. The recent discovery of anaesthetics had done much to extend and advance surgery, but there was still more to be done, and Lister was soon distressed at the high incidence of wound infections which included suppuration, erysipelas, and gangrene. In 1852 he had become a Fellow of the Royal College of Surgeons and in the following year he had taken the advice of his Professor of Physiology, William Sharpey, and spent some time studying surgical methods in Edinburgh and at a number of centres on the Continent. In Edinburgh he was impressed by the high standards of surgery compared with London, and became an assistant to James Syme. In 1860 he was appointed Professor of Surgery in the University of Glasgow. In the intervening years he had begun to study wound infection and wound healing and had had his attention drawn to an article written by Pasteur on the causes of fermentation and putrefaction by the Professor of Chemistry, Thomas Anderson.[15] Up to this time the doctrine of Liebig had prevailed, namely that putrefaction was due to oxygen in the air. Lister immediately became convinced by Pasteur's alternative theory, i.e. The Germ Theory of Putrefaction, and realised that microorganisms in the air might be responsible for the wound infections which he was encountering. From then on Lister was to show his ability as a bacteriologist. The amount and variety of his work were amazing especially when it is realised that he had no proper laboratory. Much of his earlier work on inflammation was done in his house in Edinburgh around 1857. His work on antiseptics was done during the Glasgow period (1860–9) and his bacteriological studies in his second period in Edinburgh (1869–77). All this work was done when he was pursuing an active surgical career both in private and hospital practice.[16] On the 9th August, 1867, at the Annual Meeting of the BMA in Dublin he read a paper to the Surgical Section entitled 'On the antiseptic principle in the practice of Surgery'.[17] Other surgeons were giving the method a trial and a paper was given by Hamilton at a meeting of the Medical Institution of Liverpool in 1868, reporting five cases of severe wounds which had been successfully treated. Of interest in this report is a reference to two other methods of the time of dealing with large wounds and amputations, namely (1) Paget's method of passing a current of air constantly over the part and (2) pneumatic occlusion as practiced by the French surgeons.[18]

The Franco-Prussian war broke out in 1870 and provided further experience in the treatment of wounds and emphasised their importance.

There was a high incidence of pyaemia on both sides. Buildings used to house the wounded consisted of private houses, schools, and churches, which were so constructed that efficient hygiene was well-nigh impossible.[19] Groups of English surgeons hastened to lend assistance to both sides and it appears that the German medical services were rather better than those of the French. Hospital overcrowding resulted in many cases of 'hospital gangrene'.[20] Disinfectants and antiseptics were used but did not seem to be effective. Lister had been asked to advise on the antiseptic treatment of wounds received on the battlefield and he devised a simplified method.[21] But this did not prove to be successful for the conditions were such as to preclude the satisfactory carrying out of the strict system demanded by Lister's regime.

Further details of Lister's outstanding contribution to Surgery are not necessary, for they have been ably described elsewhere.[22] Suffice it to say that during the next 20 years Lister continued his experiments with carbolic acid dressings and sprays and at the age of 65 on his retirement had his historic meeting with Pasteur at the Jubilee meeting in 1892 at the Sorbonne in Paris. From Glasgow Lister had returned to Edinburgh in 1869. In 1877 he returned to London to be Professor of Clinical Surgery at King's College, and after much opposition was able at last to convert his native city which had been so reluctant to accept his antiseptic doctrine. Like all great research workers Lister was never satisfied and was forever striving to improve his techniques. In his later years he decided to abandon the use of the carbolic spray and at the Berlin Congress in 1890 confessed his error. It illustrates well his rule of conduct expressed in a letter to Pasteur in another connection: 'Next to the promulgation of new truth the best thing I can see that a man can do is the recantation of a published error'.[23]

The next 20 years were to see a tremendous expansion of Bacteriology, but before dealing with this it will be necessary to consider some other lines of research which were in progress. In 1855 John Simon had been appointed Central Medical Officer attached to the Board of Health, and from 1858 till 1871 came under the Privy Council. It was during this latter period that he stimulated his assistants to learn more about infectious disease (see chapter 13). This group included a number of very able men and brief reference to some will give an idea of what they achieved. E. Headlam Greenhow graduated from Edinburgh and had a very versatile career. He practiced in Tynemouth with his father and in 1853 was responsible for saving the town from a cholera epidemic by vigorous application of the Public Health Act.[24] He moved to London in the same year and became Lecturer in Public Health at St. Thomas's Hospital. His main contribution was a two year 'Inquiry into the Different Proportions of Deaths produced by certain diseases in Different Districts in England'. It was the first time that a work of this kind had been attempted and John Simon thought it of sufficient importance to be presented as it was to Parliament in 1858. In subsequent years he made substantial contributions to the Annual Reports, which were submitted to the Privy Council.[25] These included his studies in diptheria and the pathology of industrial pulmonary disease.[26]

In 1837 Edward C. Seaton graduated from Edinburgh University and soon showed an interest in smallpox. He was chiefly responsible for an excellent report on vaccination made by a Committee of the Epidemiological Society, and when Simon inaugurated the systematic inspection of public vaccination Seaton was made the first inspector. In 1867 he wrote his 'Handbook on vaccination' and became the leading authority on the subject, and the subsequent improvements in the technique were largely due to him.[27]

Edward Ballard graduated from University College, London in 1844 and became Medical Officer of Health for Islington in 1856. He held this post till 1870 and in this period showed his ability as a good clinical observer, and his reports included studies on the smallpox epidemics between 1862 and 1867 as well as the cholera outbreak of 1866. He is best known for his report on the enteric fever outbreak in Holloway in 1870. In this, he was able to describe one of the first milk-borne epidemics of the disease.[26]

There were many other notable assistants including John Netton Radcliffe, a graduate of Leeds who, having served as a surgeon in the Turkish Army during the Crimean War, returned to England and became well-known as an epidemiologist. He is best remembered for his investigation of polluted water in the cholera outbreaks of 1866 in East London, and for his work on the milk-born epidemic of the same disease in 1873.[29]

When it comes to mentioning research work by Simon's assistants, the outstanding one is undoubtedly John (later Sir John) Burdon Sanderson. He received his medical education at the University of Edinburgh and obtained his MD degree in 1851. Amongst his earlier appointments he became Demonstrator to John Hughes Bennett, and this may have been responsible for his flair for research which he retained throughout his life. His main interest eventually became Physiology, but in his earlier years when he was Medical Officer of Health for Paddington from 1856 to 1867 under Simon, he was greatly interested in Public Health and infectious diseases. Simon sent him to the Danzig area to investigate an outbreak of cerebrospinal meningitis, a disease not well-recognised in Great Britain, and he made his report in 1865. In the same year he showed that cattle plague could be transmitted through the blood from an infected to a healthy animal. In 1868 at Simon's suggestion he had confirmed Villemin's work on the transmission of tuberculosis in experimental animals.[1] By now he was needing laboratory space for his experiments and we find that he had established his own private laboratory in Howland Street. Now his interest in infections was to move to the vexed questions of pyaemia and septicaemia.

For some time past there had been an idea that 'fevers' in general were the result of chemical substances similar to those produced during putrefaction. Now that there was a growing possibility of the importance of bacteria in human and animal diseases the burning question of the hour became 'the germ theory' of disease. The basis for this development had arisen many years previously when Bernard Gaspard (1788–1871) began some experiments in animals consisting of the injection of putrid substances of various kinds by intravenous, subcutaneous, intrapleural, and intraperitoneal routes. The work was commenced in 1808 and the results published between 1822 and 1824.[30] Sickness and death followed in the animals and the outstanding lesion was congestion of the alimentary tract. He also found that the condition could be transmitted from one animal to another. These results were confirmed by a number of workers including Magendie, who also found that putrid blood injected intravenously could be lethal, but was harmless when given by mouth. There the matter lay until in 1856 Virchow too confirmed these findings. Further experiments followed and Panum, a professor at Kiel, found that on filtering putrid infusions, injection of the residue produced 'putrid intoxication' (as it was then called), whereas the filtrate was without effect. Furthermore, he claimed that the residue, if boiled for 11 hours at 100°C was still active, and therefore concluded that the causative substance was neither a ferment nor a living microorganism.[31] The clinical picture in the experimental animals varied and 'putrid intoxication' was less severe than 'putrid infection'. Piorry in 1837 had introduced the terms 'septicaemia' and 'pyaemia' for these conditions, the former showing haemorrhagic alimentary mucosa and lack of coagulability of the blood; the latter, in addition to the above, was characterised by metastatic abscesses. In the succeeding years it was thought that the abscesses were primary and poured pus into the blood, hence the term 'pyaemia' which literally means 'pus in the blood'. Thus, for the next several years the question was hotly contested as to whether septicaemia and pyaemia were one or two diseases. By the late 1860s this had become more than an academic exercise. Lister was much concerned at the incidence of pyaemia in his surgical cases and in 1870 an additional source of material from the Franco-Prussian War stimulated more research. In recent years Mr. Valentine A. J. Swaine has written a most interesting article on voluntary medical assistance which was supplied to both sides by British and American men.[32] In 1863 an International Committee for the Relief of Wounded and Combatants had been founded in Geneva. With the outbreak of war in 1870 a British National Committee sent out 10 surgeons and 5 nurses to Germany. Later the number increased to 62 surgeons and 16 ladies, who were assigned equally to the German and French armies. In addition, there were many other groups including one of Bart's men with whom was associated an American surgeon, Mr. Charles Mayo, who went to the Metz area to help the Germans. The French at Sedan were given assistance by Sir William MacCormac who joined a group of eight American (including

Dr. Marion Sims) and eight English surgeons. Sir John Simon established a 200–250 bedded hospital at Bingen-on-Rhine, but it was destroyed in a storm on October 30th. In addition to medical casualties with smallpox (more prevalent in the French soldiers, many of whom were only partly vaccinated), typhus, and typhoid, it appears that the incidence of pyaemia and 'hospital gangrene' was considerable. In general the medical care on the German side seems to have been superior, and it appears that the French were not adopting the antiseptic techniques of Lister.

In the meanwhile Burdon Sanderson, with his previous experience in cerebrospinal fever in man and 'cattle plague' in animals, was ready to commence his research work on pyaemia and allied conditions in 1867. It was probably started at his private laboratory in Howland Street, and he was able to continue it when receiving further welcome additional laboratory space on his appointment as Professor-Superintendent of the Brown Institute in 1871. This work was to comprise his main interest and that of many others in the next 15 years. The following summary gives some idea of the degree of interest which the subjects excited. In 1872 Burdon Sanderson gave a report of his experiments which he had instituted in 1867 to the Pathological Society of London;[33] in 1873 he gave a paper on the subject to the Royal Medico-Chirurgical Society.[34] In 1874 a series of discussions were held on 'Pyaemia in Private Practice' at the recently founded (1867) Clinical Society of London.[35] In 1880 a report was made by a Committee of the Pathological Society of London on a survey of cases between 1869 and 1878.[36,37] This gives some idea of the activity in Great Britain, but in addition there had been some extensive research on the same subject in Germany which was summarised in the British literature.[38]

In order to appreciate the difficulties of the time in regard to pyaemia and allied conditions it will be necessary to give a few details about the research work. Soon the problem was linked with yet another problem of the time, namely the nature of the tubercle and whether it was a specific lesion or merely one aspect of chronic inflammation. As previously mentioned Burdon Sanderson had confirmed Villemin's work of 1865 on the transference of tuberculosis in experimental animals. He now turned his attention to pyaemia in 1867 and gave his first report on his results in 1872. The results were complex for there was no shortage of variables in the conditions of the experiments. Changes were induced by a variety of substances including animal or vegetable putrescent material, as well as pus from a case of pyaemia; different animals were used, viz., dogs, cats, and guinea pigs, while the route of injection was either subcutaneous, intraperitoneal, or intravenous. The general conclusions were quite surprising, namely that there were two types of infective lesions produced: (1) a pyaemic type with death in a few days and presence of metastatic abscesses; (2) a tuberculous type which was less acute and which gave rise to disseminated nodules, at first hard but later becoming caseous at their centres.

Sanderson believed that these two effects of injecting 'pyaemic fluids' were caused by damaging the blood and the 'vital functions', and that as a result the blood contained a poison which produced inflammation. The latter was responsible for the pyaemic and tuberculous reactions and he therefore referred to them as 'secondary inflammations'. The description of a tuberculous reaction does not seem to have aroused much, if any, controversy. It is true that over 50 years earlier Bayle and Laennec had described the tubercle as specific for tuberculosis, but this view was by no means universally held. It had been claimed that inoculation of many kinds of noxious matter might give rise to tubercles. Also the remarkable experiment of Cruveilhier may be remembered: he injected mercury into the femoral artery of a dog, and afterwards on dissecting the thigh found miliary tubercles in the soft parts, consisting of caseous material surrounding a minute globule of mercury.[39] Leading physicians in London such as John Elliotson and C. J. B. Williams believed in a very intimate connection between non-specific chronic inflammation and tuberculosis.[40] In 1847 Reinhardt published a detailed examination of the microscopic characters of 'tubercle' and stated that there was no difference between it and ordinary chronic inflammation. Many considered this to be the death blow to Laennec's theory of tuberculosis. Sanderson was inclined to believe that the location of the lesion, i.e. where there was much lymphoid tissue, favoured the production of a tuberculous lesion. One very interesting feature of his experiments with his assistant, Klein, was the demonstration of an enhanced reaction following passage through a second animal. But the explanation of Sanderson's tuberculous type of 'secondary inflammation' was not forthcoming for some years and in the meanwhile further developments were taking place.

In 1873 and 1874 fulminant pyaemia once more came up for discussion in a series of meetings of the Clinical Society of London, which had been recently founded in 1867. Its members were physicians, surgeons and general practitioners. It was therefore discussed by a different group and therefore from a different angle. Sanderson had always maintained that some cases of pyaemia could arise internally, presumably from lesions such as ostemelitis of the temporal and other bones. Some of the members of the Clinical Society had had considerable experience of the disease as, for instance, the senior surgeons of the large London teaching hospitals. Discussion by such men naturally ranged round the conditions which may complicate surgery and were the dread of the hospital surgeon, namely, septicaemia, pyaemia, erysipelas, and 'hospital gangrene'. The debate dealt largely with the external or environmental factors, and raised the problem as to whether the incidence of these conditions were greatest in private practice, small rural hospitals, small town hospitals or large town hospitals. The discussion did not generally support the view that pyaemia was a 'hospital disease', but surgeons recognised that overcrowding was an important factor in erysipelas and

287

'hospital gangrene'. Hospital construction was considered and an interesting application made to Lincoln County Hospital: because there were recurrent outbreaks of pyaemia in the hospital, but no cases had occurred in the town the governors decided to demolish the hospital and rebuild it.[41] In regard to the aetiology of pyaemia it was clear that the cause might be 'internal' or 'external'. Also, the mechanism of pyaemia and the formation of metastatic abscesses following septic thrombophlebitis was recognised. The situation in regard to septicaemia was that its characteristics consisted of a rapid course with scattered haemorrhages and an extreme congestion of the alimentary tract. As already mentioned, Sanderson regarded it as a circulatory upset, mediated by a 'poison'. Wounds were expected to produce pus, which was often referred to as 'laudable' or 'healthy' pus, to distinguish it from pyaemic pus. Injection of 'healthy' pus had no effect on experimental animals, but 'pyaemic' pus gave rise to pyaemia.

In view of the outstanding discrepancies, the Pathological Society of London appointed a committee to investigate 'The nature and causes of pyaemia, septicaemia, and purulent infection'. The report was issued in early 1880[42,43] and consisted of a statistical study of cases in the London hospitals between 1869 and 1878. From these cases the detailed clinical and pathological features of 156 were analysed and compared with the conditions caused by experimental injection of putrid fluids in animals. The findings were very complex but a few comments may help in trying to understand the state of knowledge at the time. In interpreting the experimental results following injection of putrid fluids into animals, Koch had recognised 'septic intoxication' as a condition induced by the injection of a large amount of material, which was followed by rapid death in a matter of hours, presumably to be explained on a chemical basis. 'Septic infection', by contrast, resulted from injection of smaller amounts and frequently caused death between two and 21 days. Koch concluded that during this interval, there was multiplication of the 'poison', which he thought might be related to bacteria multiplying in the blood. It appeared that 'septic intoxication' occurred clinically in man only rarely and that most cases were 'septic infection' and thus synonymous with septicaemia. It was thought that septicaemia and pyaemia, which occurred frequently in surgical diseases, and in post-operative and post-traumatic conditions, bore no relation to erysipelas, but were two different though similar states. However, the above conditions, i.e. septic intoxication, septic infection, septicaemia, and pyaemia were by no means clear-cut and there were cases which appeared to overlap. Septicaemia was characterized at autopsy by severe congestion of the lungs and swelling of the liver, spleen, and kidneys, while the characteristic of typical pyaemia was the presence of metastatic visceral abscesses. Had the matter rested here all would have been well but in the Committee's report pyaemia had been split up into ten sub-divisions, which ultimately turned out to be artificial and extremely confusing.

Thanks to the work of Virchow some 25 years previously the importance of thrombophlebitis and embolism had been recognized and provided a satisfactory explanation of the metastatic abscesses found in pyaemia. But the outstanding obstacle to further progress was that although bacteria of different kinds, i.e., micrococci, bacteria and others, had been encountered during these clinical and experimental studies, they were yet not recognised as the basis of these diseases. To make matters even worse, attempts were made to generalize by drawing analogies with types of infection such as anthrax which behaved in a manner peculiar to itself. Such was the work of British research workers of the time, though it would be wrong not to mention much work on similar lines which was appearing in the German literature.[44] In particular, the work of Birch-Hirschfeld was of interest. He recognised various types of micrococci in pyaemic pus and described granules in the pus cells, which would later be called 'toxic' granules and to be characteristic of many infections. He also distinguished 'healthy' pus from 'putrescent' pus, finding at the same time that injection of the former gave rise to a local abscess while the latter caused septicaemia.[45] All these discussions, important as they were, formed only part of a much wider horizon, namely, 'the role of bacteria generally in the causation of disease'. The problem of the origin of life was foremost in the days of the theory of spontaneous generation, and now the problem was the origin of disease. Discussion had been held at the French Academy but this had been theoretical and the results were sterile.[46]

The activity at the time in England is emphasized by a series of lectures given by J. Burdon Sanderson at Owen's College, Manchester on 'The occurrence of organic forms in connection with contagious and infective diseases' in 1875.[47] This was followed by a discussion on the 'Germ theory of disease' by the Pathological Society of London. It was opened by Dr. Charlton Bastian, the main opponent of the Germ Theory, and included seven main speakers. It occupied the time of the Society for the first half of 1875. The results could not be described as particularly fruitful, for it was a debate on theories and there was a serious shortage of badly-needed facts. It is however of great interest as an illustration of the last real opposition to the 'Germ theory of disease'. This theory had been clearly outlined by Henle, as far back as 1840 but had not received much acceptance until the 1860s, when the work of Pasteur and Lister added great impetus to it. A period then followed when many assumed that the demonstration of bacteria in a lesion was sufficient to establish it as the cause. Thus, when the discussion at the Pathological Society commenced, the opponents of the Germ theory, ably led by Charlton Bastian, set out to disprove it, rather than to propose an alternative explanation. As could have been anticipated, some speakers were in favour, some against, and some non-committal. There were no definite conclusions drawn but the general opinion seems to have been that the Germ theory in its present form was not acceptable. In view of the change which was to occur in the next few years with the almost universal acceptance of the theory, the reasons for this surprising turn-around might be briefly considered. At the time the striking feature of the discussion was the forceful leadership of the opponents by Charlton Bastian, who it will be remembered maintained his viewpoint of heterogenesis until his death in 1915. The two strongest proponents were Dr. T. J. Maclagen, then at Dundee, and J. Burdon Sanderson, Professor of Human Physiology at University College, London and Professor-Superintendent of the Brown Institute. Sanderson was probably the stronger of the two and he had been advocating the theory for at least four years. But on this occasion his communication was brief and he confined his remarks to facts, without indicating any of the conclusions which might follow. His lectures (referred to above) in Manchester were published in the 'British Medical Journal'[48] only a few weeks before his paper given at the Pathological Society.[49] These two communications by Burdon Sanderson provide a striking contrast to one another, and one senses a certain reluctance to take part in the discussion. If this is so, it probably relates to his fear expressed at Manchester when he stated, 'in the meantime, let us carefully guard against undue precipitation, in the process of combining the few facts that we are already in possession of, into a system'.[50] His remarks did little to strengthen the case in favour of the Germ theory and so it was left to Dr. T. J. Maclagen to play the part of the leading proponent at the next meeting of the Society. Dr. Bastian claimed to have proved that bacteria did not cause disease because fluids containing them had sometimes produced no effect and he also stated that the virulence of certain contagious mixtures diminished in direct proportion to the increase in bacterial content. Dr. Maclagen countered these with two remarkable statements, namely that (1) no advocate of the germ theory had stated that bacteria caused the phenomena of disease, and (2) that disease was caused by much smaller organisms which had not yet been seen, but which underwent degeneration, after which bacteria appeared. These arguments did not carry much weight; the rest of his communication was much more convincing, but dealt only with specific fevers. He obtained support for his theory by referring to the differing natural history of these specific fevers. The growth of millions of germs with increased nitrogen and water consumption would account for the features of the febrile state; the duration of the fever would be determined by the amount of a certain material required for the organic growth of the germs; the seat of the local lesions differed from one disease to another in that in only certain localities could 'the contagium particles find something which is requisite to their fecundation and propagation as distinguished from their organic growth'.[51] All this is highly theoretical but he did allude to a practical aspect in saying that the local site in the instance of Lister's cases was the wound. It was surprising that more was not made of the four specific diseases which most clearly showed a connection with organic forms, namely, cowpox, sheep pox, splenic fever and relapsing fever. From the accounts at the time this discussion was not very successful. There were certainly some notable absentees such as Sir William Jenner, Sir John Simon, Joseph and Lionel Beale. They could have added much though the greatest pity was the small contribution from Burdon Sanderson, who probably knew more and had done more research himself than any of the others.

But if the Germ Theory lacked support in 1875 some startling changes occurred in the next few years. In 1876 Koch demonstrated the anthrax bacillus as the cause of splenic fever and was able to explain the long survival of the organism under adverse conditions. In 1879 Pasteur discovered attenuation of the bacillus of chicken cholera. At the International Congress of Medicine in London in 1881, Koch demonstrated his solid culture technique. By 1883 the Germ Theory had become widely accepted, a striking contrast to the state of affairs eight years previously. But the really great triumph was in 1882 when Koch discovered the bacillus which caused tuberculosis. Throughout the whole of this century tuberculosis had exacted its toll and now fresh interest in the subject was aroused; it was even said 'that the subject bids fair to monopolise the attention of the scientific world' as a result of Koch's discovery.[52] In order to appreciate the importance of Koch's discovery, it will be necessary to recall some of the earlier views on tuberculosis.

One of the highlights of the French School of Pathological Anatomy was a description of the symptoms and the gross lesions of pulmonary tuberculosis, or phthisis as it was then called. For this we are indebted to Gaspard-Laurent Bayle and his friend René Laennec.[53] Laennec's description of the pathological lesions in the lung is of great interest.[54] He described the coalescence of the tuberculous lesions and the subsequent formation of cavities. In view of the rather lax use of the word 'tubercle' in the literature his definitions are useful. The smallest lesions are of the size of a millet or hemp seed and are called miliary tubercles. When smaller lesions unite they 'form more or less voluminous masses, pale yellow in colour and opaque' and are then called 'crude tubercles'. He also pointed out that these large masses may be formed without any previous development of miliary tubercles. Lastly he made an interesting comment on the latter, namely, 'they have the appearance of having all come into being on the selfsame day, and usually no single one of them is visibly in a more advanced state than any other'.[55] Apart from its pathological interest the real significance of this work was to indicate that tuberculosis of the lungs was a specific disease process and not just a variant of what might be called ordinary chronic inflammation. This viewpoint seems to have been widely accepted on the Continent, but in Great Britain it was not necessarily so. Indeed, about the middle of the century well-known physicians such as Thomas Addison, John Elliotson, and Charles J. B. Williams (a pupil of Laennec) believed chronic inflammation and tuberculosis to be identical. When in 1847 Reinhardt

291

published a detailed account of the microscopic features of 'tubercle', he asserted that there was no difference between it and chronic inflammation, and this was thought to be the death-blow to Laennec's theory.[56] In 1865 Villemin used rabbits to show that tubercle could be transmitted from one animal to another.[57] This would seem to add strength to Laennec's theory, but contemporary workers were reluctant to accept it. As a result, John Simon suggested that Burdon Sanderson should attempt to confirm it, and this he did successfully in 1868. It was then that some research work was published which bedevilled the whole problem for the next 15 years. It will be recalled that between 1867 and 1871 Burdon Sanderson was engaged in some work on pyaemia involving tissue reactions to the inoculation of a variety of 'putrid fluids'. There were two types of reaction: (1) an acute pyaemic reaction with metastatic abscessess and (2) a more chronic lesion with formation of small nodules resembling miliary tubercles. Other workers such as Cohnheim, Frankel, Wilson Fox and others confirmed that tubercles could be produced by inducing simple inflammation by the insertion of vaccine virus, threads, pieces of cork, paper and other non-tuberculous materials.[58] Many similar experiments had been done in the past as for example the production of the miliary tubercles in the lower limb following the injection of metallic mercury into the femoral artery of a dog by Cruveilhier.[59] Lebert and Wyss claimed to have produced tuberculosis in rodents by the injection of mercury and charcoal into the jugular vein.[60] With such weighty evidence the matter appeared to have been settled and it does not seem to have been discussed further during the next few years. Sanderson must have had his reservations for he concluded that nothing 'induced tuberculosis with such constancy as material taken from an undoubted tubercular source'.[61] In 1882 the whole controversy once more broke out when Koch claimed to have identified the tubercle bacillus as the specific agent which gave rise to tuberculosis. Klebs had suggested that the 'non-tuberculous' material used in the earlier experiments might have been contaminated. Cohnheim, who had obtained his results in Berlin, failed to repeat them in Kiel and Breslau, and Frankel had a similar experience when he repeated his experiments in a private house.[61] In England, at the request of Sanderson and Wilson Fox, Dr. Dawson Williams was asked to repeat their earlier experiments. This was done, there being care to avoid contamination, no antiseptics were used in the procedures, and the results were all negative. They were communicated to the Pathological Society of London on 4th December 1883, and the President expressed his gratitude to Dr. Wilson Fox and Dr. Dawson Williams for bringing the error to light.[62] The theory that tuberculosis was a specific disease now seemed established and Cohnheim lent his support. In Germany the subject was debated at the Berlin Medical Society in November 1883[63] and by the Congress of German Physicians at Wiesbaden in April 1883, where surprisingly Professor Klebs was unwilling to accept Koch's specific theory.[64] It had been a protracted struggle to establish the nature of tuberculosis and this is partly due to the ingrained belief that the disease 'ran in families' and that there were certain inherent factors which predisposed sufferers to it.

This part of the subject cannot be left without saying yet a further word on the pyaemic experiments carried out by Burdon Sanderson in 1867.[65] These results proved misleading to workers for many years. Errors in research are liable to occur, but in this case it is surprising that the 'errors' were also confirmed by men as eminent as Cohnheim and Frankel.[58] The 'tuberculoid' reactions to a large number of different 'putrid fluids' seem to have been of two kinds: (1) large lesions in the lung with characteristic caseation, and (2) miliary tubercles in the lungs, but also in the spleen and liver, and occasionally in other organs. In fact some animals had clinical tuberculosis whilst others had miliary tubercles and Burdon Sanderson himself stated that 'nothing induced tuberculosis with such certainty as material taken from an undoubted tubercular source'.[61] Cruveilhier's experiment of injecting metallic mercury into the femoral artery of the dog had shown miliary tubercles in the thigh, but there is no mention of tuberculosis and these lesions were presumably 'foreign body' in type. In more recent years Pagel investigated the tissue reactions to many organisms and materials in mice and guinea-pigs and stated 'the foreign body elicits by its mechanical and surface action the typical foreign-body giant cell and nothing else; however foreign material to which a certain chemical effect is added will provoke granulomata indistinguishable from tubercles with all intermediate forms of giant cells between the Langhans and foreign-body type'.[66] It would therefore seem possible that Burdon Sanderson's miliary tubercles were in reality modified foreign-body granulomata induced by the crude putrid materials. The animals with clinical pulminary tuberculosis might have been inoculated with contaminated material or even with tuberculous material itself.

As has been seen, the earlier studies of bacteria bore little relation to man and much of the work related to animal disease. It was only when Lister foresaw the application of Pasteur's results that bacteriology became predominantly medical. The advances were so diverse that by the end of the century it was beginning to become a subject separate from the newly-founded Pathology. To this great advance many workers contributed, but the three great names were Koch, Lister, and Pasteur. Koch, originally a general practitioner, took up laboratory studies on his return from service in the Franco-Prussian War. By meticulous technique he put bacteriology on a firm base. In 1876 he confirmed the anthrax bacillus as the cause of anthrax, and in 1882 discovered the tubercle bacillus. But his outstanding contributions were (1) his method of obtaining bacteria in pure culture; (2) his use of stains to demonstrate bacteria; and (3) the formulation of Koch's postulates. The latter could well have been the most important for at this time when many bacteria were being described, there was the great danger of assuming that the presence of bacteria automatically established them as being the cause of the disease. Lister's contribution was essentially practical and applied to Surgery. Brought up in the midst of his father's optical researches, it was natural for him to turn to the microscope and throughout his career he carried out many bacteriological researches. He was trained as a surgeon and practiced the art throughout his life and laid claim to be the father of modern surgery. Once his techniques had been accepted, surgery expanded to an enormous extent and carried with it a safety which had never been known before. Pasteur maintained his versatile career and his interest in medical problems was recognised by his election to the Paris Academy of Medicine in 1873. He pursued a different route in bacteriology from that of Koch and it is surprising that his name was never connected with the discovery of a new organism. He was a man of brilliant ideas and an astute observation was to determine his future interests. In 1879 the bacterium which caused chicken cholera was discovered by Perroncito and cultured by Toussaint. In the following year Pasteur, working on this organism, found that the virulence declined when it was kept in culture and regained it when injected into animals. He at once demonstrated the possibility of attenuated organisms in making vaccines. He had been interested for some time in the lifelong immunity which followed an attack of smallpox, and from then onwards all his energies were devoted to immunity and the prevention of disease. In the next year he was able to show the value of vaccines in the prevention of such diseases as anthrax, swine erysipelas, and rabies. In 1881 he attended the International Congress of Medicine in London, and gave a paper on 'Vaccination in relation to chicken cholera and splenic fever'.

While these remarkable events were taking place on the Continent there were some interesting developments in Great Britain even apart from the great work done by Lister. At the time when the term 'pathologist' was beginning to be freely used, the leading figure was probably W. S. Greenfield. Educated at University College, London, he became Professor-Superintendent of the Brown Institute in London (1878–1881) and Professor of Pathology at the University of Edinburgh (1881–1912). He gave one of the earliest descriptions of the histology of Hodgkin's disease, and worked out the bacteriology of woolsorter's disease in 1880.[67] Less well-known is the fact that he prepared an anthrax vaccine of attenuated organisms about a year before Pasteur.[68]

As indicated, the opposition to Lister in London had been considerable and at times he must have been glad that he brought with him his small team from Edinburgh in 1877. Chief amongst these was William Watson Cheyne (1852–1932), who as a young medical student had become fired with enthusiasm on hearing one of Lister's lectures. In 1880 he had been made Assistant Surgeon to King's College Hospital and with Rickman Godlee was one of Lister's loyalest supporters. He was also made Demonstrator of Surgical Pathology and carried out microscopic examinations on his specimens. He inaugurated and paid for the establishment of an Institute of Clinical Pathology, and had as his assistant Lenthal Cheatle.[69] In this way Clinical Pathology became recognised as a hospital department. He won the Jacksonian Prize of the Royal College of Surgeons for his essay on 'Principles, practice, history, and results of antiseptic surgery'. He became a very successful surgeon, was made Professor of Clinical Surgery, and wrote a work on 'Antiseptic Surgery' and also a 'Manual of Surgical Treatment'.[70]

Another supporter of Lister's theory was Edgar Crookshank (1858–1928), who qualified in Medicine in 1881 and had been one of Lister's dressers. Partly because of this he was selected to go to the Egyptian War where he was present at the battle of Tel-el-kebir. On the basis of his experience he wrote a detailed account of antiseptic surgery in the war. At this time he had decided to devote himself to Bacteriology and therefore visited Pasteur in Paris and Koch in Berlin.[71] On his return he published his 'Manual of Bacteriology' in 1886 and was appointed Professor of Bacteriology at King's College Hospital in the same year. It was the first Chair in the subject, and was to be the only one for many years.[72] Soon afterwards he was put in charge of the first laboratory in England for research and teaching in Comparative Pathology.[72] With the above experiences, a young man appointed to a Chair at the age of 28 would seem to be on the threshold of a most promising career. But surprisingly and inexplicably, he resigned his Chair three years later and for the remaining 42 years of his life devoted himself to local politics in Sussex and to world travel.

Like Lister and Watson Cheyne, Alexander Ogston (1844–1929) was a surgeon with a considerable interest in Bacteriology. He was a graduate of the University of Aberdeen in 1865 and studied on the Continent in Prague, Vienna, Berlin, and Paris. He was greatly impressed by Lister's work and applied his principles to bone surgery in which he took an early interest.[74] His research into suppuration was rewarded in 1882 when he discovered staphylococci by examining the pus from 100 abscesses.[75] He had a very successful surgical career, being Senior Surgeon at the Aberdeen Royal Infirmary from 1880 to 1898 and subsequently Professor of Surgery at the University in 1882. His war service was very extensive for he took part in three wars, namely, the Egyptian War, the Boer War and World War I. Participation in the latter was remarkable as he was 69 when war broke out.

With bacteriology set on a firm basis by the technical achievements of Koch, the developments between 1880 and the end of the century can only be described as phenomenal. During this short period most of the bacteria pathogenic to man were discovered. In 1883 Koch went to Egypt with the German Cholera Commission and discovered the Vibrio Cholerae. He followed up his work on tuberculosis and at the 10th International Congress in 1890 he claimed that in tuberculin he had found a remedy for the disease. Unfortunately this did not materialise though his tuberculin became useful as a diagnostic agent. In the following year the new Institute for Infectious Diseases was opened and students flocked to Berlin in even greater numbers. There were many other institutes founded in Europe but the only one which rivalled Berlin was of course the Pasteur Institute in Paris, which also became a centre for young bacteriologists to visit. This had been opened in 1889 and, because of Pasteur's interest in attenuation of bacteria, concentrated its research to a large extent on immunity. In the next few years vaccines became available for chicken cholera, swine erysipelas, anthrax and rabies. In 1883 Pasteur had organised a French Cholera Commission which, like the German one, went to Egypt. Thuillier, who had worked with Pasteur on swine erysipelas, accompanied the Commission but succumbed to cholera at the early age of 27. In 1889 Roux and Yersin demonstrated the effects of diptheria exotoxin, and in the same year Faber obtained a similar exotoxin from tetanus bacilli. In 1890 von Behring and Kitasato showed that immunity developed after the administration of diptheria exotoxin, which gave rise to an antitoxin. In late 1891 (on Christmas night) Geissler, working in von Bergmann's clinic in Berlin, successfully treated a diphtheritic child with diptheria antitoxin.

In 1894 a young Belgian bacteriologist joined the staff of the Pasteur Institute, namely, Jules Bordet (1870–1961). In 1901 he founded the Pasteur Institute in Brussels, and became the leading immunologist of the day. He worked on many aspects of immunity but is chiefly remembered for discovering the part played by heat-labile complement in haemolysis and bacteriolysis. This work paved the way for the establishment of the Wasserman test for syphilis in 1906. In his early days at the Pasteur Institute in Paris he had worked as assistant to the great Russian scientist Eli Metchnikoff (1845–1916). Metchnikoff had been educated at the University of Kharkov and had studied marine biology in Heligoland, and zoology at Giessen, Göttingen, and Munich under Leuckart, Henle, and von Siebold. In 1870 he was made Professor of Zoology and Comparative Anatomy at Odessa. In 1882, because of political troubles, he resigned his chair and became Director of the municipal bacteriological laboratory. Later he left Russia and after spending a short time in Messina he accepted an invitation from Pasteur to work at the Paris Institute in 1883, where he subsequently became sub-director.[76] At this time considerable rivalry had sprung up between the Paris and Berlin Institutes and therefore between Pasteur and Koch. As a member of the Paris Institute Metchnikoff was soon to experience opposition from the German bacteriologists. This all arose in connection with research on the basic mechanisms of immunity. It had been found that blood and tissue fluids appeared to have some inimical effects on bacteria. In 1888 these were confirmed by a British bacteriologist called Nuttall (1862–1937) working in Flugge's Institute in Göttingen. At this stage Hans Buchner (1850–1902) of Munich embarked on a long series of experiments on bactericidal substances which he named 'alexines' (from the Greek word meaning 'to defend'). Thus arose the 'humoral theory' of immunity which was accepted for a number of years.[77] However the cellular theory of immunity sponsored by Metchnikoff provided some opposition. For some years it had been known that leucocytes could engulf bacteria and in 1874 Panum had suggested that this might be a method of destroying microbes. Metchnikoff, working at first with starfish and then with certain crustaceans, observed phagocytosis by some mesodermal cells which possessed some digestive powers. He extended his observations to bacterial infections such as anthrax and erysipelas and in 1883 launched his theory which maintained that immunity was mediated by cellular rather than by humoral mechanisms.[78] This dispute lasted for at least the next ten years, and some idea of its intensity can be obtained by reading the report of the Bacteriology section at the International Congress of Hygiene and Demography held in London from the 10th–17th August, 1891.[79] In this discussion the leading proponents of the two theories were Metchnikoff for the cellular and Buchner for the humoral, while Dr. Hankin took up an intermediate position. At that time the cellular theory seems to have been in the ascendant but in the next few years the humoral theory advanced as the actions of toxins, antitoxins, and other antibodies were discovered. Amongst Metcknikoff's many interests was one in death which he believed was related to intestinal flora. When aged 70 his colleagues and friends gave a dinner in his honour, and he addressed them afterwards on the subject of 'Death'.[80] It consisted of a study of the short life of the silkworm moth, and his attempt to find the cause of death. Eight months later he himself died and his ashes are preserved in the Pasteur Institute.

With Paris and Berlin the focal points of bacteriology, one might wrongly assume that there had been little going on either in America or Great Britain. But in America the subject was being advanced by such men as Flexner and Welch, and in 1886 D. E. Salmon (1850–1914) and Theobald Smith (1859–1934), working in the Bureau of Animal Industry in Washington, showed that a vaccine of dead organisms could induce immunity against live bacteria. Live vaccines had carried with them some risk, and with this eliminated, trials with dead vaccines became increasingly more common. Theobald Smith went on to have a very successful career at Harvard, where he was Professor of Comparative Pathology (1896–1915) and at the Rockefeller Institute as Director of the Department of Animal Pathology (1915–1929).[81]

In Great Britain it is true that no school of Bacteriology developed as in France and Germany. When an institute was founded it was some years later, for the British Institute of Preventive Medicine, founded in 1891, was not engaged in active work till 1893 and later. The reason for this seems to have been the fact that the three early British contributors to the subject were not primarily bacteriologists. Also at the time there were very few trained pathologists like W. S. Greenfield, who might have been attracted to the subject. Lastly, the establishment of Chairs of Pathology and the University recognition of the subject were still in the future.

The greatest contribution from Britain came from Joseph Lister. But he could not have founded an institute whilst running a busy hospital and private surgical practice. When we realise what he did achieve, it is remarkable that he ever found time to carry out the pathological studies of wounds and his bacteriological experiments. His influence as a medical man did much to direct attention to human diseases, rather than those of animals which were largely studied in the very early days of bacteriology.

One man who has not been widely recognised is William (later Sir William) Roberts (1830–1899). The son of an Anglesey practitioner, he had studied medicine at University College, London and graduated in 1853. He had shown remarkable ability as a student and greatly benefitted by having for his teachers such men as Sharpey, Walshe, Garrod, Jenner, Quain (Jones), Hare and Erichsen. Wilson Fox and George Buchanan were amongst his contemporaries, and he was Dresser to Mr. Erichsen at the time when Joseph Lister was his House Surgeon. He subsequently went to Manchester where he spent about 30 years on the active staff of the Royal Infirmary, and also became the first Professor of Medicine at the new Victoria University. He wrote on many subjects and in 1865 published 'A Practical Treatise on Urinary and Renal Diseases' which was a great success. From the time that he was Lecturer in Pathology at Manchester, he was always interested in research and fitted up a small workroom in his home. Even when provided with laboratory space at the new Owen's College he still continued to do his experiments at home. In 1874 he published a paper on 'Biogenesis' and this took him into the controversy of spontaneous generation.[82] His further interest in this subject culminated in an address at the B.M.A meeting in Manchester, entitled 'Contagium vivum and its application to Medicine'.[83] Roberts was a strong supporter of Lister, and it was felt that this address had established the Contagium Vivum Theory on a firm basis. Roberts had conducted a number of experiments on the sterilisation by heat of hay infusions and other mixtures. Some of the results were anomalous and indeed inexplicable, as for instance, when he found that alkaline nutritive media were much more difficult to sterilise than were acid ones. These results, strange though they appeared, had been confirmed by Ferdinand Cohn in Breslau, and now a similar attempt was to be made by an Englishman named John Tyndall.

John Tyndall (1820–1893) was a physicist who became Professor of Natural Philosophy at the Royal Institution in 1853, and on the death of Faraday in 1867 he succeeded him as Resident Director. He was an outstanding research worker, who was also well-known for his clarity of exposition. His research covered many aspects of his subject, and in 1870 he was engaged in demonstrating particles in the air by means of a beam of light, and methods by which these particles could be removed. In that year he first made known his views on germs in the air, and this was the signal for a sharp reply from Dr. Charlton Bastian, who felt that a physicist should not invade the terrain which properly belonged to biologists and physicians.[84] Tyndall was able to confirm Roberts' experiments and he communicated his results to the Royal Society[85] in papers entitled 'The optical deportment of the atmosphere in relation to the phenomena of Putrefaction and Infection' and 'Further researches on the deportment and Vital Persistence of Putrefactive and Infective organisms from a physical point of view'. By now, Tyndall was involved in the midst of the spontaneous generation controversy, and his results gave the final blow to the theory. He had found that bacteria had a sensitive and a resistant phase to sterilisation by heat, and Ferdinand Cohn was one of the first to demonstrate that spores were endowed with great heat-resisting properties. In 1887 Tyndall retired from his Chair of Physics and it is sad to relate that he died in 1893 when he accidentally poisoned himself with chloral hydrate.[86]

The above gives some idea of the great achievements of a few individuals prior to the development of a concerted effort by many. This occurred when the British Institute of Preventive Medicine (later the Lister Institute) commenced its work, and an interesting event involving the first Director, Dr. Marc Armand Ruffer (1859–1916), should be told.

As already mentioned, the 1880s were characterised by some brilliant advances in immunisation, which occurred at the Pasteur Institute when vaccines were prepared against chicken cholera, swine erysipelas, anthrax, and rabies. In 1889, Emile Roux (1853–1933) and Alexandre Yersin (1863–1943), working with Pasteur in Paris, had discovered that the effects of diptheria were caused by an exotoxin derived from the bacillus. In the following year, Emil von Behring (1854–1917) and Kitasato (1852–1931), working in Koch's laboratory in Berlin, announced the discovery of antitoxin having the power of specifically neutralising diptheria exotoxin. Shortly after this, a young British pathologist of French parentage, namely, Armand Ruffer, was working in the Pasteur Institute and was taught Roux's technique of preparing diptheria antitoxin by immunising horses (1892). On Ruffer's return to England he became the first Director of the new British Institute of Preventive Medicine (see chapter 16) and it was there that diptheria antitoxin was first produced in Britain. Professor G. S. Wilson tells of an interesting happening at the time. While Ruffer was immunising a horse against diptheria, the nephew of a young physiologist called Sherrington contracted the disease. Ruffer allowed him to take some serum from this horse (which was only partly immunised), and some hours after administration the boy made a dramatic recovery (1894). It would therefore seem that Sherrington, who was later to become the leading British neurophysiologist, was the first person in Britain to administer antitoxin therapy for diptheria.[87]

Such was the state of affairs in bacteriology at the end of the 19th century and the extraordinary advances already made still continued. The study of viruses properly belongs to the next century. However, in 1871,

Tiegel had filtered anthrax bacilli and in 1884 Charles Chamberland (1851–1908), working with Pasteur, designed a filtration apparatus in the form of a hollow candle made of unglazed porcelain;[88] other types were designed at the time. This led to the description of infective agents which were called viruses, and were 'filtrable' because they could pass through a bacterial filter, or 'ultramicroscopic' because they were too small to be seen with the light microscope. This subject is raised because there were two remarkable observations made in the 19th century on viruses which are frequently overlooked. John Brown Buist was a bacteriologist in Edinburgh and a surgeon and superintendent at a smallpox hospital in the town. In 1887 he took some fluid from a vaccination, spread it on a slide and stained it with Gentian Violet. When he examined the slide under the light microscope he observed many small round granules. He thought that they were the infectious agent of the condition but he was unable to culture them. When he measured them he came to the conclusion that they were spores. His observations were overlooked for many years. But in 1904 the French bacteriologist Borrel and the German bacteriologist Paschen independently rediscovered these elementary bodies and they were subsequently referred to as 'Borrel bodies' or 'Paschen bodies'.[89]

The failure to cultivate viruses on artificial media precluded the possibility of applying Koch's postulates to the investigation. It was soon found that this difficulty could be overcome by the use of the 'virus neutralisation test'. By this technique the activity of the virus is neutralised by the action of a specific immune serum. Such a test had been carried out in 1892 by the American George M. Sternberg (1838–1915). He was a medical officer in the Federal Army and was captured at the battle of Bull Run, though he later escaped. He showed that inoculation of a calf with 'vaccination material' to which serum from an immune calf had been added failed to produce a vaccination ulcer. Sternberg must have been very versatile for he is said to have discovered phagocytosis in 1881, three years before Metchnikoff, and also to have developed modern photomicrography. He rose to become Surgeon General of the U.S. Army and was called the 'Father of American bacteriology' by no less a person than Robert Koch.[90]

REFERENCES

1  MacNulty, A. S., Fitzpatrick Lectures 1946–7, p. 38. Royal Institute of Public Health & Hygiene.
2  Bulloch, W., 'History of Bacteriology'. Oxford University Press 1938, p. 46.
3  'Lancet'. (1846) ii, pp. 549–52.
4  Bulloch, W., 'History of Bacteriology'. Oxford University Press 1938, pp. 51–2.
5  Ibid p. 3.
6  Ibid pp. 94–105.

7   Ibid p. 79.
8   'Lancet'. (1915) ii, p. 1228.
9   Bulloch, W., 'History of Bacteriology'. Oxford University Press 1938, p. 93.
10  Ann. N. Y. Acad. Sci. 1957, *69*. p. 257.
11  Wilson G. S. & Miles A. A., 'Topley & Wilson's Principles of Bacteriology and Immunity'. Williams & Wilson Co. 5th Ed. 1964, pp. 2208–9.
12  Bulloch, W., 'History of Bacteriology'. Oxford University Press 1938, p. 181.
13  Ibid p. 180.
14  'Lancet'. (1926) i, pp. 57–8, 107–9.
15  Cameron, H. E., Lister Centenary Celebration, Oct. 1927, p. 44. American College of Surgeons, Detroit, Michigan; Wellcome Historical Med. Museum.
16  Bulloch, W., 'British Medical Journal'. (1927) i, p. 655.
17  'British Medical Journal'. (1871) i, pp. 31–2.
18  Ibid (1968) i, p. 413.
19  'Lancet'. (1870) ii, pp. 922–31.
20  'British Medical Journal'. (1874) i, p. 132.
21  Cameron, H. E. Lister Centenary Celebration, Oct. 1927, p. 91. American College of Surgeons, Wellcome Historical Med. Museum.
22  Ibid p. 11.
23  Ibid pp. 50–1.
24  Lambert, R., 'Sir John Simon 1816–1904'. Macgibbon & Kee, London 1963, p. 199.
25  'British Medical Journal'. (1888) ii, pp. 1104–6.
26  Trans. Path. Soc, (1864) *65*, p. 68.
27  'British Medical Journal'. (1880) i, p. 188.
28  Ibid (1897) i, pp. 281–2.
29  Ibid (1884) ii, p. 588.
30  Bulloch, W., 'History of Bacteriology'. Oxford Univeristy Press 1938, pp. 129–30.
31  Ibid p. 132.
32  'British Medical Journal'. (1970) ii, pp. 511–14.
33  Ibid (1872) i, pp. 508–10.
34  Ibid (1873) i, pp. 601–2.
35  Ibid (1874) i, pp. 380–6.
36  Ibid (1880) i, pp. 134–6.
37  'Lancet'. (1826–7) ii, p. 243.
38  'British Medical Journal'. (1873) ii, p. 148.
39  'Lancet'. (1826–7) ii, p. 243.
40  'British Medical Journal'. (1873) ii, p. 148.
41  Ibid (1874) i, p. 195.
42  Ibid (1880) i, pp. 134–6.
43  'Lancet'. (1880) i, pp. 225–6, 503–4.
44  'British Medical Journal'. (1873) i, pp. 618–19.
45  Ibid (1873) i, p. 706.
46  Ibid (1875) i, p. 514.
47  Ibid (1875) i, pp. 69, 199, 403, 435.
48  Ibid (1875) i, p. 69.
49  Ibid (1875) i, p. 492.
50  Ibid (1875) i, p. 437.

51  Ibid (1875) i, p. 557.
52  'Lancet'. (1883) ii, p. 1002.
53  Major R. H., 'Classic Descriptions of Disease'. Charles C. Thomas, 2nd. Ed. 1939, pp. 72–5, 77–81.
54  Long, E. R., 'Selected Readings in Pathology'. Charles C. Thomas 1929, pp. 153–65.
55  Ibid pp. 162–3.
56  Parkes, E. A., 'British Medical Journal'. (1873) ii, p. 143.
57  Major, R. H., 'Classic Descriptions of Diseases'. Charles C. Thomas, 2nd Ed. 1939, pp. 75–77.
58  Green, T. H., 'Pathology & Morbid Anatomy'. Lea Bros. & Co. Philadelphia. 6th American Ed. revised Boyd S. 1899, pp. 309–10.
59  'Lancet'. (1826–7) ii, p. 243.
60  Ibid (1883) ii, p. 991.
61  Green, T. H., 'Pathology & Morbid Anatomy'. Lea Bros & Co., Philadelphia, 6th. American Ed. revised Boyd S. 1899, p. 310.
62  'Lancet'. (1883) ii, pp. 991–2.
63  Ibid (1883) ii, p. 1002.
64  Ibid (1883) i, p. 839.
65  'British Medical Journal'. (1872) i, pp. 508–9.
66  Pagel, W. Amer. Rev. of Tuberculosis. 1942, *46*, p. 301.
67  Comrie, J. D., 'History of Scottish Medicine' 1932, Vol 2, p. 697. Wellcome Historical Medical Museum Bailliere, Tiudall & Cox.
68  Greenfield, W. S., 'Lancet'. (1881) ii, p. 784.
69  'Lancet'. (1932) i, pp. 963–5.
70  'British Medical Journal'. (1932) i, pp. 821–2.
71  'Lancet'. (1928) ii, p. 41.
72  Ledingham, J. C. G., Brit. med. Bull. (1944) *2*, pp. 261–5.
73  'British Medical Journal'. (1928) ii, p. 79.
74  Ibid (1929) i, pp. 325–7.
75  Bulloch, W., 'History of Bacteriology'. Oxford Univerisity Press 1938, pp. 149–51.
76  'British Medical Journal'. (1891) ii, pp. 378–80.
77  Bulloch, W., 'History of Bacteriology'. Oxford University Press 1938, pp. 256–8.
78  Ibid pp. 259–60.
79  'British Medical Journal'. (1891) ii, pp. 378–80.
80  Ibid (1916) i, pp. 60–1.
81  Bulloch, W., 'History of Bacteriology'. Oxford University Press 1938, pp. 397–8.
82  Philosph. Trans. (1874) *164*, ii, pp. 457–77.
83  'British Medical Journal'. (1877) ii, pp. 168–73.
84  Bulloch, W., 'History of Bacteriology'. Oxford University Press 1938, pp. 109–10.
85  Philosph. Trans. (1867) *166*, i, pp. 27–74; (1877) *167*, i, pp. 149–206.
86  'Lancet'. (1893) ii, p. 1452.
87  Wilson, G. S., J. Hygiene, (1879) *82*, pp. 342–3.
88  Bulloch, W., 'History of Bacteriology'. Oxford University Press 1938, p. 230.
89  Williams, Greer, 'Virus Hunters'. Hutchinson of London 1960, pp. 51–3.
90  Ibid pp. 97–100.

# NINETEEN

# The growth of Clinical Pathology, 1910–48

## The Beginnings, 1910–27

The end of the First World War marked the commencement of a new era, and new developments in medicine soon appeared. There were great advances in such fields as Thoracic Surgery, though from our point of view developments in technological subjects such as Radiology and Pathology are more relevant. Certainly, it was soon realised that no modern hospital could provide an efficient medical service without departments of these subjects.

In England, as compared with the Continent, the recognition of Pathology as an independent discipline was delayed. Its importance was realised by physicians and surgeons, many of whom had been responsible for the advances made in the 19th century. In 1907 a London surgeon, Mr. C. B. Lockwood, had given an address to the South Midland Branch of the British Medical Association.[1] This was really a eulogy of Clinical Pathology which was described as being a dominant factor in the diagnosis of medical and surgical cases. The importance of finding the causative organism in infection was stressed and it was pointed out that early diagnosis of cancer could be made by immediate histological sections. At this time most teaching hospitals had well-developed departments of Pathology, headed by directors or by recently-appointed professors. In many cases, these heads of departments were only part-time and were often described as Assistant Physicians with charge of the laboratory. London University, unlike the provincial universities, was slow to develop links with hospital pathology. This was largely because teaching centres sprang up at the large London general hospitals, which treasured their independence and were reluctant to link up with the University. This delayed the establishment of Chairs and it was not until 1912 that the first full-time Chair of Pathology was established. This was at St. Bartholomew's Hospital, London, and other London hospitals then followed suit. In general it can be said that by the end of World War I Pathology was well-established at teaching centres throughout the country.

By contrast, the subject hardly existed in provincial non-teaching hospitals. Only a few, such as the Royal Devon and Exeter Hospital, and the Royal Sussex County Hospital, Brighton, had pathology departments in the immediate period after the First World War, and the Pathologist usually performed other duties. For example, the Princess Alice Memorial Hospital at Eastbourne was founded in 1883. In 1888 a mortuary was constructed and a Pathologist was appointed in 1899.[2] It appears that as late as 1919 (the year in which he retired) he was administering anaesthetics for such operations as tonsillectomy, and he stated that he had been doing this for 30 years.[3] But by 1920 it was realised that every general provincial hospital was going to need a department of Pathology and in most cases a full-time pathologist. The problem was to find out how this need could be met.

A glance at the medical literature of this period gives some idea of the state of affairs. The National Insurance Act of 1911, revolutionary as it had seemed at the time, had only partially succeeded in providing medical care for workers receiving a minimum wage. By the end of the first eight years many shortcomings were apparent. General practitioners did not like the scheme, and it was criticised because it provided no benefits to the dependents of the insured. Also, it provided only general practitioner care and excluded specialist opinion and special examinations or tests. In order to amend these deficiencies, a BMA sub-committee, under the chairmanship of Dr. H. B. Brackenbury and including the Insurance Commissioners, was set up. This body drew up a series of reports, the third of which was named M25 and it is this which immediately concerns us. It was of necessity very long for it dealt with the wider aspects of National Insurance, and included in particular proposals for revision of service under the act and possible extensions of the current benefits. In order to acquaint the medical profession with its findings, the Committee sent a copy of a memorandum on the report to all practitioners in May 1919.[4] It was emphasised that the proposals were at this time only tentative. The plan for obtaining the opinions of as many practitioners as possible was quite elaborate. The memorandum was first to be discussed throughout the country by local Medical and Panel Committees of every area. Representatives of the sub-committee and some Insurance Commissioners attended these group committees to provide explanations when needed. Then in London in July there was a special conference at which representatives from all local Committees met Dr. Brackenbury and his Committee to express their opinions. The discussions were considerable and on the first day extended from 10.30 in the morning till 9.30 at night. These, as well as some correspondence in the 'British Medical Journal', seem to indicate that the main interest ranged around the 'terms of service' – i.e. whether there was to be a 'capitation' or an 'attendance' fee. Many seemed to favour the latter.[5]

Among the proposals for extension of the service was the provision of pathological tests. In the correspondence referred to above (prior to the London Conference) only one letter mentioned this proposal,[6] and in the report of the discussion at the conference[5] it was not mentioned at all. This probably gives some idea of the lack of interest in clinical pathology, certainly at the practitioner level.

Some impression of the Committee's proposals for Pathology is given in a leading article published by the 'Lancet' in June 1919 and entitled 'Clinical Pathology in detail'.[7] The pathological service would be carried out by two types of laboratory, firstly 'those provided as an essential part of the equipment of clinics and other treatment centres', and secondly 'larger research laboratories associated with institutions of university rank'. The latter were already in existence but the former would have to be developed and staffed, and there was no indication of how this was to be done. Were this scheme adopted, it would seem that the bulk of the work would be done at the large institutions and would carry with it the advantages of uniformity of techniques and hopefully of results. By contrast the range of work at the smaller laboratories would be very limited and unlikely to attract the better type of pathologist. The 'Lancet' also pointed out the advantages of having local laboratories, where delays in results were less likely and where the clinician could discuss the significance of the results with the pathologist.

In the end this proposal did not come about but it did serve to stimulate some individuals already working in clinical pathology. The view-point expressed in the 'Lancet' was soon underlined by letters from H. Miller of Hamilton,[8] from 'A Bacteriologist' and from A. G. Shera[9] who had just been appointed pathologist to the Princess Alice Memorial Hospital in Eastbourne. All emphasised the necessity of developing local clinical laboratories in order to provide an efficient pathological service. Before this could be brought about there were certain difficulties to be overcome. In the first place, there were few clinical pathologists at the time and therefore some training programmes would need to be organized. On the other hand there were a number of men who during the war had been introduced to pathology in Army hospitals and would therefore be at least partly trained. Perhaps one of the greatest problems was hospital finance, for at that time the endowments on which the voluntary hospitals existed had been eroded by the great rise in prices. Many felt themselves unable to build and equip a hospital laboratory, to say nothing of providing an attractive salary for a pathologist. In spite of this, a number of local hospital laboratories were built in the next 15 years, though this development was no part of any organised plan.

During the next seven or eight years there must have been much speculation on the future of pathology, and it is unfortunate that the only clue we have to this are occasional letters and a few lectures which were published in the medical press. Two pathologists made a plea for a National Pathological Museum[10,11] illustrating chiefly the variety of histological appearances seen in tumours, both human and animal. Much more important was the emergence of two pathologists, very different in so many ways, but both of whom were to play an important part in the moulding of clinical pathology. S. C. Dyke who subsequently became the founder of the British Pathologists Association (later to become the Association of Clinical Pathologists), returned from the war in 1920, and was invited to set up a Clinical Pathology unit at St. Thomas's Hospital. In 1924 he became Pathologist and Bacteriologist to the South Staffordshire General Hospital, now the Royal Hospital, Wolverhampton.[12]

During the next few years he attempted to show practitioners the value of an intelligent use of the clinical laboratory, as when he addressed the Wolverhampton Divisions of the BMA.[13] On another occasion he read a paper to the British Hospitals Association.[14] He described the type of laboratory which should form a part of every hospital, and indicated the type of outside work which would be available to the pathologist, including tests for panel patients in the National Insurance System. Dyke believed so strongly in clinical pathology that he wanted a service which would be available to all. This would require the appointment of at least one pathologist for every hospital, who would be a specialist of rank equal to that of physicians and surgeons. Time and again he stressed the need for a close association of medicine and pathology and maintained that the clinical pathologist of the future should feel equally at home in the wards and in his own laboratory. In pursuing such an aim, his interest lay apart from the academic aspect of his subject. A man of ideas and determination his extroverted personality made his influence in his field profound.

C. Powell White provided a contrast to Dyke, and was 20 years his senior. He held a number of posts including that of Assistant Pathologist to St. Thomas's Hospital from 1903 till 1906. A man of considerable ability, he was introverted and more attached to research and the academic side of Pathology. He was greatly respected and it is interesting to find that he was the only pathologist who was appointed to office at the foundation of each of the two main pathological societies. In 1906, he became first Treasurer of the Pathological Society of Great Britain and Ireland and in 1927 the first President of the British Pathologists Association. He never occupied a Chair of Pathology and was probably most content when working at research on General Pathology as Pilkington Research Fellow in Manchester where he enjoyed working with Lorain Smith.[15] In letters to the 'Lancet' he expressed great concern about the status of Clinical Pathology and the Clinical Pathologist in the eyes of his academic colleagues.[16] He was disappointed that no university offered an honours degree in general Pathology as they did for other sciences, for he really regarded Pathology as a branch of Biology. He was also strongly opposed to the charging for work done in university departments of pathology to provide money to finance the department.[17]

Looking back at a time which would seem to have been crucial for Pathology and its future it is surprising that the amount of correspondence about it in the medical journals was so small. At this time there must have been about 400 pathologists, for in 1924 the Pathological Society debated whether the membership should not be limited to that number. But most of these were in academic work and therefore unwilling to interest themselves in this new development of Clinical Pathology. Their attitude is probably best understood by reference to some articles by A. E. Boycott, Professor of Pathology at University

College Hospital, London, and a man renowned for his outspokenness.

In 1921, Boycott spent some time studying medical education in Canada and the USA.[18] At the same time he noted the extensive use of 'Clinical Pathology'. Instead of such tests as blood counts being performed by the pathological department, they were done in the clinical department. Boycott argued that this was much better, chiefly because he regarded a test such as a blood count to be in every way similar to using a stethoscope to examine the chest. In fact, such tests really belonged to medicine but should be a part of Pathology. When a few years later he gave an address at the University of McGill, Montreal, on 'Progress in Pathology', he spoke of there being two sorts of Pathologist.[19] One group called themselves pathologists but their real heart was in Medicine; the other group was in Pathology 'because they have had it laid upon them to try to know about the reactions of live things to injury and disease'. This latter group would obviously want to avoid contact with clinical medicine and would be more attracted by Biology and Comparative Anatomy.

Apparently, Boycott's views were held by the majority of members of the Pathological Society, who would therefore have little desire to assist this rising group of clinical pathologists in their troubles. There was another important factor which separated the clinical pathologists from their academic colleagues. When the Pathological Society was formed, its sole aim was to advance Pathology as a science and never to become embroiled in medico-political issues, a policy to which it has steadily adhered over the years.

So the clinical pathologists were few in number, were unsupported by the bulk of pathologists, and they were going to need some remarkable leadership and great determination if they were to survive.

## The founding of the Association of Clinical Pathologists, 1927

New Year's day fell on a Saturday in 1927 and the 'British Medical Journal' and the 'Lancet' on that date both contained a letter which was to prove eventful.[20] It came from eleven practitioners of Pathology who announced that a meeting would be held at 2.30 p.m. on Friday the 7th of January at the London School of Medicine for Women. This meeting was 'for the purpose of considering the advisability of forming a society to represent the interests of those engaged in the practice of pathology'.

The meeting was attended by about 40 medical men and women and Dr. S. C. Dyke was in the Chair. It was decided to form a society which would be called 'The British Society of Pathologists', the aims of which would be 'to develop the application of pathology in relation to medicine, and to protect the interests of those engaged in its study and practice'; these were accepted together with a Constitution at the first Annual General Meeting on the 28th of January 1928. Membership would be open to all registered medical practitioners engaged in the study and practice of pathology. The officers of the new society were C. Powell White (President) and S. C. Dyke (Secretary) and the council members were G. Hadfield, W. Grace, J. G. Greenfield, A. Renshaw, A. G. Shera, A. F. S. Sladden, R. V. Solly and E. Wordley.[21] Surprisingly this announcement excited no correspondence except one letter in the BMJ[22] which stressed the importance of post-mortems with forensic problems being carried out by pathologists and not general practitioners, a topic which was to be widely discussed during the next 15 years. This absence of correspondence might be interpreted as lack of interest but it should be pointed out that at that time the vast majority of letters to the BMJ were related to scientific matters and not to medical politics.

The news of the formation of the new society must have travelled quickly for on the 5th of October 1929 the Council was informed that the Secretary had been elected to Honorary Membership of the American Association of Clinical Pathologists. The Council agreed to ask the Annual General Meeting for permission to reciprocate by electing the American Secretary (Dr. Giordano) to Honorary Membership of the British Society of Pathologists.

But in Great Britain the formation of the new society should not have occasioned much surprise because for some years individual pathologists had been voicing their discontent. The British Medical Association had received a number of letters from pathologists and as a result had appointed a special Committee to discuss problems of Pathological Laboratories and Private Practitioners of Pathology. The BMA Council had regarded the matter of such importance that it appointed a special committee instead of referring it to one or more of its Standing Committees. The BMA considered the report of the Committee in December 1926[23] and referred it to their Representative Committee in 1927.[24] These discussions indicate that the main grievance of pathologists was that they needed protection. While the findings and recommendations of the BMA committee showed a great deal of sympathy with the pathologists, the new society which had been formed thought that the BMA had not gone far enough. So they asked the BMA if they would set up a new Consulting Pathologists Group to deal with the problems that they faced. The BMA agreed to do this and the group was formed at an inaugural meeting on the 2nd of March 1928. A subsequent meeting of the Group was held in Cardiff on the 25th of July.[25] The British Society of Pathologists was well satisfied with this as all the members of the Group were members of their new society. About 40 attended the Cardiff meeting when the total membership was about 77. Conditions for membership were as follows: 'Every member of the Association' (i.e., the BMA) '(not being a member of the Public Health Service) who is working in an institutional or private pathological laboratory engaged in examining and reporting on specimens for clinical purposes is *ipso facto* a member of the Group'.[26] The following committee members were elected: S. C. Dyke (Wolverhampton), J. G. Greenfield (London), I. Walker Hall (Bristol), A. Renshaw (Manchester), A. F. S. Sladden (Swansea), and C. Powell White (Manchester). With the formation of their society and also the BMA Group the pathologists felt ready to try to redress the wrongs about which they were complaining. According to the Year Book of the Society for 1929, the secretary at a meeting on the 29th of January recorded the Society's satisfaction at the formation of the BMA group and added that the Group would deal mainly with politico-economic matters and that the Society would concentrate more on the academic and scientific sides. In retrospect it seems surprising that this statement should come from a Society whose origin was essentially political. However it was a wise decision, for the backing of the BMA would undoubtedly be an important factor in any future reforms or changes which the Society might wish to make.

With this brief introduction to the Society it is now important to consider the problems of the private pathologists in more detail. At about this time it was becoming increasingly obvious that pathology was going to play a large part in the development of clinical medicine, and a large number of pathologists was going to be needed. The teaching or university hospitals already had their pathologists and their laboratories and were well able to carry out the diagnostic pathological tests on their patients. Some had even gone further and set up 'clinical research departments' in which they carried out pathological tests for other hospitals and practitioners on a fee basis. For example, in 1927 it was stated that St. Bartholomew's Hospital, London had had such a department for well over 20 years.[27] In non-teaching hospitals in many parts of the country there were few pathologists and in other parts no service was available at all. It was in these areas that the private pathologist was needed. But unlike a private practitioner who could 'put up his plate' and practice with the minimum of equipment, the private pathologist could not afford to equip a laboratory for himself (even in those days!) at the outset of his career. The logical solution was that the voluntary hospital should provide the laboratory, but many felt unable to finance the employment of a pathologist. So a compromise was reached whereby the hospital provided a laboratory and allowed the pathologist to use it for work on his private patients who paid him a fee. The pathologist in return paid the hospital for the use of its laboratory. In theory this sounds simple and logical but it gave rise to many acrimonious disputes between the pathologist and not only the hospital administrators but also his clinical colleagues. For instance, some hospitals claimed that the fees did not belong to the pathologist and that he should only receive a proportion of them. At this stage the pathologist who was concerned with his private practice suddenly found himself threatened and in need of protection, and this was the state of affairs and indeed the main reason for the foundation of the British Society of Pathologists.

The threats to the pathologist came from three different quarters. First there was the teaching hospital which in some cases carried out tests for other non-teaching institutions as well as for local authorities and practitioners, and for this they received fees. The fees that they charged were low and as a result of this in some areas they received work which should have gone to the private pathologist in the locality. In 1931 the Society (by then the Association of Clinical Pathologists) agreed that under certain circumstances university and teaching hospitals might have to carry out work for other hospitals, local authorities, or practitioners, but that they should not be permitted to advertise such a service. Secondly, there was the case of the 'County Laboratories'. These were laboratories which had been set up by Local Government authorities, and were concerned in carrying out pathological tests to detect infectious disease, i.e. they were used for public health purposes. In areas where there was no private pathologist or pathological service they extended their range of tests and provided clinical diagnostic examinations for patients, chiefly those of insurance practitioners. Unfortunately, they did not stop at this and in some cases were openly in competition with the laboratories of voluntary hospitals. In 1926 a leading article appeared in the BMJ under the title of 'The Country Pathological Service'.[28] This was in all probability written by S. C. Dyke. It drew attention[8] to the activities of these Country Laboratories which were of course subsidised by Local Government Funds. The situation was particularly bad in South Staffordshire where the County Laboratory was in the same grounds as the Voluntary Hospital; the latter's pathologist was Dr. S. C. Dyke who literally had a rival on his doorstep! The third source of anxiety was in many ways the most serious as it concerned the establishment of laboratories by commercial firms who carried out pathological tests at a very low rate. This rate was so low that no private pathologist could compete with it. Even worse, these firms were advertising the performance of such tests in the medical press. The pathologists claimed that the commercial side of the firm was being publicised by the advertisements for pathological tests. Indeed a large part of the discussion at the original BMA Committee was concerned with this very point and the pathologists were urging that the BMJ should refuse such advertisements. The pathologist was of course at a disadvantage for he was not permitted to advertise, though he was allowed to notify practitioners in his neighbourhood of the services which he was able to provide. The BMA was unwilling to agree but favoured restriction of the laboratory belonging to the firm by recommending that it must be under the direction of a registered medical practitioner, and that such a person must also sign the reports. When the resolutions of the original BMA Pathological Committee were made known there was a prompt reaction from the Medical Superintendent (a registered medical practitioner) of a commercial firm called 'Virol'. He protested at what he regarded as a sweeping condemnation of commercial laboratories. He pointed out that the pathological laboratories of Virol had been established about 14 years

310

ago (1913) and had carried out tests for a large number of practitioners who otherwise could not have got them performed. He also stated that this aspect of the firm was entirely separate financially from the firm itself and that any profits were ploughed back for the purpose of research in Clinical Pathology.[29]

From the above summary the complexity of the problems of the private pathologist can easily be seen. The one thing that is absolutely clear is that the pathological services throughout the country were sadly deficient. One aspect of the above which was very clearly recognized by Dyke was the question of whether the private pathologist of the future was to be based at a voluntary hospital or whether he might become an employee of a Local Government Authority at one of their County laboratories. On this point he was quite rightly adamant. Over and over again he stressed the importance of close co-operation and consultation between clinician and pathologist, and maintained that the County Laboratory was only concerned with a relatively narrow field of medicine.[28,30,31] In an article entitled 'Wholesale Pathology' the point was emphasized by condemning the practice of pathology by post which was likened to a slot machine.[32] We have evidence that 'postal pathology' was much in vogue at the time from an appeal in the BMJ in 1923 by the Postmaster General, in which he laid down stringent regulations for the packaging of pathological specimens sent by post.[33]

In January 1930 the name of the society was changed to the 'Association of Clinical Pathologists' (ACP) and it is still so known today. It was often described as a 'breakaway group' from the Pathological Society of Great Britain and Ireland. It is probably true that the members of the Association were not at all anxious to sever their connections with the Pathological Society which had been founded in 1906. But the older society was essentially one related to Histopathology and Bacteriology and as the leading members were in the academic field they failed to see and understand the difficulties which faced the clinical pathologist. Also their aims were entirely scientific and they were unwilling to get involved in medical politics. From this point onwards the two societies drifted further and further apart and it was not till over 30 years later that they were ever to co-operate, namely in the foundation of the College of Pathologists.

Before dealing with ACP activities in its early years, it would be well to mention the difficulties in acceptance which Pathology has faced. Nowadays, it is a commonplace to say that Pathology is both a basic science and a clinical subject. In past years it would seem that some medical people thought that it was neither! In 1928 Powell White drew attention[34] to the fact that the universities would not accept Pathology as a subject for a science degree as they had accepted Anatomy and Physiology, and he pointed this out to the Pathological Society. He also stated that 'when the University of London took over University College it refused to take over the department of pathology as an integral part of the College on the same terms as the departments of anatomy and physiology'. This was probably because they did not recognize pathology as a science, and regarded it simply as something to be taught to medical students. At that early date there were few who visualized anyone taking on pathology as his life's work. In a parallel way the clinicians of earlier times were reluctant to accept the pathologist as a colleague, many regarding him merely as a servant. Some clinicians (and some academic pathologists!) even refused to call anyone working in clinical pathology a pathologist. The status of a pathologist at the turn of the century had been very low, but thereafter progressively improved, so that at the formation of the National Health Service in 1948 senior pathologists were granted the same consultant status as other specialists.

We can now consider how this embryo group of clinical pathologists addressed themselves to their current problems. They certainly knew what they wanted and the expedition with which they set about their tasks is in retrospect most commendable.

## Progress of the ACP up to World War II, 1927–37

Meetings of the ACP were held twice a year, the winter one being in London and the summer one in the provinces. It says much for the enthusiasm of the society that during the first 10 years only one meeting (Plymouth, 1932) had to be cancelled for lack of support. Many of the scientific papers were aimed at providing practical help for the pathologist in his daily work. At the summer meeting in Chester in 1928, the main topic was a general one on 'techniques of blood examination'. At that time it was decided to produce 'Broadsheets' on reliable standard methods for certain pathological examinations, and the first of these appeared towards the end of 1928. They are still issued and it is safe to say that this venture was one of the most helpful and far-sighted ever conceived by the Association. Many of the specimens received by patho-logists (especially some sent by post) were unsuitable for examination and the Association soon realised the importance of 'educating' general prac-titioners in the proper use of pathological services. Thus in 1930 it was decided to draw up a small pamphlet for practitioners on 'When and how to collect specimens for laboratory diagnosis'. The necessary medical staffing to enable good work to be done came up for discussion and in the same year it was decided that a medically-qualified pathologist would be needed for every hospital with over 200 beds.[35] At the same time the BMA Consultant Pathologists Group drew up a scale of fees for pathological tests which would be applicable to National Health Insurance patients, and the British Medical Association gave its approval.

One other topic which concerned the ACP Council was the question of forensic work. At the time many autopsies were carried out by general practitioners. The Association insisted that these should only be done by experienced pathologists and in 1929 tried to get special fees for such autopsies. In 1931 the Director of Public Prosecutions agreed to a proposal of the ACP to provide a panel of recognised pathologists experienced in forensic work, and much was to be heard of this later.

In these early days there were few clinical pathologists and some of these had become interested in the subject through experiences during World War I, probably mostly related to tropical diseases. There were virtually no programmes for training in the teaching schools though some workers in the pathological laboratories, on failing to obtain a permanent academic post, drifted into one of the few posts available in non-teaching provincial departments. Even in the early 1930s some took up such posts without any training at all and, as it were, 'learned on the job'. Help was not forthcoming from the academic pathologists for most were not in sympathy with the aims of the Association. As a result there was little progress made in the field of training. Specialist status was only likely to be obtained by a qualification such as the Membership of the Royal College of Physicians or the Fellowship of the Royal College of Surgeons, two examinations which were clearly not designed for pathologists. The only appropriate examination available at the time was the MD in Pathology given by the University of London, and obtained by only a few academic pathologists. Accordingly, the ACP Council (largely motivated by Dyke) sent letters in 1928 to the Deans of the Faculties of Medicine of the Universities of England, Wales, Scotland, and Northern Ireland, and to the Royal Colleges of Physicians of London and Edinburgh, pointing out the need for a Diploma in Clinical Pathology.[36] The Universities of Oxford, London, and Manchester and the Royal College of Physicians of London, appointed committees to consider the matter, and the University of London and the Royal College of Physicians of London asked for further information. Hopes ran high when in 1931 London University announced that it would provide an examination for a Diploma in Clinical Pathology (DCP). The ACP at once objected to one of the regulations, namely that, as part of the candidate's training, he must spend at least one year 'as a whole-time worker under the supervision of the head of the pathological department of one of the colleges or schools of the University of London'. In the discussions which followed, the University agreed to award, in addition, an External Diploma for those who had not trained in a pathology department of their university. Finally in 1935[37] the University advertised the Diploma which was open to graduates in Medicine and to registered medical practitioners. The examination subjects were (1) Morbid Anatomy and Histology, (2) Bacteriology and Serology, and (3) Biochemistry, and the examination was to be held in October. It is interesting to note that even as late as 1935 no mention is made of Haematology as a separate subject.

One event in 1934, which was to be of importance in connection with the DCP in the future, was an announcement that it was expected that the new British Postgraduate Medical School at Hammersmith would be opened for students in October.[38] This school had been given recognition for an initial two year period by the University of London, and was to include a Department of Pathology, the first professor being Edgar H. Kettle.

No account of the early days of the ACP would be complete without reference to an address given in 1937 by the retiring secretary Dr. S. C. Dyke.[39] It was entitled 'The future status of the clinical pathologist' and gave a very clear picture of what the ideal clinical pathologist should be. A good knowledge of the working of his laboratory was essential and he should also know the limitations of his methods. In this regard he was indeed a specialist because of his special knowledge. But once more Dyke emphasized the aspect dear to his heart and one which motivated him throughout his career. The clinical pathologist must have a first-class knowledge of medicine so that he felt just as much at home in the wards as in his laboratory. By his experience he should have a sufficient knowledge of the natural history of disease and thus be worthy of consultation by his clinical colleagues. To attain such ideals would not be easy, but one who did so would command respect and be unlikely to lack at least equal status amongst other members of the consultant medical staff. Good training was essential and Dyke was much heartened by the institution of the Diploma of Clinical Pathology by the University of London. He thought that in the future it would become the hallmark of a well-trained pathologist just as the 'Fellowship' was the hallmark of a well-trained surgeon. This, however, was not to be, for this Diploma became localized at the Postgraduate School, Hammersmith and few external candidates attempted it. It soon had a rival which again had limited success, namely the Diploma in Pathology instituted by the Conjoint Board. A feeling grew that a Diploma was not good enough to provide equal status for the pathologist compared with his clinical colleagues who had Membership or Fellowship of their Royal Colleges. This attitude was to persist and remain unsolved until the founding of the College of Pathologists over 25 years later in 1963. But Dyke had steered the clinical pathologist on the right course and he relied on what might be called 'his Association' to maintain it.

It is surprising that Dyke's address excited no correspondence at all. The leading articles of the issue made no comment, and were devoted to 'The limitation of hearing aids' and 'Mental disease in London'. Such was the status of Clinical Pathology in those days! But in spite of this a number of addresses, many by ACP members, attempted to draw attention to the importance of Clinical Pathology in modern medicine, as will be seen from the following examples:

(1) 'The Status of Pathology' – a Presidential address to the British Pathologists Association (1928)[40]
(2) 'Clinical Pathology as an aid to the practitioner' by R. C. Matson to the Guildford Division of the BMA (1928)[41]

(3) 'The work and responsibilities of the Pathologist' by Sir Bernard Spilsbury. The second Stephen Paget Memorial Lecture (1928)[42]

(4) 'The Clinical Pathologist and Toxicologist in Medical practice' by Sir William Willcox to a joint meeting of the Manchester Medical and Pathological Societies (1929)[43]

(5) 'The use and abuse of the hospital pathological laboratory' by S. C. Dyke to the Worcester Medical Society (1932)[44]

(6) 'The Pathologist in Medicine' – a commentary on 'The Laboratory; its place in the modern world' by Stark Murray (1934)[45]

At the 1930 summer meeting of the ACP in Cheltenham, a physician, Dr. J. R. Collins, gave an address on 'Sins of the Pathologist'[46] and it is a great pity that a talk with this attractive title does not appear to have been published.

Dyke was convinced that Clinical Pathology was inseparable from Clinical Medicine and that the Clinical Pathologist must be based in the laboratory of a General Hospital. His great fear was that the pathologist might drift into County Laboratories and become part of Public Health. The other corollary was that the Clinical Pathologist, in order to hold his own with his fellow specialists, must have a basic training in Clinical Medicine as well as a mastery of the use of laboratory investigations. The question of status was a pressing one, for many pathologists in the provinces were being asked to work under conditions which were decidedly sub-standard. The author (GJC) well remembers sometime in 1936 or 1937 a discussion which followed a special ACP Dinner. It was attended by about 40 pathologists, was chaired by Dyke, Greenfield and Cuthbert Dukes, and had a physician and surgeon as honoured guests. When pathologists were invited to report on their working conditions and their relationship with their colleagues, the exchanges grew very heated. The surprising thing to an onlooker was the variation of experience from pathologist to pathologist, and although some were well-satisfied, there were quite a few who seemed to have much to complain about. If Dyke's suggestions on training were adopted, the pathologist was going to earn his status the hard way, for in addition to obtaining a Diploma in Clinical Pathology, it was suggested that he might want to have a specialist qualification in General Medicine, presumably the MD or the MRCP. Dyke was much heartened by the co-operation of the University of London in providing its Diploma, but the ACP Council had expressed concern that no one had so far taken the examination. Its future was to be very different from that which was anticipated, as will be seen later.

When it came to the question of an ideal training, Dyke felt that this must be done at a General Hospital where laboratory investigations, clinical data, and autopsy findings could be correlated. He very much feared the danger of specialisation at too early a stage. He was obviously much influenced by his own experience at the Royal Hospital, Wolver-hampton, where the Assistant Pathologist was also the Resident Medical Officer and could promote the liaison between laboratory and bedside which Dyke so much desired. It might be mentioned that this hospital must have been one of the earliest of the provincial hospitals to make use of Pathology. Dr. C. A. MacMunn, who graduated in 1872, was the first pathologist, being appointed Honorary Pathologist and Physician to the General Hospital (as it was then called) probably in the late 1870s or the early 1880s.[47] He was greatly interested in the use of the spectroscope in physiology, writing books on 'The Spectroscope in Medicine', and later 'The Clinical Chemistry of Urine'. In 1913–14 the Pathologist to the Royal Hospital was Dr. William Boyd, who became world-famous as an author of textbooks on Pathology and who held three Chairs of Pathology in Canada. In 1924 Dyke was appointed to the post and remained in it till he retired in 1952 and was succeeded by A. G. Marshall.

In these ten formative years the ACP had much to its credit. It had moved towards organizing a complete national service of clinical pathology. Clinical pathologists were few at the time of its inauguration for there were only 77 members of the BMA Consulting Pathologists Group. By the time that Dyke retired from the Secretaryship of the ACP there were probably about 250. The Association had pressed for better training for young pathologists and had sought to ensure, by the issue of many Broadsheets, that reliable technical methods were employed. They had been successful in campaigning for a recognized qualification in clinical pathology. At the time of the founding of the Association probably the only examination in Pathology was the MD given by the University of London and taken by only a few academic pathologists. The services of pathologists had been made known to general practitioners, and pamphlets distributed to them explaining the proper methods of submitting specimens for pathological examination. The situation in regard to post-mortems involving forensic problems had improved a great deal and the general practitioner had given way to the pathologist. Most important of all they had established that the place for the Clinical Pathologist was in the laboratory of a Hospital and not in one under a Public Health Authority. They had ensured a measure of protection to the private pathologist and thus provided a future for him as a specialist in line with specialists in other branches of medicine.

## Wartime developments, 1938–48

The groundwork of the ACP had been well-laid by the end of the first ten years, but the period which followed included the years of World War II. As a result many plans made were of necessity postponed and the ACP membership was disrupted when a number of its members left the country to play their part in the Services abroad. However the ACP continued to meet twice a year, except in 1940 when both meetings were cancelled. The summer meeting due to be held in Bristol in 1944 was also cancelled, in response to a request by the Government to curtail travel as much as possible.

In the immediate pre-war years the growing importance of Haematology was indicated by a whole session on the subject at the January meeting in 1938.[48] More important still, in view of the possibility of war, was the session on Blood Transfusion in June 1937.[49]

Although the war might be thought of as a deterrent to the progress of Pathology it was in fact responsible for many advances, some of which arose in a surprising way.

In 1934 the Committee of Imperial Defence had started discussions on the methods of protection which might be needed in the event of bacteriological warfare, and in 1936 appointed a sub-committee to study this problem. It soon became clear that the existing bacteriological services would be quite unable to deal with such a problem to say nothing of epidemics which might result from population movement following evacuation of towns. They recommended that supplementary services should be instituted and that the Medical Research Council (MRC) be responsible for their organisation. This was agreed and the new service was called the 'Emergency Public Health Laboratory Service'.[50] While the MRC was to run this service in England and Wales generally, control for the London area would be exercised by the Emergency Medical Service (EMS) operating directly under the Ministry of Health. Preparations were hastily made in 1938 and 1939, and the service was ready to go into action in August 1939, one week before the outbreak of war. The detailed organisation of the service has been well-described by G. S. Wilson.[50,51] Modifications of the plan had to be made because of the unexpected course of the first year when the expected aerial bombardment did not take place. It was soon found that the expertise available at these emergency laboratories could provide medical officers of health with facilities which they had never had before, and many voluntary hospital bacteriological departments were glad to use them as consultants. Thus the service rapidly became an integral part of the public health organisation, and in 1944 the Ministry of Health sought permission to continue the system on a peace-time basis as the Public Health Laboratory Service and to extend it to the whole of England and Wales. The Medical Research Council agreed to administer this for an initial period of five years. The aim was to develop a national service for public health and epidemiology. Further progress was now made by the institution of a five-year training period for those wishing to follow a career in public health bacteriology.[51] It seems certain that this extension of the subject also benefitted bacteriology as a whole and raised its status. However, it has been emphasized that Public Health Bacteriology and Hospital or Clinical Bacteriology are two separate branches of Pathology, the one serving the community, and the other the individual, even though the two subjects may sometimes come together in a combined laboratory.

Another wartime institution which did much to improve coverage of Pathology throughout the country was the Emergency Medical Service (EMS). The development of Clinical Pathology in this system progressed during the war but did not proceed as rapidly as Public Health Bacteriology, presumably because it was thought that the problem was less urgent. In the early months of the war the provision of Clinical Pathology in the London area was organised by the EMS. It was based on a system of sectors, each centering on a large teaching hospital. Certain laboratories later known as 'designated' were selected to be under the Ministry of Health through the Sector Pathologists.[52] In June 1942 the Ministry of Health produced Circular 2658, giving plans for the organisation of a Clinical Pathology Service in the provinces.[53] This plan was similar to that in London and involved the recognition of 'area' laboratories which would carry out work for their own hospital, for some other hospitals and also for general practitioners. Smaller hospitals would have only sideroom laboratories, and would not have immediate and continuous supervision by a medically qualified pathologist. The grouping of hospitals was made by a hospital officer with the aid of an honorary consultant pathologist, who was ideally a member of the staff of a university pathological department. This scheme, practised throughout the war, did much to improve the facilities for Clinical Pathology throughout the country and was a definite step towards providing a national service in the subject.

Lastly a few words should be said about the development of the Emergency Blood Transfusion Service. A voluntary service was set up in the early 1920s, and later became the British Red Cross Transfusion Service – the first of its kind in the world. Between the world wars Blood Transfusion slowly advanced, but in the immediate pre-war years, namely 1938 and 1939, it began to accelerate. Such progress as was known is well described in an article by L. W. Proger,[54] on which we have freely drawn. Many advances had been made from experience in the Spanish Civil War in the use of transfusion for the treatment of both military and civilian air-raid casualties. Thus, in 1938, the Medical Research Council undertook to organise an Emergency Blood Transfusion Service. London, having special problems of its own, was to be served with blood from four depots on the outskirts of the city and the southwestern part of the country was to be supplied by the Army Transfusion Service which was stationed in that area. With the collapse of France in 1940 and the return of the British Expeditionary Force, it became clear that the whole of the British Isles was vulnerable, and that a complete service was needed. Accordingly, nine Regional Blood Transfusion Officers were appointed to cover the rest of England and Wales.

Technical advances were soon forthcoming as a result of research carried out in America and Great Britain. Blood substitutes such as plasma could be given without the fear of blood group incompatibility, and dried plasma solved a storage problem since it could be kept for several months without deterioration. These and many other developments formed the basis of the sophisticated methods now employed in a modern Blood Bank Unit.

To return to the Association of Clinical Pathologists, it appears that its main activity during the war years was the setting up of a National Service in Clinical Pathology. As far back as 1934 the Council had started to draw up a plan for such a service which would be centered round the laboratories of the voluntary hospitals. By 1939 the immediate prospect of war had modified this approach and the Council discussed with the British Medical Association 'Pathological services in time of emergency'. Dyke wrote a memorandum on 'the civilian requirements of pathology in the event of an outbreak of hostilities', while the Association had some correspondence with the Medical Research Council on the advisability of organising Blood Donors on a national basis. Discussions continued and in 1940 included 'a nationally organised pathological service on a regional basis'.

In July 1939 the Ministry of Health announced the Emergency Medical Service and invited applications to serve in it in the event of war.[55] The Presidents of the Royal Colleges urged doctors to support this service. When planning the pathological aspect of this service Sir Philip Panton was to play the leading part. Between December 1940 and December 1942 Dyke wrote three letters to the ACP Council dealing amongst other matters with the part played by clinical pathologists in the EMS. During this period, he foresaw that what was the EMS today might well be a national health service tomorrow. He was therefore greatly concerned that the EMS pathological service should be developed on the right lines and also be suitably remunerated. He stated his views in 1941 in an article entitled 'Towards a National Service'. Many others must have had similar views, for at this time the Beveridge Committee was in session. In December 1942, Sir William Beveridge published his report for a comprehensive National Health Service. In the following year the Royal College of Physicians invited the ACP to send a representative (1) to meetings which would consider the Beveridge Report and the White Paper on a National Health Service and (2) to sit on the Central Advisory Medical Council to consider specialist and consultant status with special reference to the proposed establishment of a register of specialists by the GMC. Dyke was appropriately named to be the representative in each instance. The ACP Council discussed the White Paper and made certain comments. But in 1943 the ACP Council was able to submit a draft memorandum on 'A National Pathological Service' for discussion by their members. In 1947 it was amended and was entitled 'A National Service in Clinical Pathology'. It was approved by the Membership of the Association, and the British

Medical Association largely adopted it as a basis for discussion with the Minister. The Secretary of the ACP wrote to the Minister and no doubt included a copy of the memorandum.

The intense discussions and debates on the Health Service have been well documented elsewhere and it remains only to say that the new service came into effect on the 5th July, 1948. By coincidence the Association of Clinical Pathologists came of age in the same year. In January 1948 the ACP held its 21st birthday dinner at the Piccadilly Hotel, London, when the President, Dr. Cuthbert E. Dukes gave the toast of 'The Past, in honour and gratitude'.[56]

REFERENCES

1 Lockwood, C. B., 'British Medical Journal'. (1907) ii, pp. 493–5.
2 Surtees, S. J., (personal communication).
3 Gabbett, H. S., 'British Medical Journal'. (1919) ii, p. 152.
4 'British Medical Journal'. (1919) i, pp. 616–17, Leading article.
5 Ibid (1919) ii, Suppl. pp. 23–35.
6 Rigby, R. H., 'British Medical Journal'. (1919) ii, pp. 58–9.
7 'Lancet'. (1919) i, p. 1088 Leading article.
8 Miller, Hugh, 'British Medical Journal'. (1919) ii, p. 222.
9 Shera, A. G., Ibid (1919) ii, pp. 287–8.
10 Shaw, E. H., 'Lancet'. (1923) ii, p. 364.
11 Clarke, J. Jackson, Ibid (1923) ii, pp. 484–5.
12 'Lancet'. (1975) i, p. 703 Obituary Notice.
13 Dyke, S. C., 'British Medical Journal'. (1925) ii, pp. 934–6.
14 Dyke, S. C. 'Lancet'. (1926) ii, p. 363.
15 Dean, H. R., J. Path. Bact. (1931) 34, pp. 581–5. Obituary Notice.
16 Powell, White C., 'Lancet'. (1923) ii, p. 536.
17 Ibid (1926) ii, p. 520.
18 Boycott, A. E., Ibid (1921) ii, pp. 773–75.
19 Ibid (1924) ii, pp. 997–1000.
20 'Lancet'. (1927) i, p. 38.
21 Ibid (1927) i, p. 204.
22 Rees, F., 'British Medical Journal'. (1927) i, p. 856.
23 'British Medical Journal'. (1927) Suppl. Vol. 1, p. 2.
24 'Lancet'. (1927) ii, p. 189.
25 'British Medical Journal'. (1928) Suppl. Vol. 2, p. 95.
26 Ibid (1928) Suppl. Vol. 2, p. 1.
27 Ibid (1927) Suppl. Vol. 1, p. 4.
28 'British Medical Journal'. (1926) i, p. 143. Leading article.
29 Gordon, A. K., 'Lancet'. (1927) ii, p. 306.
30 Dyke, S. C., 'British Medical Journal'. (1925) ii, p. 934.
31 Dyke, S. C. 'Lancet'. (1926) ii, p. 363.
32 'British Medical Journal'. (1926) i, p. 205. Leading article.
33 Ibid (1923) i, p. 265. Medical news.
34 White, C. Powell, 'Lancet'. (1928) i, p. 381.
35 A.C.P. Year Book 1929.

36  A.C.P. Year Book 1928.
37  'Lancet'. (1935) ii, p. 533.
38  'British Medical Journal'. (1934) i, p. 220.
39  Dyke, S. C., 'Lancet'. (1937) i, pp. 365–7.
40  White, C. Powell, 'Lancet'. (1928) i, pp. 381–3.
41  Matson, R. C., 'British Medical Journal'. (1928) i, p. 897.
42  Spilsbury, Sir Bernard, 'British Medical Journal'. (1928) i, pp. 1079–80.
43  Willcox, Sir W., 'British Medical Journal'. (1929) i, pp. 453–4.
44  Dyke, S. C., 'Lancet'. (1932) ii, pp. 107–10.
45  'British Medical Journal'. (1934) i, p. 902.
46  Ibid (1930) ii, p. 20.
47  Ibid (1911) i, p. 531. Obituary notice.
48  Ibid (1938) i, p. 353.
49  Ibid (1937) i, p. 1329.
50  Wilson, G. S., 'British Medical Journal'. (1948) i, p. 678.
51  Wilson, G. S. 'Brit. med. Bulletin'. (1951) 7, pp. 147–153.
52  'British Medical Journal'. (1940) ii, p. 475.
53  'Lancet'. (1942) ii, p. 44.
54  Proger, L. W., 'British Medical Journal'. (1942) ii, pp. 252–3.
55  'Lancet'. (1939) ii, p. 268.
56  'British Medical Journal'. (1948) i, p. 280.

# TWENTY

# Problems of training and qualifications 1947–52

All developments after the war were based on the earlier growth of clinical pathology. Up to the turn of the century much of the Pathology available in hospitals was carried out by part-time clinicians. The next 20–30 years saw the advent of the full-time pathologist who, in provincial hospitals, was responsible for all aspects of the subject. However his basic training, such as it was, related mostly to Morbid Anatomy and Histology, thus making him a valuable asset to his clinical colleagues. Because the Morbid Anatomist was 'there first', an idea developed that when he was provided with colleagues in other branches of Pathology, the chief must always be the Morbid Anatomist. It was only after the war that this contention was seriously challenged.

In 1870, as already mentioned, there were few laboratories in existence except Sir John Simon's at St. Thomas's and the private laboratories of Sir John Burdon Sanderson and Lionel Beale. The Brown Institute, opened in the following year, provided badly-needed space for research. But by the turn of the century, Bacteriology had burst on the scene and laboratories for it were in great demand, both for diagnosis of disease and for the production of immune sera. So rapid was the development of Bacteriology that it might well have swept Morbid Anatomy off its feet. In the event there were demands for separate departments of bacteriology, and also for university chairs in the subject. But Bacteriology did not develop as a single subject because it arose in two different fields. John Simon had encouraged research in infective diseases before bacteria were discovered. The latter now became incorporated into the research and became part of what may be called Public Health Bacteriology. This was provided by local government authorities and concerned itself with the health of the community. The range of bacteriology carried out in these departments was not large and they were chiefly responsible for helping the local Medical Officer of Health. By contrast, the hospital bacteriologist was much busier, now that the diagnostic use of the subject had been recognised, and he was serving the sick individual. Thus the two types of bacteriologists pursued their different paths and it was only during World War II that there was some measure of co-operation. During the war the public health bacteriology was organised by the Emergency Public Health Laboratory service, and the hospital bacteriology by the Emergency Medical Services (see chapter 19). This worked so well that when the National Health Service was instituted a similar plan was adopted.

In the London teaching hospitals the organisation of a pathological service was far from satisfactory. In one hospital, the autopsies were carried out by junior members of the clinical staff until the early 1930s. On the surgical side they reported on the biopsies and other surgical specimens. There were academic departments of Morbid Anatomy, Bacteriology and Chemical Pathology. In addition there was a 'Clinical Laboratory' staffed by a Clinical Pathologist with three or four junior clinical assistants, who were often filling in time whilst awaiting an appointment on the Honorary Staff of the hospital. This Clinical Laboratory carried out the, at the time, simple haematology, the routine bacteriology and a few simple chemical tests. One might well ask what the staff of the academic department of Pathology did; they of course did the undergraduate teaching and some research. But as can be imagined this system did not work well. For instance there were some specialised examinations in bacteriology which were not carried out in the Clinical Laboratory, and these were referred to the academic department. It became a question as to whether a test was 'easy' or 'difficult', for this would determine where it would be examined, and as can easily be imagined there was not always unanimity on this matter. It was not until the middle 1930s that this incongruous state of affairs was rectified.

For showing the proper pattern for a modern Pathology Department we owe much to Professor E. H. Kettle. He had seen more than enough of the old system, when the clinicians dominated Pathology, during his tenure of the Chair in that subject at two London teaching hospitals. For this reason, when appointed to the Chair of Pathology at the newly-founded British Postgraduate Medical School at Hammersmith, he divided his department into four sections which operated independently under a sub-departmental head, and covered Morbid Anatomy, Chemical Pathology, Bacteriology, and Haematology.

The two main problems facing the ACP at this time were to design a suitable course of training for young pathologists and to provide a qualification which would give them the status of a specialist. It will be remembered that the University of London had offered a Diploma in Clinical Pathology in the early 1930s at the request of the Association. But for various reasons this examination was not readily accepted by pathologists. There were two successful candidates in 1936,[1] one in 1938,[2] and four in 1939.[3] This state of affairs persisted till 1949, only an occasional success being reported. In 1950 there was a sudden change when there were 20 successful candidates – 15 for an Academic and 5 for an External Diploma.[4] This sudden change resulted from the establishment of a course for the examination at the British Postgraduate Medical School. It is not known exactly how this association of the DCP with Hammersmith came into being. According to Harrison[5] the first organised course was held in 1945, and he taught on the subsequent courses from 1946. It is not known whether the Hammersmith course came into being because none other was available, or whether the Board of Studies of London University in Pathology (founded in 1941)[6] had any hand in it. As a result the DCP became known as 'the Hammersmith

Diploma', and it did not solve the ACP's problem because there were few young men who could afford to take a year off without pay to attend the course. The only encouraging sign was that in 1948 the Worcester Royal Infirmary and in 1949 the Leicester and the North Staffordshire Royal Infirmaries were recognised as study centres for the DCP.

In the immediate post-war period the ACP was flourishing, its membership increasing, and its meetings much improved in quality. The BMA Pathology Group Committee elected new members in 1946, namely Prof. G. R. Cameron, Prof. D. F. Cappell, C. E. Dukes, S. C. Dyke, R. W. Fairbrother, J. G. Greenfield, R. J. V. Pulvertaft, A. F. S. Sladden and Sir Lionel Whitby. It seemed that the Association was ready for action. However, as the junior society they were reluctant to go ahead without the support of their senior colleagues, namely the Pathological Society of Great Britain and Ireland. But so far no such co-operation was forthcoming. With the possibility of a National Health Service in the near future, the ACP felt that it should be ready to negotiate attractive terms of employment for its members. Accordingly, in 1946 they invited the Pathological Society to form a joint committee for the purpose. The Society declined to do so, for according to their constitution their aim was only to advance the science of Pathology. The ACP was forced to 'go it alone', and in August 1946, following discussions by the ACP Council, the secretary sent a letter to the Minister of Health. In it were a number of suggestions which the Council felt were essential for the satisfactory organisation of a National Service in Clinical Pathology. In 1948 Cuthbert Dukes gave a Presidential Address entitled 'Human relationships in Clinical Pathology'. In it there was a decided attempt to pour oil on troubled waters. Dukes refused to regard the ACP as a breakaway group, and paid great tribute to the founders and members of the Pathological Society. He went on to say that the leaders of each of the societies had its own special function to perform in relation to the advancement of Pathology, and that one might help the other. He added that there should be one society concerned chiefly with pure science, and another with applied science. Of great interest was his comment that recently many men in senior academic posts in Pathology had joined the Association of Clinical Pathologists. This was true and the trend continued over the next few years, by which time the majority of senior members of the Pathological Society were also members of the ACP. It seems likely that Cuthbert Dukes and W. H. MacMenemey were largely responsible for this desirable state of affairs.

With no support coming from the Pathological Society in spite of the above movement, hopes turned towards the Royal College of Physicians. It was true that this body had shown little interest in Pathology over the years, but the future might be better. This optimistic view arose when it was decided by the Minister of Health that, just as the Royal College of Surgeons of England would speak for the Anaesthetists in the National

Service, so the Royal College of Physicians of London should represent the Pathologists.

Accordingly on the 23rd January, 1947 the ACP appointed a subcommittee on Training and Qualifications, the two most urgent matters in the setting up of a National Service in Clinical Pathology. The constitution of the Sub-Committee was E. N. Allott (Chairman), S. C. Dyke, R. W. Fairbrother, J. G. Greenfield and W. H. MacMenemey. This body is often referred to as the Allott Committee and it was encouraged to seek the co-operation of the Royal College of Physicians. The Committee acted rapidly and issued its first report in August 1947. The training recommendations were:

(1) a minimum of 5 years post-registration experience unless the candidate had previously obtained a first or second-class honours degree in one of the medical sciences or a degree of Doctor of Philosophy. In such cases 4 years' experience would be adequate.

(2) a minimum of 1 year post-registration general clinical training, including at least six months as a resident house physician in general medical wards.

(3) a minimum of 3 years laboratory training, of which it was thought desirable that 1 year should be spent in a university science department and 2 years in approved laboratories of clinical pathology.

(4) the possession of a higher degree or diploma in medicine, e.g., M.D. or M.R.C.P.

Its second report was brought to the ACP Council in January 1948 and was based on the replies to a questionnaire sent to ACP members. The result may be summarised as follows:

(1) There was general agreement about the need for a higher qualification.

(2) Some thought that it should be carried out by the ACP in conjunction with a College or University.

(3) Others thought that there was a need for a College of Pathologists conducting its own examinations at 'Membership' level.

It seems likely that this was the first occasion when the possibility of an independent College was seriously mooted. These recommendations were sent to the Royal Colleges, the BMA, the Pathological Society of Great Britain and Ireland, the 'Lancet', and the 'BMJ'. The 'Lancet'[8] and 'BMJ'[9] commented briefly on them.

The Council considered that the committee was sufficiently important to remain in being. It therefore came to be called 'The Standing Committee on Training and Qualifications', though it was decided in January 1950 to omit 'and qualifications'. In the event this Committee remained in existence until 24th June, 1955 when it was disbanded.

In January 1948 the Council decided to turn to the RCP for help, and the secretary was asked to negotiate the setting up of an RCP Standing Committee of Pathology. This the RCP agreed to do, and nominated 17 members who were either Fellows or Members of the College. Of these, 13 were also members of the Association of Clinical Pathologists (see below). The ACP members in general found it unsatisfactory, for they had no power of nomination to this committee, all the control being retained within the RCP. It would seem that this approach to the RCP was motivated by a hope that the Physicians would modify their MRCP examination and make it suitable for pathologists. If this could be brought about, it would do much for the status of the pathologist,or so it was hoped. As will be seen later the question of the MRCP for pathologists bedevilled all the future discussions and was eventually the rock on which a possible Faculty of Pathologists in the Royal College of Physicians finally foundered.

In constituting his Committee the President of the RCP had consulted the Pathological Society and the Association of Clinical Pathologists, and had then nominated the following as members of the new Standing Committee on Pathology. The President of the College with J. H. Dible, G. S. Wilson, Sir Lionel Whitby, S. C. Dyke, E. N. Allott, R. J. V. Pulvertaft, W. G. Barnard, G. Payling Wright, T. F. Hewer, S. P. Bedson, W. H. MacMenemey, A. H. T. Robb-Smith, Sir Philip Panton, A. W. Downie, A. F. S. Sladden, and the Registrar. This was approved by the RCP Comitia in July 1948.

The terms of reference were 'to enquire into the training and recognition of medical specialists in Pathology, and to make recommendations covering this branch of medical practice in the future'. Between July 1948 and October 1949 the Committee met four times and on the 27th October submitted a report to the RCP Comitia (Minute XV). The Committee soon realised that there were many types of pathologist, and the question arose as to whether any recommended course of training should apply to all, or only to a certain group. It was decided to make the recommendations general and applicable to all. There was to be a one-year period of clinical training after registration. At this stage a higher qualification in General Medicine or Surgery would be useful and either the MRCP (London) or the FRCS (England) was recommended. The training period in Pathology would extend over five years, the major part being in a teaching hospital. The report ended with a number of recommendations designed to assist Committees of Appointment in deciding whether applicants for posts in Pathology could be recognised as trained Pathologists. In view of what lay ahead the most important decision was the proposed institution of a Diploma in Pathology set up by the two Royal Colleges. This examination (the Conjoint Dip. Path.) would probably be taken after three years general training in all branches of Pathology, and prior to the final two years when the trainee might study in a specialised branch of his choice. On 27th July, 1950 the RCP

Comitia (Minute XXI) approved proposals from the Conjoint Examining Board for the setting up of a Diploma in Pathology. This was received with no great enthusiasm by the ACP, for they were offered no voice in the conduct of the examination. The members of the Conjoint Examining Board who came to the decision were Dr. C. M. Hinds Howell (Chairman), Sir Adolphe Abrahams, Sir Harold Boldero, Mr. L. E. Norbury, Mr. P. H. Mitchener, Mr. Geoffrey Keynes, and the Presidents of the Royal College of Physicians and the Royal College of Surgeons, and it is noteworthy that there was no representative from Pathology. Such was the birth of the ill-fated Diploma of Pathology which was never a success, and as time went on it was more and more realised that it did not provide the increase in status which the Clinical Pathologist was seeking. Apparently the majority of candidates came from foreign medical schools. It would seem that having produced the above report, the Committee felt that the job had been done, for we have no record of further activity until 1958. In fact as one pathologist aptly put it – 'it was a Standing Committee, which had never stood but had only lain down!'

But if the RCP Standing Committee was accused of idleness the same could not be said of the ACP. Ever since the idea of an independent College or a Faculty attached to the Royal College of Physicians had been suggested, it was constantly under discussion. In the early 1950s, largely due to MacMenemey, a number of branches of the ACP were formed throughout the country, and over the next 10 years they were to play an important role in expressing the views of ACP members.

At the January ACP meeting in 1950, the question was raised about methods of formation of 'A College, Faculty, or Institution'. A sub-committee of J. G. Greenfield, E. M. Darmady, and C. G. Signy was appointed to look into the matter. Following an interim report at the 1950 Summer meeting in Leeds, a full report was brought to Council in December 1950. It was found that the ACP would have to take legal steps to ensure the right to speak and act on behalf of Pathology. In brief, to achieve this one of the following steps would be necessary:

(1) Affiliation to an existing Royal College.
(2) Incorporation, by which it might become an independent Faculty or College.
(3) Application for a Royal Charter without any previous incorporation.

From a practical standpoint, 'Incorporation' was the method of choice. Thus, when in the immediate future application was made for incorporation of the ACP many ordinary members thought that the Association was doing so as a preliminary step towards transformation into a College or Faculty of Pathology.

The year 1951 was an important one. The President, Sir Lionel Whitby, gave his address on 'Whither Pathology'.[10] Unlike many other communications of the time, it dealt with the future of Pathology rather than the organisation of the subject within the Faculty of General Medicine. He visualised Haematology and Chemical Pathology as the growing parts of Pathology in the future. But significantly he added in the last sentence that, if the Association adhered to the clinical rather than the technical aspect of Pathology, 'the Association will have strong and natural links with its legitimate parent – the Royal College of Physicians'.

The ACP Spring meeting in 1952 was held at Portsmouth and is important to us because of an address given by W. H. MacMenemey and entitled 'Does the Pathologist need a Faculty?' By this time the question of College or Faculty was being freely discussed and had stimulated some correspondence in the weekly medical journals. Already it was becoming clear that a younger age group favoured the foundation of an independent College, while older members advocated an affiliation with the Royal College of Physicians. The more senior pathologists soon grew alarmed at the growing support for a College and one might hazard a guess that MacMenemey (a strong RCP Faculty supporter) hoped that his address would prevent the tail wagging the dog! This article was a very useful one and stated the grievances of pathologists very clearly. He pointed out that the question of status no longer arose since all specialists were given equal status under the National Health Service. The existing diplomas, i.e., DCP and Dip. Path., were unsuitable, and in no way comparable with the Diplomas of the Royal Colleges. Probably quite rightly, he rejected the idea of modifying the MRCP for pathologists to make it more suitable for them. He was insistent that pathologists should remain attached to the College of Physicians, the body 'appropriate' for them. The real problem was that the Royal College of Physicians was a College of General Physicians, and admission to it was by an examination in General Medicine. MacMenemey wanted the Clinical Pathologist to be regarded as a general physician, as well as a Pathologist. Aware of the feeling amongst younger pathologists that the RCP was not interested in them, he tried to vindicate the College by mentioning one or two ways in which it had helped, e.g. the formation of the Standing Committee in Pathology by the President, Lord Moran. One can understand the attitude of the younger pathologists. They were told that they should be attached to the RCP, a body which they could only join by passing an examination in a subject not specifically theirs. The RCP would speak for Pathology, but need not necessarily say what pathologists desired. In fact one ACP member said that the ACP would obtain its hearing not by right, but through the goodwill of others. MacMenemey conceded this point and indicated that it would be largely remedied by the expediency of incorporation – and this may explain the Council's action of application for incorporation in 1952, which has been already mentioned.

Before proceeding further a word should be said to explain the difficulties of the RCP. There is no doubt that many members of the College of Physicians were genuinely anxious to help pathologists, but many pathologists doubted the intentions of the presidents of this period. The College dared not make examination concessions to the pathologists, for if they did so they would certainly be inundated with requests for similar concessions from the many other branches of medicine. The difficulties of a general college catering for the wants of specialised bodies, becoming more numerous every day, had long been realised. As long ago as 1910 Dr. (later Sir) William Hale White proposed a Committee to reconsider the MRCP examination. However this remained an examination in Clinical Medicine only, in an era when Medicine was expanding so rapidly. As a result there were many men distinguished in allied fields such as Pathology, Public Health, Tropical Medicine, and Physiology who never entered the College. Sir William wisely felt that the College would gain in prestige only if it attracted the best representatives of all branches of Medicine. This far-sighted view-point was supported by eminent men such as the physiologist E. H. Starling, and during his presidency (1931–38) Lord Dawson of Penn did much to encourage the admission to the College of representatives of every facet of Medicine. But in the 1950s the College was still one of General Medicine, and the MRCP was in theory not a mark of proficiency in a speciality, but an indication of the suitability of an individual for further training as a physician. This reminds one of the 'general versus special' problem in regard to hospitals. In the past century when special hospitals were appearing, physicians and surgeons on appointment to the staff of a large London teaching hospital were requested to resign any appointment that they might have at a special hospital!

To return to the activities of the ACP at the January meeting in 1951 the physician Sir Henry Cohen gave a paper on 'The limitations of laboratory investigation'.[11] In it he stated that what one needed to know about a laboratory test included:

(1)  what was it done on?
(2)  who did it?
(3)  how was it done?
(4)  when was it done?

In 1950 the words 'and qualifications' were omitted from the title of the ACP Training Committee, which was subsequently called 'The Standing Committee on Training', but continued to debate the problems of qualifications. The question of the suitability of the Dip. Path. was frequently discussed and at a meeting in January 1952 a memorandum was drawn up stating many ways in which the examination could be modified in order to raise it to the level of the MRCP or FRCS. It was about this time that confidence in the RCP started to wane. The ACP Standing Committee had voiced its dissatisfaction with the Dip.Path. and its concern about the working conditions of pathologists, to the RCP

Standing Committee. But the latter committee never met and on one occasion it appears that the ACP Chairman of Council referred the criticisms of the Dip.Path. back to the ACP Standing Committee. The ACP now showing more concern, asked that the RCP Committee meet every six months. They submitted specific questions to the RCP Committee, but all was to no avail. As a result the ACP was being driven to consider the setting up of their own examinations, and of course to give it status the formation of either an independent College or a Faculty would be needed. The turning point really came at the Exeter meeting in March 1953. It should be mentioned that in the previous year the Association had commenced to hold its meetings in Spring and Autumn rather than in Winter and Summer as heretofore. The feature of the Exeter programme was a debate 'that this meeting would welcome the institution of a college or faculty of pathologists'. It was a spirited debate and when in the late afternoon a vote was taken the motion was carried by 47 to 19. It was felt by many that this vote was not representative, because at the time of the vote many had already left the meeting. It seems that the poor entry into Pathology at the time had led many to believe that it would be improved if a suitable examination could be provided. Certainly one great problem in advising young pathologists was to indicate what examination to take. Again, the purpose of the examination was debated. The DCP and Dip.Path. dealt with technical ability; the MRCP was not an examination in Pathology. In retrospect there were some outstanding difficulties. If the examination was to be a test in Clinical Pathology it would be unsuitable for other types of pathologist. Did members want a Faculty of Pathology or only one of Clinical Pathology? Most appeared to want the examination to cover all of pathology, a mammoth task both for examiners or examinees! Should the examination be like the MRCP, a test of suitability for future training, or should it be a hall-mark of a trained pathologist? Some maintained that what made a man a good pathologist was experience, and that this could not be obtained by examinations.

It was interesting that in the course of the debate both Dyke and Darmady emphasised that steps towards obtaining 'incorporation' of the ACP had nothing whatever to do with the formation of a Faculty or College. An account of the debate at Exeter was sent to every ACP member.

By 1953 the ACP Standing Committee on the Training of Clinical Pathologists had discussed the question of a Faculty and issued a report to the Council (document C8/53). The Council, no doubt surprised at the result of the debate at Exeter, held a joint meeting with the Training Committee on the 18th June. As a basis for discussion the secretary provided a memorandum, in which he set out a proposal for the formation of a Faculty affiliated to the Royal College of Physicians. Following a further meeting the Council decided that there was a *prima facie* case for investigating further the possibility of a Faculty or College. At the

General Meeting of the Association in October 1953 it was decided to form an independent ad hoc Committee which was subsequently referred to as the Hadfield Committee.

The terms of reference were:

(1) to consider the advantages and disadvantages of a college or faculty of pathologists.
(2) to consider whether such a college or faculty should represent all pathologists or only clinical pathologists.
(3) if a faculty, to explore the alternative merits of being affiliated to one or more existing colleges or of being an independent body.
(4) to work out the details, and in particular to investigate the practicability of qualifying examinations.

The constitution of the Committee was: Professor Hadfield (Chairman), E. N. Allott, S. P. Bedson, E. M. Darmady, R. W. Fairbrother, F. Hampson, A. Sachs and Joan Taylor. Professors J. H. Dible, A. C. Lendrum, and J. W. Orr were nominated as observers by the Pathological Society, and Cuthbert Dukes and W. H. MacMenemey of the ACP attended at the Chairman's request. This committee amassed a large amount of evidence regarding the views of members on the above matters, by asking for written statements or by interviewing pathologists and taking verbal statements. Informal discussions between individuals and the Committee were frequent. It met on six occasions between December 1953 and June 1954. In March 1954 an interim report was issued which recognised the need for an academic organisation in pathology, but thought that the institution of a College of Pathologists was neither practicable nor desirable. The committee asked permission to explore the possibility of forming a faculty affiliated to one or both of the two Royal Colleges. A full report of the Committee's work was given in June 1954, and it was noted that according to the President of the RCP a Faculty affiliated to his College might be possible but he did not advise it at a time of such rapid change as the present.

The Hadfield Committee had first of all appealed to all ACP members to express their personal views on establishing a College or Faculty, as well as a suitable examination for pathologists. Later they asked Past Presidents, Past Council Members of the last two years, and present Council Members to give their opinions. The Committee had done some excellent work in a very short time, and the final report was based on an analysis of 129 letters. Comments on these communications and the Sheffield Memorandum will be dealt with in the next chapter.

One point on the nomenclature of the committees should be made. The Hadfield Committee was an ad hoc committee which was sometimes called the Ad Hoc Committee on Academic Affairs. It should not be confused with the later Standing Committee of Academic Affairs which was formed in 1955 and was under the Chairmanship of Professor D. F. Cappell (see chapter 21).

There were other important activities of the Association which must be mentioned. Dyke, having founded the Association successfully in 1927, was stimulated to get world-wide recognition for Clinical Pathology. In 1943 he founded a European Association, the first meeting being held at the Royal Society of Medicine on the 26th and 27th of November.[12] It was attended by a number of refugee pathologists and was followed by further meetings in Oxford[13] in June 1944 and in London[14] in January 1945. Dyke was anxious that there should also be unity with America where there was a growing Association. The final step was taken at the first meeting of the 'Societe francaise de Biologie Clinique' in Paris in 1947, when a 'World Federation of Associations of Clinical Pathology' was formed and Dyke elected as the first President.[15] It was defined as 'an international association of societies devoted to that branch of Medicine known in Great Britain and the United States as Clinical Pathology'.

There were two important events in Britain. In 1945 the first issue of the 'Proceedings of the Association of Clinical Pathologists'[16] appeared and this was later to be continued as the 'Journal of Clinical Pathology'. Under the able editorship of C. Gordon Signy, during the next 30 years it achieved remarkable success. In one of its early issues three prizes of £50, £30, and £20 were offered for a design of a pathological department.[17] The laboratory should serve a population of 200,000 to 300,000. It should provide 'clinical pathology for an area or group hospital, and for the general practitioners of the area including domiciliary services, and bacteriology for local authorities in public health'. Five entries were received, none of them from Pathologists, and the ACP considered that all were disappointing. It was agreed to select one for either the 2nd or 3rd prize but we were not told who was successful. Two names were mentioned, namely Hayton and Hopps, but it is not known whether or not they were the winners or who they were.

In 1946 Clinical Pathology received academic recognition when R. J. V. Pulvertaft was elected by the University of London to the first chair in the subject.[18] It is said that following this event Pulvertaft was asked, 'What is Clinical Pathology?' His reply, in his own laconic way, was to the effect that it was like love or conversion – it could not be defined but could only be experienced!

In the same year the Institute of Medical Laboratory Technicians asked the Association if Fellows of the Institute might be made eligible for Associate membership of the Association. This was turned down because the Association then and again in future years always insisted that its members should be medically qualified.

In the post-war years there was a very rapid growth in the membership of the ACP. The meetings had greatly improved, but the responsibility for their organisation had become onerous. Thus, in 1953 it was agreed to appoint a Meeting Secretary and J. N. Cumings was selected. At this time papers on similar subjects became grouped together, and this was a very necessary step in view of the growing specialisation within the subject. This matter is mentioned because this procedure contrasted strongly with that at meetings of the Pathological Society. Until late in the 1960s it was always the policy of this society to take the papers in the exact order in which they had been submitted. As a result few papers on similar aspects of the subject ran consecutively.

The Association found itself drawn into many different channels in pathology, and was forced to appoint a number of special committees to carry out the work. Increasing specialisation made Committees on Histopathology, Chemical Pathology and Haematology (1949) essential. For some years the Association had been negotiating with Coroners to ensure that forensic work should be carried out by pathologists with suitable training. In January 1949 the Committee on Coroners' Necropsies (set up in 1946) became reconstituted as the Committee on Forensic Pathology. In 1951 a Technical Methods Committee came into being in order to recommence the issuing of Broadsheets (on pathological techniques) which had been discontinued since the early months of World War II. In 1952 the Ethics and Professional Affairs Committee made its appearance. With the growth of Clinical Pathology, the young pathologist found himself faced with a wide variety of problems often concerned with laboratory administration. These might involve negotiating with his clinical colleagues, hospital committees or local authorities. The Ethics and Professional Affairs Committee was much used as an advisory body, but was never able to act on behalf of the individual pathologist.

From these examples some idea of ACP activity can be gleaned and it was certainly a comfort for the clinical pathologist to know that he had the Association behind him. There was in fact an additional body to protect him as the ACP was closely associated with the Pathology Committee of the British Medical Association, where problems of a medico-political nature could be adequately dealt with.

The formation of ACP branches throughout the country was a feature of the immediate post-war years, and these received immediate acceptance. Bearing the mark of MacMenemey's originality many of these regions were given pre-Norman Conquest names such as the Northumbrian, the East and West Mercian, the East Saxon, Cambrian and Wessex. One member who seemed less pleased was heard to say to a fellow member, 'who do you belong to – the posterior Druids?' These branches held meetings once or twice a year. Young pathologists were encouraged to report their research work even if at the time it was incomplete. Papers of special merit were earmarked for a programme at the national meetings. The social side was no less important and a corporate spirit developed between members of a branch and also between neighbouring branches. At times when a vital matter was under discussion it was not uncommon for the Council to refer it to the branches for their opinions. As can be imagined the branches became stronger and as will be seen later they played a very decisive part in influencing the future of Clinical Pathology.

REFERENCES

1  'Lancet'. London (1936) i, p. 58.
2  Ibid (1938) ii, p. 1552.
3  Ibid (1939) ii, p. 1007.
4  Ibid (1950) ii, p. 545.
5  Harrison, C. V., (personal communication).
6  'British Medical Journal'. (1941) i, p. 422.
7  'Lancet'. London (1947) ii.
8  'Lancet'. London (1947) ii, p. 219.
9  'British Medical Journal'. (1947) ii, p. 218.
10  Whitby, Sir Lionel, J. Clin. Path. (1951) 4, pp. 129–136.
11  Cohen, Sir Henry. Ibid (1951) 4, p. 115.
12  'British Medical Journal'. (1943) ii, pp. 826–7.
13  Ibid (1944) ii, pp. 287–8.
14  Ibid (1945) i, p. 379.
15  Ibid (1947) ii, p. 1006.
16  Ibid (1945) ii, p. 498.
17  J. Clin. Path. (1948) 1, p. 179.
18  'British Medical Journal'. (1946) ii, p. 248.

# TWENTY ONE
# College or Faculty? 1952–58

By 1952 the paramount need was a suitable examination for trained pathologists. The Conjoint Board had instituted the Diploma of Pathology which was generally considered to be unsatisfactory. Certain alterations had been suggested, but no action had been taken because Professor J. H. Dible had advised against an approach on this matter being made to the RCP Standing Committee of Pathology. Many members of the ACP began to feel that pathologists would be forced to set up their own examination. In March 1953 the ACP Council received a letter from the East Mercian Branch proposing that 'a Faculty of Clinical Pathologists be set up linked with the Royal Colleges of Physicians and Surgeons'. In 1952 the ACP Secretary had reported that he had had unofficial talks with Sir Russell Brain, the RCP President. It appeared that the Secretary was to talk also with the RCS President, Sir Cecil Wakeley. The wording is equivocal and it is not clear whether he was asked to discuss matters with Wakeley or whether he asked permission to do so. However, there is no record of any results from any such conversations. Following their preliminary report in March 1954, the Hadfield Committee was empowered to have talks with the Presidents of the Royal Colleges on the future organisation of Pathologists and the provision of a specialist examination. As stated in the last chapter, in June 1954 the ACP Council was told that the RCP President's personal advice was against the formation of a Faculty linked with the RCP 'at a time when such rapid changes were taking place'. There is no record of the reaction of the President of the RCS, if indeed he was approached.

At this time, although many pathologists advocated affiliation with the Physicians, there was a lesser number who favoured the Surgeons. In the post-war years the activity of the RCS stood out in contrast to that of the RCP. The then President of the RCS, Sir Alfred (later Lord) Webb Johnson had made his College into a postgraduate teaching centre, with departments of Anatomy, Pathology, and Physiology. In 1945 Rupert A. Willis had been appointed Professor of Pathology and was succeeded by Geoffrey Hadfield in 1948, and George J. Cunningham (an ACP member) in 1955. Some pathologists thought they would have a better standing in a College which had recognised the importance of their subject by having a special department. It should be mentioned that in the post-war years Sir Alfred Webb Johnson attempted to establish a large medical centre in Lincoln's Inn Fields, where the Surgeons had their Royal College. At this time the RCP was contemplating leaving their premises in Pall Mall East, and Webb Johnson invited them and the Royal College of Obstetricians and Gynaecologists to join him in Lincoln's Inn Fields, to create a single academy of medicine. It is sad to say that the Physicians refused and a golden opportunity was lost. Shortly afterwards the Physicians and Obstetricians moved to new sites in Regent's Park.

Throughout 1954 discussions on the organisation of pathologists continued, and the ACP Committee on Training made a critical report on the Diploma of Pathology examination. They decided to 'leave it on the table' for six months and this seems to have been the prelude to the disbanding of the committee in June 1955.

But the Hadfield Committee on Academic Affairs had still much work to do, and it was January 1955 before its final report was presented to the ACP Council. They had 129 letters to analyse as well as many new communications from senior pathologists. In addition, there was an event which, many believed, greatly influenced opinion amongst pathologists. In February 1954 five pathologists in Sheffield, namely E. K. Blackburn, J. Colquhoun, J. L. Edwards, Arthur Jordan, and C. G. Paine, sent a printed memorandum specifically produced for the Hadfield Committee.

This document was a remarkable one, a forthright and cogently argued case for the establishment of a College or independent Faculty of Pathologists. It was circulated to all ACP members and doubtless influenced the feelings of many. It must have come as a shock to the Hadfield Committee for at about this time it had ascertained that out of 28 members, mostly senior including some part presidents and Council members, only seven were in favour of establishing a new body (E. M. Darmady, Arthur Jordan, J. O. Oliver, R. J. V. Pulvertaft, A. Sachs, Joan Taylor, and C. Taylor). The Sheffield memorandum was comprehensive and discussed the pros and cons of a College or Faculty. It favoured an independent College, went into its constitution, and even worked out how it could be financed. The latter was of great importance for in many of the discussions at this time opponents of a College, and even some who favoured it, dismissed it without further consideration because it was thought to be impossible to finance. The Sheffield group must have soon run into the difficulties of outlining a scheme agreeable to all types of pathologist. It was probably this, and their appreciation of the special needs of hospital pathologists, that led them to propose a College or Faculty confined to Clinical Pathologists. One thing not mentioned was the future of the ACP and one presumes that it would have been transformed into the new body and would thus disappear in name.

The Hadfield Committee continued its work throughout 1954 and it should be noted that in the Interim Report it stated 'that it recognised the need for an academic organisation in Pathology, but that the institution of a College of Pathologists was neither practicable nor desirable'. The final report of the Committee to the ACP Council was delivered in January 1955, and based on 129 letters, the Sheffield Memorandum, and a number of statements from senior pathologists including past

Presidents and Council members of the ACP. It was decided that an abbreviated report (a formidable task) should be compiled by Dr. Cuthbert Dukes (the ACP Chairman of Council) and sent to all members in preparation for discussion at the Annual General Meeting of the ACP later in the year. The report appeared in March 1955 and concluded with the following statement: 'We have here the opinions of 33 experienced pathologists, representatives of many branches of pathology, each exceptionally well qualified to express an opinion with respect to the academic needs of pathologists'.

Such an observation, although factually correct, should not pass without comment, for it implies that there was some measure of agreement amongst pathologists. A reading of the evidence given to the Committee shows that the reverse is the case. There was very little support amongst senior and especially academic pathologists for either a Faculty or a College, but pathologists were still split down the middle and the great divergence of views made the writing of the report most difficult. The Chairman divided the report into five sections as follows:

(1) Views of observers and members of the Hadfield Committee.
(2) Comments by past presidents and members of Council of the ACP. In these two sections the secretary made abstracts from any contribution which appeared to be an individual's most distinctive contribution.
(3) The discussion of these documents by the Committee.
(4) The decisions of the Committee.
(5) Epilogue.

Thus, the Hadfield Committee expressed no corporate view, and it did little to clarify what was a very complex situation. One important proposal emerged during the discussions of the Committee. Anxious to have a qualification of status the ACP had asked the RCP to modify the MRCP to make it suitable for pathologists. But at that time and indeed in later years the RCP felt that their Membership was a special one to be reserved for Physicians. In the contributions to the Hadfield Committee by Douglas Collins and R. J. B. Pulvertaft mention was made of a proposed new examination. It would be called a Mastership in Pathology, and is said to have been proposed by the President of the Royal College of Physicians. This would be awarded by the RCP but be distinct from the Membership, and holders of it would not be eligible for election to the Fellowship. One new suggestion emerged, namely that a Board of Pathology be established to provide the required examination, presumably similar to that in existence in the U.S.A.

The Council spent the whole of the morning of Saturday, 29th January, 1955, discussing the findings of the Hadfield Committee. The unrest which existed in the ACP was chiefly confined to the younger members. It was from this group that a demand issued for a faculty or college of pathology and a recognised higher examination in the subject.

Senior pathologists remained unconvinced that any such actions were necessary. When it came to the question of affiliation of a faculty to either or both of the Royal Colleges, there was virtually no support, as it was agreed by all that pathologists must at all costs maintain their independence. Once more an impasse had been reached and so the discussion returned to improvement in the training of pathologists, a practical proposition and therefore much more attractive. An extension of 'refresher courses' for pathologists was desirable, and these activities could be well taken care of by an Academic Affairs Committee. It should be mentioned that about 1950 Cuthbert Dukes, who later became ACP Adviser in Postgraduate Education, had already started the Refresher Courses (chiefly in special histopathology) which met with instant success. In October 1952 Dr. G. K. McGowan, acting for the Committee on Chemical Pathology, organised the first Refresher Course in this subject and this met with an equal success.

After so much discussion the decisions of the Council sound disappointingly negative. No further action was to be taken at the present time in regard to the formation of a College or Faculty of Pathology. There were no proposals about the specialist examination, but there were many members who believed that a Mastership of the Royal College of Physicians would in the end prove to be the solution. The one positive proposal was the formation of a new Academic Affairs Committee. At the Annual General Meeting in September 1955 the ad hoc Hadfield Committee and the Allott Committee on Training were disbanded and replaced by a Standing Committee on Academic Affairs with D. F. Cappell as Chairman and E. M. Darmady as Secretary. It was intended that this new committee should keep all academic matters under constant review, and might perhaps placate many younger pathologists who had been clamouring for some action.

The Academic Affairs Committee consisted of the following:

| | |
|---|---|
| D. F. Cappell (Chairman) | W. H. Fulton |
| E. N. Allott | M. Haines |
| G. Archer | F. Hampson |
| A. C. P. Campbell | J. W. Heggie |
| F. E. Camps | A. Jordan |
| R. Cruickshank | J. B. Manning |
| E. M. Darmady | W. H. MacMenemey |
| C. E. Dukes | R. J. V. Pulvertaft |
| R. W. Fairbrother | A. G. Signy |
| J. S. Faulds | W. St. C. Symmers |

Shortly after its formation, the names of G. J. Cunningham and Joan Taylor were added.

The Council recommended the following tasks for the new committee, namely:

(1) to consider the advantages and disadvantages of a college or faculty of pathologists.

(2) to consider if such a college or faculty should represent all pathologists or only clinical pathologists.

(3) if a faculty, to explore the alternative merits of being affiliated to one or more existing colleges, or of being an independent body.

(4) to work out the details and in particular to investigate the practicability of qualifying examinations.

The Council was evidently anxious to establish that the pathologists of the future should be a consultant and not merely a super-technician.

Between September 1955 and June 1958 the new Committee on Academic Affairs held at least 12 meetings and issued reports from time to time as will be seen. It faced many problems, the most immediate of which were to determine a suitable examination for pathologists, and a body suitable to sponsor it. At this time there was much pressure, some of it generated by the Sheffield Memorandum, from younger pathologists for the formation of an independent college. Older members felt that only one side of the problem had been expounded, and that an attempt should be made to present to the younger pathologists the case for a Faculty affiliated to the Royal College of Physicians. Although the RCP had shown little enthusiasm for such a project, MacMenemy, the ACP Secretary, felt there was still hope as evidenced by a long letter which he wrote to the President of the RCP (Sir Russell Brain) in which he stated the problems facing pathologists (13th June, 1955).

It seems clear that at this time the Royal College of Physicians would

(1) modify the Diploma in Pathology if the pathologists desired it.

(2) raise no objection to setting up a new higher examination or Mastership of Pathology in the RCP but that it could not be used as a stepping stone to the Fellowship.

(3) that it would not agree to modifying the MRCP to make it more suitable for pathologists.

MacMenemey in his letter to Sir Russell Brain had expressed pleasure at the possibility that the RCP might be able to supply accommodation for a Secretariat of the ACP. He mentioned that future ACP meetings would probably be held at the Royal College of Surgeons and it seems certain that he felt this would be the way to have a foot in each camp!

The Academic Affairs Committee commenced by discussing the report on the Diploma of Pathology previously issued by the ACP Committee on the Training of Clinical Pathologists. It hoped that the approving committee, namely the Conjoint Board, would be advised by a joint committee of the RCP and ACP, rather than by the Standing Committee of the RCP. It also suggested that a list of approved laboratories for training be prepared and reviewed annually.

The year 1956 was noteworthy for three events. Firstly on the 18th February the ACP at last became incorporated under the Companies Act of 1948, and again some wondered whether this was going to be the first step towards the foundation of an independent Faculty or College.

Secondly, there was a meeting between senior officials of the RCP and representatives from the Academic Affairs Committee. The reaction of the RCP to an examination for pathologists remained unchanged (see above).

Thirdly, the ACP Council received a report from the Committee on Academic Affairs on the 4th October. This indicated that most of the committee's time had been spent on training. There was a report on the training of Chemical Pathologists and a memorandum outlining the principles underlying the training of Forensic Pathologists. When it came to the question of training Morbid Anatomists, it was felt that no examination could test a candidate's ability and that the aim should be to find out whether he or she was suitable for a senior trainee appointment. The Committee also felt that there should be no single examination which would be a *sine qua non* for a consultant post in pathology. This point of view is understandable but it was not helpful to senior pathologists who were constantly being approached by trainees to know which examination they ought to take. When it came to a consideration of the examinations available at the time, the DCP was said to be unsuitable, the MRCP (Edinburgh) the best (as part of the exam could be taken in Pathology), and the Conjoint Dip.Path. perhaps suitable if certain changes (detailed in the report) were instituted. There was little or no support for the proposed Mastership of the RCP and it was obvious that confidence in this body was low. The report recommended 'that it would be unprofitable to pursue further with the RCP the question of setting up higher qualifications in Pathology'. In regard to the Dip.Path. examination, the ACP would be willing to assist the Conjoint Board in assessing the suitability of laboratories for training for the examination.

The work of the Committee for the years 1956–57 was outlined in a second report to the Council. There had already been reference to the enthusiastic reception of the postgraduate Refresher Courses. The possible appointment of a Dean had been suggested and on the 28th June 1957 it was decided to appoint Dr. Cuthbert Dukes as ACP Advisor in Postgraduate Studies. The subjects dealt with in the first report had been investigated in greater depth, but the basic approach in the second was similar. Suggestions for the training of Forensic Pathologists were in fact given in much greater detail. One new proposal was for a junior grade of ACP membership. The new grade would be provided for trainees no earlier than in the second year of training. These Associate members would have many privileges but would not be allowed to participate in the organisation and administration of the Association nor to vote at business meetings. Council discussed the matter but did not agree to adopt it.

In February 1957 Professor R. J. V. Pulvertaft resigned from the Academic Affairs Committee and his place was taken by Professor C. H. Gray.

The year of 1958 was in many ways a momentous one and there were signs of steady progress by the Academic Affairs Committee. In January the ACP Council received some proposals to improve the standard of training and to set up a supervisory body. The document was a lengthy one and almost certainly drawn up by the Secretary of the Committee. With so many divergent views it was soon realised that only a compromise solution was practicable. Much old ground was gone over again, but in the case of the examination it became clear that the only one which would satisfy pathologists would be one which was instituted by pathologists. In retrospect, it seems that although it was thought that the ACP was the ideal body to sponsor it, yet there was a certain reluctance because it was felt that the ACP was not primarily an academic body. But ironically the ACP seemed to be the only body which was really interested in the education of pathologists, but did not have the necessary facilities. The point on which there was some degree of unanimity was on the pattern of training and each group which had so far made recommendations on this subject agreed that trainee pathologists should

(1) receive a basic all-round training in Pathology, including technical methods.
(2) acquire a basic knowledge of general medicine in its widest sense.
(3) be trained in a laboratory of high standing in the profession or alternatively that the laboratories should be limited in the time that the candidates should stay with them.
(4) undertake and publish some original work.
(5) obtain a degree in pathology.

In regard to what an appropriate examination should be, there was as yet no conclusion. A Board of Pathology was again suggested (like that operating in the USA) in order to organise the examination. The passing of the examination and the completion of the training programme might be linked up with the proposed two-tiered membership already mentioned, and qualify an individual for Full Membership of the Association.

The pros and cons of a Faculty, either affiliated to the RCP or independent, were discussed and a proposal for its financing was made. The workings of Faculties already in existence were outlined with their advantages and disadvantages. Strangely enough, no mention was made of the possibility of an independent College.

In April 1958 two documents prepared by the Academic Affairs Committee were submitted to Council at the meeting in Dublin. One was an historical summary of events leading up to the present memorandum of the Committee and this will not be considered further. The other

341

(Document C6/58) was a memorandum concerning examinations in Pathology. Here little progress had been made and once more it contained a criticism of the present examinations available. A senior member of the Association (Cuthbert Dukes) doubted the need for any examination and thought that the ACP should concentrate on postgraduate teaching courses. Once more an outline of a type of examination was given. Finally, it was recommended that the Association approach the Pathological Society and the Royal Medical Colleges with a view to setting up a Board or other organisation for the institution of postgraduate qualifications in Pathology. If this materialised it would be necessary to decide how the supervising and examining body should be appointed. There appeared to be three alternatives for setting up the examining body, viz,

    (i)   by the Association of Clinical Pathologists.
    (ii)  by a new board outside the ACP with representatives from the Royal Colleges and the Pathological Society.
    (iii) under the aegis of the existing examining boards.

Finally, at the June meeting of Council, a report was received from the Academic Affairs Committee (Document C12/58) on its work for the year 1957–1958. From this time the Committee held no further meetings, for reasons which will subsequently be given. It should perhaps be mentioned that the Chairman, Professor D. F. Cappell, drew up two documents, namely:

    (i)   'Abstracts from the deliberations of the Committee on Academic Affairs 1955–1958'.
    (ii)  'D. F. Cappell's comments on the possible examinations for a higher qualification in Pathology'.

These documents were dated the 13th and 20th November, 1961, and as far as is known no action was taken. But by this time there had been other important developments.

In 1957, the Presidency of the Royal College of Physicians had been taken over by Robert Platt, a nephrologist with a very good experimental department in Manchester, who had considerable sympathy with pathologists and was much more willing to help them than were his predecessors. He no doubt also realised the advantages of keeping pathologists within his College. At the ACP Council meeting on 31st January, 1958, it was announced that the President of the RCP had written a letter stating that he proposed to reconstitute the Pathological Committee of the College which had not met for many years. He asked the Association to supply him with the names of possible members. It was understood that it was not necessary that all the members should be Fellows or Members of the College. The Council suggested the following names:

E. N. Allott
Sir Samuel Bedson
D. F. Cappell
R. Cruickshank
G. J. Cunningham
J. S. Faulds
F. Hampson
A. Jordan

N. H. Martin
W. H. MacMenemey
G. R. Osborn
R. J. V. Pulvertaft
A. G. Signy
Joan Taylor
G. Payling Wright

From what has been recently stated it might be supposed that the formation of an independent College of Pathologists had been dismissed once and for all. This may have been true as far as senior members of the ACP were concerned, but it was far from being the case with the more junior members. They were clamouring for some action to be taken and were strong believers in a College. At this time the ACP branches became very active and the pros and cons of Faculty versus College were constantly under debate. It was probably the first instance of the effect of the branches on the policy of the Association. Council became somewhat concerned when just prior to the June 1958 meeting demands were received from four branches (The Channel Coast, East Saxon, Thames Valley and the Wessex) that Council consider the possibility of setting up an independent College. Council therefore discussed the matter with results that caused universal surprise.

It should be recalled that at a Council Meeting in 1955 there had been a short discussion on whether or not it was appropriate to consider the setting up of a separate organisation in pathology such as an independent College or an affiliated Faculty. Speaking from memory, the author (G.J.C) recalls that when a vote was taken there was a majority of 14 to 3 against taking any such action. Yet only three years later when a similar vote was taken it was unanimously agreed that 'steps should be taken forthwith to discuss the way in which a College of Pathology might be inaugurated and to consider the functions of such a body'. This unanimity was a decided change of heart and included Council members such as J. N. Cumings, A. G. Marshall, and E. N. Davey, all of whom had previously been strong opponents. It was decided that a Working Party be set up 'to consider the formation and functions of a College of Pathology'. The constitution of the Working Party was:

Professor G. J. Cunningham (Chairman)
Professor D. F. Cappell
Professor J. N. Cumings
A. Jordan
Joan Taylor

The Chairman of Council (E. N. Allott) and the Secretary (F. Hampson) were *ex officio* members.

343

After the formation of the Cunningham Working Party, in June 1958, the Standing Committee on Academic Affairs ceased to meet and was, to use the words of one Council member, 'put into cold storage!'

## REFERENCES

The information in this chapter was obtained mainly from ACP Council Minutes, Year Books, and Reports of Annual Meetings.

# TWENTY TWO

# How the College was formed 1958–64

The Cunningham Working Party, well aware of the urgency of its task, held its first meeting on the 16th July 1958, and its fourth and final one on the 18th September. The final report was sent out to Council Members at the end of September and a short statement was made by the Chairman to members of the Association at the Annual General Meeting. In summary the report included:

(1) An analysis of the present situation in Pathology.
(2) The basic reasons for the formation of a College with a list of its possible functions.
(3) The division of functions between a College and existing pathological bodies.
(4) The detailed procedure for the formation of a College.

In the various discussions which had taken place at this time it became clear that opponents of the scheme for an independent college, as well as some of its supporters, dismissed the idea because of the excessive cost. This was only valid if the aim was to put up a building comparable with those of the existing Royal Colleges. The argument was fallacious because a College like that of the Obstetricians and Gynaecologists had started in a very modest way in a house with limited staff and accommodation. It was therefore essential to try to settle this matter one way or another. Accordingly, the Chairman approached a firm of Chartered Surveyors and inspected three properties in the West End of London which were at the time available. One of these (which was in Portman Square) was selected for detailed study and it was calculated that a sum slightly in excess of £5000 per annum would be needed to cover the rent and the running costs. It would have to be a modest start, but it was clear that if pathologists considered that an independent college would be advantageous, then they should not be deterred by financial considerations. The cost of purchasing freehold property was out of the question. It may be mentioned that at this time an excellent building on the Embankment and owned by the Incorporated Accountants was for sale at what was considered to be a reasonable price of £170,000. The annual costs of maintenance would have been about £20,000. It is of interest that this site was almost certainly the one on which the Conjoint Laboratories of the Royal Colleges of Physicians and Surgeons were erected in the late 1880s.

On 2nd October, 1958, a few days after the Working Party had submitted its report, Dr. Cuthbert E. Dukes gave the third Foundation Lecture to the Association. This lecture was given every three years, the first in 1952 by the ACP Founder, Dr. S. C. Dyke, and the second by J. G. Greenfield in 1955. It provided a contrast to the prevalent discussions on the organisation of pathologists. In it, the title of which was 'Motives in Pathology', Dukes examined the reasons for entering Clinical Pathology, the aims of the ACP and the motives of clinicians using laboratory tests. The choice of Faculty or College was not mentioned and Dukes's motive was obviously an attempt to close the ranks of members of the ACP. It seems likely that it did not attract the attention which it deserved because of more pressing considerations and it does not appear to have been published in the medical press.

During the period of activity of the Working Party the Chairman circularised 54 pathologists, asking for their confidential opinions about the desirability of forming a College, the functions it could perform and the possible effects on the Pathological Society and the Association of Clinical Pathologists. The 48 replies received were most enlightening and did much to facilitate the discussions of the Working Party. There was substantial though not overwhelming support for an independent College. Many favoured it but, as indicated above, seemed overawed at the size of the venture and the expense which would be incurred. Most were convinced that the training of pathologists needed defining and some sort of supervision instituted; a recognised examination was essential. As to the future of the existing societies, none feared for the Pathological Society whilst the vast majority were convinced that with the formation of a College the Association of Clinical Pathologists would become redundant and disappear. The opening comment of one member of the Working Party at its first meeting was that 'he hoped that this was not going to be a burial party for the ACP'.

More important even than this report was a memorandum which it was proposed to circulate to all ACP Members together with a voting form, in which they were asked whether they approved of a College and, if so, whether they would agree to give 10 guineas as a gift, pay an entrance fee of £10 on becoming a Member and pay an annual subscription of three guineas per annum should this be found necessary. It was further suggested that unless a substantial majority opinion of support was obtained it would not be worthwhile proceeding with the venture. It was agreed that for a valid result 75% of members must vote and that there must be a 75% majority of those voting.

At the Annual General Meeting which followed Dr. W. H. McMenemey gave his Presidential Address on assuming office. This address was entitled 'The future position of the Pathologist in Medicine', and was published in the 'Lancet' of October 18th.[1] It reviewed the historical background of pathology and pointed out that pathologists were already represented by the ACP so far as the Ministry of Health was concerned, and that, if the RCP could be persuaded to provide a special MRCP examination for pathologists with a smaller clinical content, then it should not be necessary to set up a new College.

In spite of this Council proceeded to collect the views of ACP members and the closing date for the vote was the 30th November 1958.

The result showed that 74% of all members had voted and of these 77.4% had approved the principle of setting up a College of Pathologists. However, only 69.7% had answered 'Yes' to all questions and thus agreed to an entrance fee of ten guineas and an annual subscription of three guineas. Although these figures were slightly below the required ones, at the ACP Council Meeting in December 1958 it was decided that they were sufficient to proceed with the proposal.

One argument in favour of an independent college was the size of the potential membership, and the following figures were obtained from the 'British Medical Journal'.[2] The number of Consultants on the 31st December, 1957 was:

| | |
|---|---|
| General Surgery | 999 |
| General Medicine | 965 |
| Anaesthetics | 852 |
| Pathology | 723 |
| Obstetrics | 500 |
| Radiology | 493 |
| Radiotherapy | 134 |

There was one great difficulty which faced the ACP. If they did proceed with the formation of an independent college, they could not 'go it alone' and a united front amongst pathologists was essential. This would mean the co-operation of the Pathological Society. It was anticipated that there would be some opposition judging from some unofficial conversations with its senior members.

At the ACP Council Meeting in December 1958, the Chairman was asked to write to Professor G. L. Montgomery (Secretary of the Pathological Society), explaining the recent vote and giving the results. He further proposed that a working party consisting of four members of each society be formed to obtain a broader census of opinion among all pathologists; that the terms of reference be as wide as possible and might include the formation of a College of Pathology; and that a wider poll be taken to include members of the Pathological Society. This would mean a joint action by the two societies and its importance can be imagined when the following facts are realised. The Pathological Society was the senior and older body, and consisted of more members than the ACP, 1380 in May 1961, which included non-medicals such as scientific research workers, veterinary, dental, and other pathologists. The ACP, by contrast, included only those who were medically qualified; the membership numbered about 1000.

The Committee of the Pathological Society considered these proposals at their meeting in January 1959. They declined to join the proposed working party and were unwilling to conduct a vote amongst their members. However they finally, after much discussion, agreed to a compromise. They were willing to supply the ACP with the names of their members, and consented to the ACP conducting the poll. The ACP would draw up a memorandum on the purpose of the poll and a suitable voting paper. These were to be submitted to the Secretary of the Pathological Society for approval. This the ACP agreed to do and requested the Cunningham Working Party to hold an additional meeting in order to draw up the necessary documents. This took place on the 6th March, 1959 and the draft documents were approved. The voting paper was essentially similar to that sent to ACP members, except that Path Society Members who were also ACP members and had voted previously were asked to identify themselves. The closing date for the poll was 15th May, 1959, so that the results could be discussed by the ACP Council in June and by the Committee of the Pathological Society in July. The poll showed that there was a voting response of only a little under 53% from Members of the Pathological Society who had not already voted as members of the ACP and of these 53% approved of a college in principle. Only 20% agreed also to the proposed financial provisions.

At the ACP Council in June 1959 a shock item on the Agenda was an announcement that, as a result of some informal discussions with the President of the RCP, it now appeared that the Royal College of Physicians was prepared to offer a Faculty to the Pathologists. To anyone conversant with the inner workings of the ACP Council and the Royal College of Physicians it would not have been so surprising, as will be explained.

During his period of office as ACP Secretary McMenemey, himself a Fellow of the RCP, aimed at keeping the President well informed of the problems faced by hospital pathologists. This is well illustrated by a long letter written to Sir Russell Brain on 13th June, 1955. It related to the recent formation of the Standing Committee on Academic Affairs with Professor D. F. Cappell as Chairman, and gave some indications of the various matters which would be discussed. Of considerable interest is the statement that ACP members have heard 'with interest that there would probably be no difficulty in instituting a Mastership in Pathology if an examination higher than the D.Path. was considered desirable, or an affiliated faculty with full autonomy in examinations and adequate representation on the College Council; they know too that your personal advice is against the formation of a faculty at present'. McMenemey also referred to 'the suggestion that the ACP Secretariat might be housed in the College' and he asked certain questions related to this possibility. McMenemey always maintained that the President was 'interested' but there was little sign of any activity during Sir Russell's term of office which terminated in 1957. He was succeeded by Sir Robert Platt and before long it became clear that relationships between the ACP Officers and the RCP President had become much closer. Sir Robert must have soon become aware of the problems facing hospital pathologists, the main one at the time being the need for a suitable examination. The deficiencies of the existing examinations have been discussed in a previous chapter. As also previously mentioned, he proposed the reconstitution of the RCP Pathology Committee which had not met for eight years. The ACP Council submitted 15 names at the request of the President who selected 11 to serve on the Committee in addition to himself and the Registrar of the RCP. This body was appointed by the Comitia on 24th April, 1958 (two months before the appointment of the Cunningham Working Party, and seven months before the first ACP vote). At the same time the ACP Council agreed to ask the new RCP Committee 'to consider modifying the Diploma in Pathology examination' in order to make it into 'an introductory diploma to be taken at a relatively early stage in training' and to 'institute preliminary discussions with interested bodies about postgraduate qualifications in Pathology'.

The RCP Committee met on two occasions and brought out a draft report of certain proposals. There is no record of its reception by the ACP or whether the recommendations were adopted, but any such events probably happened during the year 1958. Thus, by the time (June 1959) that a Faculty within the RCP was a possibility, the examination for pathologists became only part of a wider issue, namely, their organisation within the profession. At the time some very senior pathologists were closely allied to the RCP as Fellows, and it would seem that they were anxious to strengthen the rather tenuous bonds which linked pathologists to the RCP. At the ACP Council in June 1958, it became clear that the result of the vote of the Pathological Society had strengthened the case for an independent college. But many members were impressed by the encouraging news from the President of the RCP. It was therefore decided that

(1) the Council should have further discussions with the RCP President, their representatives being the Chairman of Council (E. N. Allott), the Secretary (F. Hampson), and the President-Elect (J. N. Cumings).

(2) an Extraordinary Council Meeting should be held on 22nd September 1958 solely to discuss the question of Faculty or College.

The Committee of the Pathological Society received the voting figures, but expressed no surprise 'as the voting had followed the pattern of the ACP's earlier poll of its members'. The proposal from the RCP was mentioned, but it was agreed that no action was called for at the moment.

At the extraordinary meeting of Council on 22nd September, a memorandum was provided by the Secretary, indicating that the President of the RCP had introduced 'a new and major factor into the situation' by offering an organisation of pathologists within the RCP. He had agreed that it would be reasonable that the passing of an examination approved by pathologists in this organisation should confer eligibility for election to the Fellowship of the College with rights equal to those of physicians. The document listed advantages and disadvantages of a separate College of Pathologists and some problems to be solved in connection with its founding, together with a list of advantages and disadvantages of a Faculty within the RCP. The Chairman of Council pointed out that those members of the two pathological organisations who had voted for a College had done so in ignorance of the new offer by the PRCP and stressed the friendly and co-operative reception which he and his colleagues had received from the President.

The effect of this counter-proposal was to cause a sharp division of opinion amongst Council members. It had been conveyed by a letter from the PRCP and it was said that the Comitia had indicated its support for such a project. Moreover, the ACP members who had met the President informally had been greatly impressed by the warmth of their reception. It was obvious that such a proposal must be examined further and Council agreed to accept the invitation of the President to discussions; this was welcomed particularly by the older members. Others (mostly younger) were dismayed for they felt that this rather belated offer would place the College proposal, for which there was so much support, in jeopardy. Obviously there were many things to be discussed before any decision could be made. The Council therefore decided (presumably to pacify the supporters of an independent college) to appoint a committee – the Ways and Means Committee. This has often been referred to as the Working Party, but it is incorrect and renders it liable to be confused with the original Cunningham Working Party which gave its final report to the Council in 1958.

The Ways and Means Committee consisted of G. J. Cunningham (Chairman), E. N. Allott, N. H. Ashton, D. F. Cappell, J. N. Cumings, F. Hampson, A. Jordan, G. R. Osborn, and Joan Taylor. The primary purpose of this Committee was to explore further the ways and means of setting up a College of Pathologists. In retrospect it was clearly handicapped by having to deal with the proposals made by the RCP as a matter of urgency before it could get on with its primary purpose. Furthermore, it became evident that many of its members were very anxious to avail themselves of the offer made by the President of the RCP. The Committee had its first meeting on the rather appropriate 5th day of November 1959. The fifth and final meeting was held on 29th January, 1960 and a report submitted to the ACP Council a few days later. This report was discussed at a special meeting of Council on 12th February, 1960. It should be noted that in preparing this report the Chairman not only had the help of his committee members, but also the views of about 20 junior pathologists who, at his invitation, had submitted their opinions. A number of Branch Secretaries also provided information about local discussions which had been held.

Because it had been arranged that members of the ACP should meet the President and representatives of the RCP to discuss the Faculty proposals on 17th December, 1959, the first two meetings of the Ways and Means Committee were devoted to formulating definite proposals to submit to the RCP. This took up much time and as a result no mention was made at either meeting of the Ways and Means Committee of setting up a College of Pathologists. At the outset the Committee was anxious to keep the Pathological Society fully informed and the ACP Chairman of Council was asked to approach the Secretary of the Pathological Society to find out whether they would agree to D. F. Cappell and G. J. Cunningham acting as their observers, as both were at that time members of the Pathological Society Committee. In the event the Pathological Society agreed to send A. W. Downie as an observer though the only meetings he attended were the ones with the RCP representatives. For the purposes of the first meeting with the RCP representatives the Ways and Means Committee appointed E. N. Allott (ACP Chairman of Council), J. N. Cumings (ACP President), G. J. Cunningham (Chairman of the Ways and Means Committee), and F. Hampson (ACP Secretary) to act as their representatives. At this meeting held on 17th December 1959 at the RCP the President (Sir Robert Platt) was in the Chair. The RCP was represented by Sir Harold Boldero (Registrar), A. M. Cooke, E. R. Boland, W. N. Mann, and J. S. Richardson. R. R. Bomford was unable to attend. Of the ACP representatives, F. Hampson was absent. A. W. Downie represented the Pathological Society as an observer. The meeting was very cordial and it was clear that the RCP President was anxious to meet the requests of the ACP representatives. It appeared that, under the conditions proposed, pathologists would have the maximum amount of independence and control that could be expected by a Faculty existing in another College. The RCP would not agree to offer an MRCP to pathologists as they wished to reserve this for physicians. They agreed to the examination for pathologists (say Membership of the Faculty of Pathology or MFP) being equal to the MRCP. This equality would be based on the eligibility of its Members to be elected to the Fellowship in the same way as Members of the Royal College of Physicians. The ACP representatives, in order to safeguard themselves, asked for a proportional number of Fellows (pathologists) to be elected each year. The RCP representatives could not agree to this, presumably because they feared that their governing body, the Comitia, might in future be swamped by pathologists. They argued that it would be better to have no fixed number as the pathologists might have a greater number elected! This seemed to be the one discordant note and at least one ACP representative disliked the idea of a pathologist being given seniority on the recommendation of a body consisting largely of physicians; he felt that if pathologists were to be approved for seniority this should be decided by pathologists. The general terms having been formulated, it was decided to leave the financial details for a future meeting. Reports of the meeting were drawn up by the RCP and ACP agreed and exchanged.

On the 12th of February 1960, Council held a special meeting to receive the report of the Cunningham Ways and Means Committee which included information, not only about the formation of a College, but also relating to the formation of a Faculty within the RCP. Council also received a document summarising discussions with representatives of the RCP, from which it appeared likely that a Faculty could be established which would:

1. Advise the College on all matters relevant to pathology (but the RCP would not be precluded from seeking advice from other sources).
2. Be governed by a Council elected by pathologists (with cross representation with the Council of the RCP).
3. Control examinations for membership of the Faculty (but the examiners to include one or more members nominated by the RCP).
4. Be formed by nominating about 300 pathologists as founder members (much less than the existing complement of consultant pathologists).
5. Have its members eligible for Fellowship of the RCP in the same way as Members of the RCP.

Financial matters were not discussed.

The Chairman felt that the Ways and Means Committee could not go any further with its primary object until the offer of the RCP had been dealt with. It was at this meeting that the deep division of opinion really became manifest. The main point at issue was whether discussions with the RCP should or should not be continued. The general feeling was that it might be discourteous to break off negotiations when the ACP representatives had been in receipt of a considerable amount of goodwill on the part of the RCP. A motion that discussions should continue was proposed by N. H. Ashton, seconded by W. P. Stamm, and carried by 12 votes to 4. The Chairman of the Ways and Means Committee hoped that any decision to continue negotiations would in no way commit the Association to any future course of action and was assured that this would not be so. For the 2nd meeting with the RCP representatives, two additional ACP representatives, namely Joan Taylor and W. P. Stamm, were appointed.

At the meeting held on the 22nd February, 1960 the RCP President (Sir Robert Platt) was in the Chair. All representatives were present and also the observer (A. W. Downie) from the Pathological Society. Again the discussions were most cordial and the general terms of the Faculty were outlined. Some accommodation would be made available. The RCP would handle the finance and be prepared to bear any losses such as might occur in the initial years. The question of the admission of non-medical members was raised and the RCP President could see no reason why they should not be admitted on modified terms. The question of election of pathologists to the FRCP remained as before. The possibility of pathologists having their own Fellowship, i.e., F.F.P., was raised, but the RCP representatives were unwilling to agree to this. They felt that they did not want the pathologists to become a separate body within the College but to be as fully incorporated in the life of the College as possible. In discussing the next steps the RCP President said he would have to bring the matter before the Comitia for approval. He could not do this until the pathologists had finally decided that they wanted a Faculty and he would have to be assured that this opinion was backed by a substantial majority. It was therefore decided that nothing further could be done until the matter had been further discussed by the ACP Council.

For this purpose a special meeting of the ACP Council was held on 11th March, 1960. An invitation had been extended to representatives from the Branches to express their views to Council at the conclusion of the Council meeting. The recent meeting with representatives of the RCP was discussed and the two new representatives of the ACP, Joan Taylor and Stamm, stated that they had been most impressed by the proposals of the RCP and were in favour of continuing negotiations. Of the other ACP representatives, Cunningham remained unconvinced and was still in favour of a College. It became obvious that there was much support in Council for a Faculty with the RCP and it was decided that when the final proposals were formulated all ACP members must be asked their opinion. In the meanwhile the following was proposed by the President (J. N. Cumings) and seconded by G. Stewart Smith:

'It was resolved to record that the Council supports the proposal of the President of the RCP of London to set up a Faculty of Pathology within the College.

The Council will continue to discuss the organisation of such a Faculty with representatives of the Royal College of Physicians and, provided they are fully satisfied with the final proposals, they will recommend that the inauguration of the Faculty be supported by the Association. All members of the Association will then be asked to express their opinion on the final proposals by completing a voting paper'.

This resolution was carried by 11 votes to 2 (Signy and McGowan; the latter's name is not included amongst those present, but his name is included among those who spoke. Cunningham, who had ceased to be a member of Council but attended as Chairman of the Ways and Means Committee, did not have a vote).

This decision was remarkable in that it showed that the Council had completely reversed its opinion twice in the course of two years. It also brought to an end the existence of the Ways and Means Committee without having even started on its primary task. In any case further work could hardly have been done as the Chairman was the only one who was still in favour of a College!

The discussion with the Branch representatives, which followed the Council Meeting, took on a different pattern and the majority stated that their members were not in favour of a Faculty with the RCP. This indeed was symbolic of the diversity of opinion within the Association.

During the past six months the Association had been split down the middle and this was to continue throughout the remainder of 1960.

At the ACP Council meeting in April 1960 the Secretary produced a memorandum setting out the case for a Faculty within the RCP for discussion. With modifications this was accepted as the official case for a Faculty, and G. J. Cunningham and G. K. McGowan were asked to draw up a similar document setting out the case for an independent College. McGowan asked that when the time came to vote, ACP members should not be asked to vote simply for or against a Faculty, but should be given a choice between College, Faculty, or neither. This matter was left to be discussed in relation to the poll.

At the July meeting there was a change of view. It was decided that the Secretary's memorandum should form a factual statement setting out the background of the situation, and labelled A. It would form part of a small booklet entitled 'The future organisation of Pathology'. The contents would be:

A. An historical survey of discussions which had been conducted in recent years (drawn up by the ACP Secretary and approved by Council).

B. A statement of the case for an independent College (drawn up by Cunningham and McGowan).

C. A statement of the case for a dependent Faculty of the RCP (drawn up by Blackburn and Jordan).

D. A statement of the terms of the proposed Faculty based on the discussions between the ACP and RCP representatives at their meetings.

This booklet was to be accompanied by an explanatory leaflet and a voting paper.

Documents A,B,C, and D were circulated to all ACP members in August 1960. At a special Council meeting in September the voting paper was amended and approved. A letter had been sent to the Pathological Society asking permission to send the above documents to their members. However, at a private business meeting in Dublin in July 1960 the Society was unwilling to agree to this until there had been an opportunity for further discussion at their meeting in January 1961. This decision was unfortunately not conveyed to the ACP in time to prevent the voting papers being sent to ACP members, who received them in October 1960 and were requested to return their votes not later than 19th November. The voting paper as sent out read as follows:

A 1 I am in favour of the establishment of an independent College of Pathology.

A 2 I am in favour of the establishment of a Faculty or Division of Pathology within the Royal College of Physicians of London provided that it is formed in accordance with the terms set out in 'Document D'.

A 3    I am in favour of either of the courses mentioned in A 1 and A 2 and have no strong preference for one as opposed to the other.

A 4    I am opposed both to the formation of an independent College and a Faculty or Division with the Royal College of Physicians of London.

It was agreed to send out an accompanying statement from Council with the voting paper. This was very carefully worded in order to obtain unanimity, and informed members of the unanimous opinion of Council that 'if a Faculty of Pathology is to be set up, the present proposed terms are as satisfactory as could be possibly accepted' and that they were 'such that they could well be accepted by Members of the Association'. This was very different from saying that it was the unanimous opinion of Council that it preferred a Faculty on these terms to a College of Pathologists.

It was about this time that the feelings of the protagonists reached fever pitch. There had been a particularly stormy ACP business meeting at the end of September and there were leading articles in the 'BMJ'[3,4] and the 'Lancet'.[5,6,7,8] The Widdicombe File, a popular feature of the latter, dealt with the College of Pathologists on five occasions.[9] Although mostly leaning slightly towards a Faculty rather than an independent College, these articles were on balance impartial. For an account of the current basic problems the articles written in 1959 could hardly have been bettered.[9] The receipt of the voting paper and its accompanying documents provoked an outburst. The 'explanatory note' from the Council can be seen in the Appendix I. In it, it will be seen that the two paragraphs referring to the Faculty with the RCP were printed in bold type, and the qualifying clause (if a Faculty is to be set up) was omitted so that, to many people at least, it appeared that Council had unanimously supported an RCP Faculty as opposed to a College of Pathologists. Furthermore, the envelope also contained a reprint of Professor Cappell's Presidential Address 'Pathologists at the Crossroads' ('Lancet' 1960, ii, 863); in this he made clear his preference for a Faculty with the RCP, indicated that the financial problems of a College of Pathologists were likely to be formidable, and concluded:

'These proposals (of the RCP) appear to me to be generous and to indicate a sincere and genuine desire on the part of the Royal College of Physicians to receive into their sodality the general body of pathologists in this country. It is for you to decide whether you wish to be associated with an ancient and honourable college with great prestige and influence, whose examinations are likely to receive immediate recognition, or whether you prefer to stand alone either to establish an independent College of Pathologists, with full realisation of the delays that this would involve both in setting up an examination and obtaining recognition of it, or to refrain from action altogether, indifferent to the challenge of the future'.

When these documents were received G. K. McGowan, believing them to be an unauthorised attempt to influence the vote, sent off an indignant letter to all branch secretaries of the ACP, with copies to the officers of the ACP, in the following terms (see Appendix II).

Many members, particularly those of the younger group, felt that there was an attempt to coerce them into voting for a Faculty, but even if this is untrue, there is no doubt that the inclusion of the paragraphs in heavy type was discreditable. Some, favouring a College, were certain that the vote would be prejudiced against them and they called for immediate action. The heat of feeling can be judged from some of the suggestions which were made. One group proposed submitting a vote of censure on the ACP Council. Another group, feeling that the College protagonists had no organisation, tried to collect 50 individuals who would give £10 towards the setting up of such an organisation with secretarial facilities and in that way sow the seeds of an independent College. In the end all decided to wait for the result of the poll and it may well be that the above event had the reverse effect and gained votes for the College.

Council met again in December, when voting papers had been returned. The Chairman referred to McGowan's letter sent to Branch Secretaries, and stated that the inclusion of the Presidential Address with the voting paper 'had been due to a misunderstanding', but on whose part was not made clear. Some suggested that the publisher had included it in order to save postage! With regard to the way in which Council's recommendation on the RCP Faculty was expressed, he justified this on the grounds that 'whilst some members of the Association had been adamant that the Council must remain impartial, others had been equally firm in stating that it was the duty of Council to lead'; he did not state who was responsible for the italics. The discussion took place in an atmosphere of some embarrassment but, as the results of the voting were generally known, nobody felt inclined to indulge in any witch-hunting. It was agreed that members of the ACP should be informed that the inclusion of the presidential address was due to a misunderstanding, and that the wording of the paragraphs in the covering letter was an accurate record of what had been agreed: the significance of the italics was ignored.

The results of the Ballot of ACP members were then given. Of the 838 votes cast (72% of the membership), 49.5% were in favour of an independent College, compared with 41.8% in favour of the proposed Faculty within the RCP; 552 or just over 66% were willing to support whichever body was favoured by the majority. Council therefore resolved to set up a new Joint Advisory Committee charged with the promotion of an independent College of Pathology consisting of Dr. A. G. Signy (convenor), Professor N. H. Ashton, Professor T. Crawford, Dr. B. W. Lacey, and Dr. G. K. McGowan, and to invite the Pathological Society to appoint up to five of its members to serve on it. It was agreed to inform the Secretary of the Pathological Society that the offer to conduct a poll of opinion among their members was no longer appropriate and should be withdrawn. It was further agreed to express the appreciation of Council to the President of the RCP for the generous offer made by his College. Council carried a motion expressing their complete confidence in the Secretary, Dr. F. Hampson, and thanked him for all the work entailed in the organisation of the memorandum. This motion was wholly appropriate, as private enquiries made it clear that Dr. Hampson was not personally responsible for the aspects of the referendum which had come under criticism. As Secretary he must have been involved, but presumably acted under the instructions of the Chairman of Council or the President. G. K. McGowan subsequently sent round a further letter to Branch Secretaries, making it clear that the matters to which he took exception should not be attributed to the Secretary.

A few days later, Dr. Allott resigned as Chairman of Council, on the grounds that the majority in favour of a College was in his view too small to justify Council's decision to proceed with setting up such a body, and that there should have been assurance of support from the Pathological Society. Many were saddened by this decision, for his contributions to the ACP and to Pathology in general had been great. Shortly afterwards W. P. Stamm too resigned from the ACP Council.

Professor Cappell's Presidential address may have upset some College supporters at the time of the final voting but it had even wider repercussions. It revealed another rift in the ranks of Clinical Pathologists when, during the last two months of 1960, it sparked off a spate of letters from Clinical Biochemists who considered they were underprivileged, and demanded at least equality with the pathologists.[10]

In the inevitable discussions which followed, the Faculty supporters could not understand why so many were opposed to what appeared to be a most attractive offer. It is possible that the offer was so generous that it aroused unjustified suspicions. Certainly a number of pathologists disliked the RCP system of election to the Fellowship, aware that many physicians themselves considered the system to be unfair. Whatever the reason it is clear that the age factor was the major one which split the Association, the younger members tending to favour a College and the older ones, already FRCP or confidently expecting to become so, a Faculty.

Meanwhile, the Pathological Society had been proceeding slowly in the wake of the ACP. In January 1960 its Committee had decided by eleven votes to two that it would take no part in the attempts to form a College, though at the Business Meeting on the following day it was apparent that there was more support for participation amongst the general membership. At the meeting of the Committee on January 1961 it was moved that the Committee was in favour of taking part in discussions regarding the formation of a College of Pathology, and the motion was carried by eight votes to five. The results of the ACP ballot were brought before the business meeting of the Society. It was decided that the Society too would conduct a poll of their members. The documents and voting paper were sent out in March with an explanatory leaflet and the closing date for the ballot was fixed for 4th April, 1961. The result of this was similar to that obtained by the ACP. Of the members 59.2% had already voted in the ACP ballot. Of those that had not previously voted (256), 50.4% were in favour of a College and 34% for a Faculty. The Committee of the Pathological Society had decided at the January 1961 meeting that it would not nominate its representatives to the Joint Advisory Committee until after the results of the ballot became known. Accordingly, at an extraordinary meeting on 30th May 1961 the following were proposed: G. J. Cunningham, J. D. A. Gray, J. W. Howie, A. C. Thackray and Janet Vaughan. Janet Vaughan asked for her name to be withdrawn and at the July meeting of the Pathological Society Committee it was agreed that she be replaced by Joan Taylor. It was further suggested that the secretaries of the ACP and Pathological Society should attend *ex officio* – namely F. Hampson and G. L. Montgomery respectively.

The ACP members of the Joint Advisory Committee met in January and in March 1961 with A. G. Signy in the Chair, and considered the functions of the College, method of foundation, membership, accommodation, finance, higher qualification, constitution and timetable. As soon as it was known that the Pathological Society had agreed to poll its members, it was agreed to adjourn the committee until the results of the voting were known.

From this point things started to move rapidly and the Joint Advisory Committee held three meetings on the 20th September, 20th November, and 6th December. On each occasion A. W. Downie attended in place of G. L. Montgomery, and D. F. Cappell was present by invitation. In December 1961 a report was issued. The terms of reference had been:

'To examine the position as expeditiously as possible in the light of the voting and to make recommendations on the course to be adopted. Those recommendations are to be made to the Society and to the Association; they are to be specific and practicable proposals, not couched in vague general terms'.

The report dealt with premises, grades of membership, higher qualification, and finance. The name of the new organisation would be 'The College of Pathologists'. It recommended that the parent bodies should meet again to discuss further action after they had considered the report. The Committee was also of the opinion that having, if they so decided, obtained the support of their general membership for such a course, the two organisations together should call a meeting at which the formal decision to establish a College of Pathologists could be taken and the first officers of the College appointed.

It should be noted that the goodwill of the RCP remained in evidence when its president, Sir Robert Platt, generously offered accommodation for the new College.

The governing bodies of the two organisations accepted the report of this Joint Committee. They decided to set up a Steering Committee with representatives from both bodies. Representing the Pathological Society were: Professor A. W. Downie, Professor J. W. Howie, Professor G. L. Montgomery, Professor C. L. Oakley, and Professor R. W. Scarff. Representing the Association of Clinical Pathologists were: Professor D. F. Cappell, Professor T. Crawford, Dr. F. Hampson, Dr. A. G. Signy, and Dr. G. Stewart Smith.

The Steering Committee was to act in accordance with the recommendations set out in the Joint Committee's report.

This new Steering Committee at its first meeting agreed that its first duty must be to ascertain the support which now existed for a College of Pathologists constituted on the lines suggested in the report of the Joint Committee. To this end a questionnaire was circulated and all members of the two Societies were asked to complete and return it without delay. Those members who intended to apply for foundation membership of the new College were asked to pay a part of the entrance fee when they returned the questionnaire.

It was emphasised in an explanatory note that the Committee required firm evidence of adequate support before they undertook to call a meeting for the purpose of forming the new College. They recommended that the sum payable by Founder Members should be about £50, apart from any annual subscription which might be required. Half of this sum, i.e. £25, was requested from those intending to become Founder Members, to accompany the reply to the questionnaire.

The Steering Committee met on the 24th May to consider the result of the questionnaire and reported the results in early July 1962. By the 7th May, the closing date, of the 2072 papers distributed to members 1091 (53%) had been returned. At that date 1006 (92%) members had expressed either unqualified approval or approval in principle and 63 (6k%) had stated that they were opposed to the formation of a new College on the lines suggested; 685 members had subscribed the sum of £25 which had been asked for from those intending to apply for Founder-membership. When the Committee met on May 24th the number of subscribers had risen to 727.

The Steering Committee were unanimously of the opinion that this support amply justified the formation of a College of Pathologists.

It was therefore decided to call a meeting in London on June 21st, 1962, at a time and place to be announced shortly, to which all those who had sent subscriptions would be invited. At this time the formal resolution that a College of Pathologists be founded would be put to the meeting. The meeting would then be asked to approve the appointment of provisional Officer-bearers and Council members who would be charged with the duty of preparing a draft constitution for the new College. When this had been done the provisional Office-bearers would then call a general meeting of all interested pathologists at which the proposed constitution would be submitted for approval.

The meeting was held at the Royal School of Hygiene and Tropical Medicine. The election of the following Office-bearers and Council Members was approved.

| | | |
|---|---|---|
| *President:* | Sir Roy Cameron | |
| *Vice-president:* | Prof. J. W. Howie | |
| *Registrar:* | Prof. T. Crawford | |
| *Hon. Treasurer:* | F. Hampson | |
| *Council:* | Prof. D. F. Cappell | Prof. N. H. Martin |
| | Prof. G. J. Cunningham | Dr. M. G. Nelson |
| | Dr. E. M. Darmady | Prof. C. L. Oakley |
| | Prof. A. W. Downie | Prof. R. W. Scarff |
| | Prof. J. Gough | Dr. A. G. Signy |
| | Dr. A. J. McCall | Dr. G. Stewart Smith |
| | Dr. G. K. McGowan | Dr. Joan Taylor |

The Provisional Council met four times during 1962 and studied a wide variety of topics including the drawing up of a Constitution for the new College, and also designing the pattern of a new examination which would consist of two parts, a Primary and a Final. On 5th January it had called another meeting of subscribers whose numbers had now reached over 1,000. Pathologists had closed ranks behind the College and many were happy to see that even Allott and Stamm had joined. The Memorandum and Articles of Association were approved and would be submitted to the Board of Trade. On the 12th December, 1963 the College was incorporated under the Companies Act of 1948 and registered as The College of Pathologists Ltd. In early 1964 permission was granted to drop the 'Ltd'. In March 1963 the first definitive council was elected. Plans proceeded rapidly for the first examination of the Membership, the Primary being held in April 1964 and the Final in the autumn of that year. Some accommodation had been found in 12 Grosvenor Crescent, which was later transferred to 16 Park Crescent and finally to 2 Carlton House Terrace, (see below), the present home of the College.

It was a memorable day, the 18th November 1964, when the First Annual General Meeting of the College was held. The Foundation Lecture was given by the President, Professor Sir Roy Cameron FRS on 'The Twilight World of Change and Decay', and the College dinner was held in the Hastings Hall of the British Medical Association, Tavistock Square. Already the College was flourishing and already the number of Members and Fellows had risen to 1530.

From this time onwards the College proceeded from strength to strength.[11] The first examinations were immediately accepted by Appointment committees. By 1965 the College had taken over from the

Royal College of Physicians as the 'appropriate body' to represent pathologists within the National Health Service and to make recommendations on merit awards. In 1967 the College, which had been running its affairs from modest rented accommodation, received a generous donation from the industrialist Sir Michael Sobell and was able to purchase a lease in a prestigious building at 2 Carlton House Terrace, which however required considerable repairs of war damage. In the same year the College applied for a Royal Charter, the procedures for which took just about as long as the repairs to the new building. In 1970 the College became the Royal College of Pathologists, and the newly refurbished accommodation was opened by Her Majesty Queen Elizabeth on December 10th.

The foundation of the College was a triumph, which belied all the fears of the 'older and wiser heads' who had originally opposed it. It also achieved the remarkable fact of bringing together the Association of Clinical Pathologists and the Pathological Society for the first time in their joint existence of more than 30 years.

REFERENCES

1   McMenemey, W. H., 'Lancet'. (1958) ii, pp. 841–4.
2   'British Medical Journal'. (1958) ii, Suppl. p. 139.
3   'British Medical Journal'. (1959) i, pp. 1299; 1171–2.
4   Ibid i, pp. 1271; 1258–9; 1267–8; 1820.
5   'Lancet'. (1958) ii, pp. 835–6.
6   Ibid (1959) i, pp. 884; 984; ii, p. 409.
7   Ibid (1960) i, p. 1297; ii, pp. 1028; 1084.
8   Ibid (1961) i, pp. 1385–6; ii, pp. 97–8.
9   Ibid Widdicombe File, (1959) ii, pp. 231–3; (1960) i, p. 1242; ii, pp. 921–2; 1025–6; 1094.
10  Ibid (1960) ii, pp. 985; 1033–4; 1091–2; 1147–8; 1192–3; 1251–2.
11  Foster, W. D., 'Pathology as a Profession in Great Britain, and the Early History of the Royal College of Pathologists' Chap IX, Undated, Publ. The Royal College of Pathologists, London.

Much of the material in this chapter has been obtained from the Council Minutes of the ACP, the Minutes of the Pathological Society of Great Britain and Ireland, and personal communications (through the agency of Dr. G. K. McGowan) from Dr. A. M. Cooke who was at the time a member of the Comitia of the RCP.

# TWENTY THREE

# Pathology in the 1960s

The activity of the ACP between 1958 and 1961 has been given in some detail, partly because of the vital part which the ACP played in founding the College, but also because at this time the author was directly involved in much that went on. If left at this stage the story would be incomplete and scant justice done to other important happenings. By filling in some of these it is hoped that the picture of Pathology in the Sixties might emerge with some measure of coherence.

The newly-founded College had more than enough to do as a matter of urgency and busied itself with drawing up a constitution, organising the Membership Examination, and giving attention to the recognition of laboratories suitable for the training of pathologists. It was soon realised that this latter might become a powerful weapon in inducing the Ministry of Health to improve some of the sadly-deficient working conditions of the hospital pathologist.

It was very different with the ACP which over the years had become involved in many medico-political issues, often with the co-operation of the Pathological Committee of the British Medical Association. When it came to negotiating with outside bodies such as the Ministry, the College was bound to take over and many pathologists were beginning to ask what functions would be left for the ACP to perform. In mentioning some of its other activities it should be emphasised once more that from its inauguration the Association had always studied the needs of the hospital pathologist and aimed at giving him assistance. A case in point was the Ethics and Professional Affairs Committee (formed in 1952) which offered him advice on current problems in the running of his laboratory. The width of interest of the Association can be appreciated when it is realised that there were about eight committees in addition to the Council, and it also had representation on about a dozen outside bodies. But if the ACP appeared to be in danger of withering away, bereft of many of its functions, there were two factors which were to keep it alive, namely the Branches and Education.

1. By the early sixties there were twelve Branches of the ACP in Great Britain and Ireland, which met twice a year. They were organised by Branch Secretaries, who disseminated information on ACP affairs to their members and reported members' views back to Council. The Branches also promoted a corporate spirit among pathologists in their areas. When the College was formed, the importance of such an organisation to keep the centre in touch with the periphery and vice versa was quickly realised, and the ACP encouraged the use of the Branches for this purpose. In due course the College appointed Advisers in each Branch Region and it became usual for their business meetings to start with ACP business conducted by the Branch Secretary, and to

362

continue with College business conducted by the College Adviser.

2. *Training*. This function of the ACP depended partly on the papers read at national (and branch) meetings. The ACP Council was anxious to improve their quality by appointing their first Meeting's Secretary, namely J. N. Cummings, in 1953. He held the post till 1957 when it was taken over by G. J. Cunningham with M. Sandler as assistant, and this state of affairs prevailed until 1965 when Cunningham became President. During this period it is generally believed that there was much improvement, and if this is so it was largely due to the help given to the Meetings Secretary by the Committees on Histopathology, Microbiology, Haematology and Chemical Pathology. More important were the Refresher Courses instituted in the early 1950s by Cuthbert E. Dukes who became Advisor in Postgraduate Studies. Dukes could never have realised how important his excellent idea was to be. It had been successful right from the start, and developed in a most surprising way. When started, the courses were mainly histopathological and related to problems in the special divisions of the subject. In 1960 Dukes resigned and was succeeded by G. J. Cunningham, who held the post till 1968 with R. C. B. Pugh as his Assistant. During this period the number of courses increased from 13 to 30. Also their scope was broadened and included subjects other than histopathological. With the foundation of the College and the institution of its Membership examination, the Advisor soon wondered who was going to provide educational facilities for the candidates. It will be remembered that during the debates on a Faculty of Pathology, the question arose as to whether this should be affiliated to the Royal College of Physicians or the Royal College of Surgeons. At that time the two colleges were functioning in a very different way. Both were giving Diplomas in their speciality, but the Surgeons were running courses for their diploma, namely at the College for the Primary, and at certain hospitals for the Final. The Physicians were plainly contemptuous of such a policy, which to them smacked of money-making and they in no way attempted to hide their feelings. The basic question was therefore 'Which road was the College of Pathologists going to take?' This matter was so vital that the ACP Advisor, C. J. Cunningham, approached the Registrar of the College of Pathologists and asked him which policy his College would adopt. He was assured that in no circumstances would courses be provided by the College for the Membership examination. The Advisor therefore felt free to organise a number of courses suitable for trainees and this proved to be a very successful venture. He was himself well-placed to observe any changes in educational policy of the College, for at the time he was not only on the College Council but was also a member of their Education Committee.

Courses for trainees were launched in 1963–4 and once the Membership Examination had started the demand became very great. An ACP Education Committee came into being in 1965 and within a year or so more than 100 trainees were registered on payment of a small fee. Under this scheme each one was supplied with a list of courses available, sent a quarterly Newsletter, and provided with a badge which would gain him (or her) admission to the ACP national meetings. There was much enthusiasm at the time, and the founder of the Association (Dr. S. C. Dyke) expressed pleasant surprise at the prospect of education becoming one of the main functions of the ACP.

With increasing specialisation the need for information on reliable technical procedures became paramount for the hospital pathologist. To provide for this a Committee on Technical Methods was appointed with the responsibility of reviving the Broadsheets which had been so successful in the pre-war years.

The Forensic Committee, which had been in existence for almost 20 years, was still active. It had done much to raise the standard of forensic work and had negotiated for its proper remuneration. In many instances there were also improvements in mortuary conditions, which in the past had been frequently appalling.

One venture proved to be unsuccessful. It happened in the years following the introduction of the Health Service. The first event was the formation in January 1948 of a Joint Committee of the ACP and the Biochemical Society. To meet the dissatisfaction of the hospital biochemists this committee was to discuss the training and qualifications suitable for these workers. The ACP representatives were R. J. V. Pulvertaft, E. N. Allott, N. F. Maclagen, and A. H. T. Robb-Smith. In spite of a number of meetings, by May 1949 no agreement had been reached on either salary, qualifications, or the relationship between Hospital Biochemists and Chemical Pathologists. Each body therefore sent its views to the Ministry of Health. The ACP then appointed a Committee on Chemical Pathology and a Joint Standing Committee with the Biochemical Society, and in 1950 the Royal Institute of Chemistry was given representation on the latter. The Minister agreed that this committee was the appropriate body to speak for Hospital Biochemists. Discussions went on and the question of admitting hospital biochemists without a medical qualification to membership of the ACP was raised. In January 1952 the Committee on Chemical Pathology asked Council to consider the question of Associate Membership for the Biochemists. The proposal came too late, for by the time it was discussed it became known that the hospital biochemists were planning to form an Association of Clinical Biochemists (ACB). By March 1953 this had become a reality and the newly-formed ACB intimated to the ACP that it would probably take over the functions of the Joint Committee. This decision was received with great regret by the chemical pathologists of the ACP, who had always hoped that it would have been possible to include hospital biochemists within the ACP. Doubtless several problems were solved by the formation of the ACB. There remained difficulties as yet not remedied, for the correspondence from some Hospital Biochemists at the time of the Final Vote for a College of Pathologists in November 1960 seemed to indicate that all was still not well. However the ACP decided to make the best of it and in April 1954 nominated four members to form a Joint Committee with the ACB. In October 1955 the ACB accepted an invitation to take part in a joint session at the ACP meeting. In future years it became customary to hold such sessions on the Saturday of the Autumn ACP meeting in London. The aspirations of Hospital Biochemists were realised when the College agreed to accept them as full members and provided a modified examination for them to take.

Such were some of the ACP activities at this time, and during the early years of the College it still seemed to be flourishing with its new and growing educational responsibilities. It was now approaching its 50th Birthday.

No reference to Pathology in the 1960s would be complete without some mention of other societies contributing by their activities to advances in the subject. To do justice to the numerous societies, small either because of their local nature or because of the narrowness of their sub-speciality, would be beyond the scope of this review. Consideration will therefore be confined to the main national bodies in existence at the time.

Sufficient has been said of the Association of Clinical Pathologists and its branches. The value of the British Medical Association has been considerable. It makes scientific contributions to Pathology at its annual meetings and the value of its medico-political activities, often in association with the ACP, have been unquestionable. The Pathology Section of the Royal Society of Medicine meets regularly and is well-esteemed for its scientific sessions.

As could have been foretold, the Pathological Society has continued in its traditional way, holding its summer and winter meetings, and seems to have emerged unscathed by its exposure to medical politics when it took part in the formation of the College. The sixties were to see a modernising of the format of the meetings and a somewhat belated attempt to widen the scope of the society. In spite of this its chief appeal is still confined to those engaged in research and have an academic approach to the subject. It has never wavered in its original intention to be solely a scientific society, but the author (G.J.C.) looks back with some nostalgia to the meetings of the thirties when specialisation was as yet young and each member could enjoy most of the papers.

In 1960 the British Division of the International Academy of Pathology came into being and its growing influence merits some historical details. Towards the end of 1906 (the year in which the Pathological Society was founded) there came into existence in North America a body known as the International Association of Medical Museums. Its foundation was largely due to the activities of Maude E. Abbott who became Secretary-Treasurer, and it held its first meeting on 15th May 1907. Born in Canada in 1869, she had graduated BA at McGill University. At that time this university did not accept women students of medicine so she obtained her MD degree at Bishop's College, Lennoxville, in 1894 and studied at Zurich, Vienna, and Edinburgh prior to taking the Diploma of the Scottish Conjoint Board. Most of her life was spent on the staff of McGill University where she held several posts including that of Curator of the Medical Museum and finally that of Assistant Professor of Medical Research. Her enthusiasm for museums was tremendous but she became best known for her Atlas of Congenital Heart Disease, a subject inspired in her by Sir William Osler. From 1907 until 1938 she acted as editor of the 'Bulletin of the Association of Medical Museums' and the 'Journal of Technical Methods'. The Association flourished in an era when every medical school had its own museum, and there were divisions of the Association in certain countries including North America, Canada and Great Britain. Maude Abbott died in 1940 and by this time museums were beginning to lose their popularity. The upsets caused by World War II were the final straw and by about 1955 there was left but one division (the North American-Canadian) and there were less than 50 members. A meeting was held to disband the Association, but Harold L. Stewart of the National Cancer Institute suggested that it should be revived under a new name – the International Academy of Pathology. It was pointed out that the purpose of museums was teaching and if this was less in vogue now, the academy could progress by using modern methods. A young pathologist working at the US Armed Forces Institute of Pathology, F. K. Mostofi, was made Secretary-Treasurer and by his efforts the Academy progressed with remarkable speed, and by 1960 had over 2,000 American and Canadian members. But one thing had been overlooked, namely that an 'international' body had been formed which consisted solely of North American members. When this anomaly was realised a European (G. J. Cunningham) was invited to sit on the 'American-Canadian' Council. The new type of meeting which the Academy had designed included one day which was devoted entirely to the discussion of a single subject. One of the earlier subjects was 'the red cell' and this part of the programme became known as 'the long course'. In addition there were short courses lasting half-a-day and mostly on histopathological subjects, not unlike the refresher courses given by Dukes to ACP members. The rest of the programme was devoted to papers submitted by members. It was an ingenious format and calculated to appeal to a wide public. Academic pathologists liked the 'long course' because the approach was at least partly from the basic science point of view. The short courses were invaluable for the practicing hospital pathologist.

The Academy's next concern was to make it truly international and plans were made to form divisions in foreign countries, initially by holding an Academy-type meeting in Europe to see how it was received. In 1958 F. K. Mostofi wrote to the Secretary of the Pathological Society proposing a joint meeting either to precede or follow the International Cancer Congress which would be held in London at the end of June. The

Committee of the Pathological Society declined the invitation, and in a discussion the status of the International Academy was questioned. The secretaries were asked to make some enquiries about it but it is not known whether this was done. However, it is noted that in the latter part of 1958, 'An International Committee on Pathology' was formed and Dr. Chapman Binford is listed as the representative of the International Academy of Pathology.

It was a difficult time for the Academy to negotiate with the British pathologists or societies, obsessed as they were with the question of a Faculty or College. Accordingly, the Academy turned to the European representative on its Council (G. J. Cunningham), who agreed to run an Academy-type meeting at the Royal College of Surgeons of England in June 1960, with some help from the Americans. It was a semi-official meeting, in that it was organised solely by the representative and three relatively junior assistants, namely Dr. Lucille Bitensky, Dr. John Pead, and Dr. David Pratt. It was a great success, being attended by about 400 people, and was directly responsible for the formation, later in the year, of the British Division of the Academy which 60 pathologists agreed to join. The main difference between this society and those already in existence lay in the younger age of its members and hence of its Council. The first President was in his early fifties (C. V. Harrison), and always noted for being particularly sprightly for his age! The great advantage of the Division was the relatively small size of its early meetings. The short courses were popular for they took the form of seminars with the distribution of histological slides. No attempt was made to have a 'membership drive', but the numbers steadily increased. The format of its meetings contrasted with those of the other societies. The Pathological Society meeting for many years consisted of a number of papers submitted by members and arranged in the order of receipt. The ACP found itself forced to group together papers on similar subjects for at least part of the meeting. Some of these were given by invitation. From the outset the Academy decided that special topics should be chosen and that all the speakers would be invited, a policy which did much to ensure the high quality of the programme.

In the immediate post-war years a close link had been forged between British and Dutch pathologists, thanks to the efforts of the Pathological Society, and meetings were held in Holland at regular intervals. In the sixties the Academy too was joined by several Dutch and Belgian pathologists who sponsored meetings in their countries. The Secretary of the Academy (David Pratt) introduced a number of innovations such as hiring a bus to take members to and from the meetings. This was particularly welcome in the case of foreign meetings, and for the British meetings it became customary for the bus to call at London Airport to collect Dutch and Belgian members. This is no place to enlarge further on activities of the British Division, and it will suffice to say that at present there are over 500 members.

It is thus clear that Pathology in Great Britain is well served by meetings of the three main societies. As regards publications the Journal of Pathology maintains its customary high standard and is published monthly. The Journal of Clinical Pathology has improved steadily over the years and had added to the status of the ACP: published by the BMA, in recent years it has become one of its most successful ventures. The formation of the International Academy of Pathology was accompanied by the production of a journal, 'Laboratory Investigation'. This has always been produced in America and is at present the official publication of the US-Canadian Division. In 1977 the British Division launched a new journal, namely 'Histopathology'; of a high standard and published bi-monthly, it already seems assured of success.

As seen in this short history, British Pathology has come a long way over the years and especially during this century. At times the growth of knowledge seems to have been haphazard and indeed fortuitous. By its quality it can now hold its own anywhere in the world.

If one were asked to name the one unique feature of present-day Pathology in Britain, it would have to be the College of Pathologists. It is as yet young but its progress has been phenomenal. It says much for the band of young pathologists who never wavered in their support nor weakened in their belief. The financial bogey quoted at so many of the discussions has been successfully laid.

We needed a qualification of high status and we were told that its recognition would be long forthcoming. One pessimist estimated this at 50 years and even the author (G.J.C) thought that it would be ten! Yet within five years it had become generally accepted. Already its quarters occupy a dignified site in pleasant surroundings. For this remarkable success the Officers and the Council must be warmly commended. To have received the title of 'The Royal College of Pathologists' so soon is something of which Members and Fellows may justly feel proud.

REFERENCES

Most of the material in this chapter has been obtained from ACP Year Books, Council Minutes, and personal notes made at the time by the author.

# Appendix I

At a special meeting on September 23rd, 1960, the ACP Council met to discuss documents which were to accompany the voting papers. It was agreed that these should include an introductory note from Council. It had been decided that Council should not express a preference for either College or Faculty because there was no unanimity, although a large majority was in favour of a Faculty. It was however agreed that a favourable mention should be made of the terms which the Royal College of Physicians had offered for a Faculty. The following resolution was passed unanimously.

Minute 4. *Document to accompany the Voting Paper.*

It was agreed that an introductory note should be sent to all members along with the Voting Paper. The Council were unanimously agreed that if a Faculty in Pathology is to be set up the present proposed terms are as favourable as could be expected and it was agreed to inform members of this opinion of the Council in the introductory note. It was further agreed to inform them of the unanimous opinion of the meeting that the proposed terms and conditions of formation of a Faculty were such that they could well be accepted by members of the Association.

In the event Council's note was circulated in the following form.

ASSOCIATION OF CLINICAL PATHOLOGISTS

All members of the Association will have received a booklet concerned with the possible future organisation of Pathology. In it the arguments in favour of an independent College of Pathology are stated and also those in favour of a Faculty or Division of Pathology within the Royal College of Physicians of London. These documents were prepared at the request of Council by two of its members in each case and they represent the views of those particular members. It contains also a document (Document 'D') setting out the terms on which a Faculty within the Royal College of Physicians might be established, as they have been agreed between our representatives and representatives of that College. In connection with this last document, Council wish to make it clear that the expression 'Other Consultants' in para 5 (ii) on p.13 means all other consultants. This booklet was circulated to members before Document 'D' had been received by Council. The proposals of the Royal College of Physicians as set out in Document 'D' were considered by Council at a special meeting on Sept 23rd 1960.

**This meeting was unanimously of the opinion that the terms agreed with representatives of the Royal College of Physicians for the formation of a Faculty or Division are such that they could not be bettered by any College which was considering the formation of a Faculty.**

**It was accordingly decided unanimously that Council should inform members that it believes that the offer of the Royal College of Physicians could well be accepted by members of the Association.**

## Appendix I

All members are now urged to complete the voting paper by placing a tick in *one only* of the spaces in section A and in the space in Section B if appropriate. The voting paper must be returned to Dr. F. Hampson, Royal Berkshire Hospital, Reading *not later than November 19th* 1960.

# Appendix II

Dear Dr Hampson,

The ACP circular which accompanies the voting paper contains two paragraphs in heavy print. It appears to some of my colleagues and to me that their wording combined with the printing will convey to many members the impression that the Council unanimously wishes members to vote for a Faculty with the College of Physicians.

As one who was a member of Council and present throughout the meeting at which the circular was planned, I would like it to be known that any such conclusion would be incorrect. The unanimous decision was simply to inform members that the offer from the R.C.P. was as good as any which was likely to be offered by any college and that it was considered to be a perfectly acceptable solution for those who would be satisfied with an attached Faculty. It was clearly understood that the Council would not attempt to recommend one choice rather than another. Owing to the lateness of the hour the exact wording was left to the Secretary, and because he considered that it would be impracticable to get the wording approved by Council and also printed in time to accompany the voting paper, I and presumably other Council members never saw the circular until it appeared with the voting paper.

There was no suggestion at the meeting that any other document should be circulated with the voting paper.

You will be able to judge for yourself whether the document does or does not convey what the Council agreed. You will also be able to judge whether the Presidential Address favours one side more than another and whether it was an appropriate document to send round with the voting paper, especially when both sides had an opportunity of stating their views in a previous pamphlet. It is now too late for Council to take any steps in these matters, but if your Branch has yet to hold a meeting before the date fixed for the return of the voting paper I shall be grateful if you will bring these points to the notice of your members.

*Let me make it very clear that I do not wish to impute any unworthy motives to those who prepared and circulated these documents.* It may well be, for instance, that the circulation of the Presidential Address was an error for which the Printer was solely responsible. I am concerned however to correct any false impression which may have been caused.

Yours sincerely,
G.K. McGowan.

To The Secretary of the ACP, with copies to Officers and Members of Council and all Branch Secretaries.

# Index

Abbott, Maud E. 365
Aberdeen University and medical school
126
Academic Affairs Committee (Cappell) 338,
339, 340, 341, 342
Acland, Henry Wentworth 98–100
ACP Joint Committee with ACB 365
ACP Joint Committee with Biochemical
Society 364
ACP role after Foundation of College 362
Addison 42
Aitkin, William 232, 233
American Association of Clinical
Pathologists 308, 312
Anderson's College, Glasgow 125–126
Ankylostomiasis 273–275
Anthrax organisms 281
Anti-vivisection 198–202
Apothecaries Company, London 11, 14
Apothecaries Hall, Dublin 122–123
Army medical schools 231, 232, 234
Arnott, Neil 204, 205–206
Ashanti campaign 229
Association of Clinical Biochemists (ACB)
364
Association of Clinical Pathologists, (ACP)
311
Autopsies, early 26

Bacteriophage 256
Baillie, Matthew 2
Basic sciences 70
Bassi Agostine 271
Bastian, Charlton 280, 289, 290
Bayle, G.L. 5
Beale, Lionel Smith 246
Belfast medical school 190
Bence Jones, Henry 246–247
Bentham, Jeremy 55
Bernard, Claude 238–239
Bert, Paul 240–241
Beveridge Report 319
Bichat 7
Biermayer, Lorenz 59, 80
Bilharz, Theodore 273
Bird, Golding 44
Blastema theory 83
BMA Consulting Pathologists Group 308,
312, 324
Boerhaave, Hermann 71, 74–75
Books on Pathology 30–39, 52
Bordet, Jules 296
Bostock, J. 32

Boxwell, William 190
Boycott, A.E. 306–307
Boyd, J.S.K. 234
Branches (ACP) 333, 353
Bright, Richard 43
Bristowe, John Syer 218–219
British Medical Association (BMA) 65–66
British Society of Pathologists 307, 311
Broadsheets 312
Broussais 7, 8
Brown Institute 251–256
Brown-Sequard, Charles Edouard 239–240
Bruce, David 233, 234, 235
Brücke, Ernst Wilhelm von 242
Budd, William 220
Burma campaign 229

Carswell, R. 42, 59
Chadwick, Edwin 55, 56, 57, 204, 206
Cheyne, J. 46
Cheyne, William Watson 294
China wars 229
Clark, William 107
Clift, William 53
Clinical laboratory organisation 321–322
Cohnheim, Julius 65, 223
College accommodation 361
College of Pathologists 325, 327, 343, 345
Colles, Abraham 46
Committee on Academic Affairs (ACP),
(Hadfield) 331, 336, 337
Committees, specialist (ACP) 333
Conjoint Diploma 257
Conjoint Examination 258, 262
Conjoint Laboratories 257–262
Cooper, Astley 12, 45
Cooper, Bransby 18, 19
Corrigan, D.J. 46
County Laboratories 310
Crases, theory of 84
Crimean War 229–231
Cruikshank, Edgar 295
Cruveilhier 8, 42, 59
Cullen, William 125, 133, 134
Cummings, J.N. 333
Cunningham, G.J. 366–367

Dean, H.R. 113
Delépine, Sheridan 66–67, 185–186
Diphtheria 216, 255, 261
Diploma in Clinical Pathology 313,
323–324
Dispensary system, London 14

# Index

Dreschfeld, Julius 185
Dreyer, Georges 103–105
Dubini, Angelo 273
Dublin University College 192
Dukes, Cuthbert 324, 338, 340, 345–346
Dundee University College and medical school 124
Dupuytren 8, 17, 42, 59
Dyke, S.C. 305–306, 307, 308, 309, 311, 314–316, 332

Edinburgh University and medical school 129–136
Emergency Blood Transfusion Service 318
Emergency Medical Service 319
Emergency Public Health Laboratory Service 317
Epidemics 54–55, 208, 210, 211, 230, 277
European Association of Clinical Pathologists 332

Faculty of RCP 327, 335, 339, 342, 349–353
Faculty of RCS 335
Fermentation, germ theory 278–279
Florey, Howard 105
Flourens, Marie Jean Pierre 238
Forensic Pathology 312–313
Foster, Michael 111, 112

Germ theory 291
Germany, early universities 84
Germany, university hospitals 84, 88
Glasgow University and medical school 124–126
Graves 45
Greenfield, William S. 254, 294, 349
Greenhow, Edward Headlam 216–217, 283
Griesinger, Wilhelm 273
Gruby, David 271

Hamilton, D.J. 42
Harrison, James B. 60, 61
Harwood, Busick 106
Haviland, John 106, 108
Helmholtz, Hermann Ludwig von 242–243
Henle, Jacob 90
Herbert, Sidney 231
Heterogenia 279
Histological techniques 91
Hodgkin, Thomas 19, 43–44
Hofman, August Wilhelm von 244
Holland, P.D.J. 190
Homogenia 279, 280
Horsley, Victor 235
Hughes Bennett 53, 133, 135, 245–246

Humboldt, Karl Wilhelm, Baron von 87
Humphrey, George Murray 108, 109, 110, 111–112
Hunter, William and John 1, 2, 13, 195

Immunity 296, 299
Incorporation of ACP 340
Institutes of Medicine 60, 133
International Academy of Pathology 366
International Academy, British Division 367
International Association of Medical Museums 365

Jenner Institute 266
Joint Advisory Committee (ACP & Path. Soc.) on College 356, 358
Journal of Pathology and Bacteriology 69, 260
Journal of Clinical Pathology 332

Kay-Shuttleworth, James 55, 205
Kettle E.H. 323
Klebs, Edwin 65
Klein, Emanuel 200, 252, 253
Koch 291, 293, 295

Laboratory medicine 70
Laboratories 322
Laennec 7
Larrey 5, 17
Leishman, W.B. 234
Leuckart, Rudolf 272
Lewis, Timothy 235
Leyden medical school 74
Liebig, Justus von 243–245
Lister Institute 262–267
Lister, Joseph 281–283, 294
Lobstein, J.M. 42, 59
Loraine Smith, James 186–187, 190
Ludwig, Carl 241
Lyons, R.D. 232

MacFadyean, Allan 265, 266
MacLagen, T.J. 290
Magendie, Francois 196, 198, 237–238
Manchester medical school 184
Manson, Patrick 273, 275–276
Maria Theresa, Empress 75–76
McGrigor, James 227–229
McMenemy, W.H. 328, 339, 346
McWeeney, Edmund Joseph 192
Medical Laboratory Technicians 332
Medical Officers of Health 206–207, 212, 214
Medical Research Council 317

Medical Schools, private 13, 120–121
Mediciner 126
Meeting of Subscribers to College 359–360
Meetings Secretary (ACP) 333
Metchnikoff, Elie 65, 222, 296, 297
Miles, Thomas 189
Mostofi, F.K. 366
Muir, Robert 188
Müller, Johannes 89, 197
Munro, Alexander, primus 130–132
Munro, Alexander, secundus 132, 134
Munro, Alexander, tertius 132, 134
Munro, John 131
Murchison, Charles 218
Museums 1, 28, 53, 66, 120, 130

National Health Service 319–320, 324
National Insurance Act 304
National University, Dublin 119
Natural History School 195
Nature Philosophy School 195
Nightingale, Florence 231

Ogston, Alexander 295
Owen, Richard 53
O'Sullivan, Alexander Charles 192

Paget, George 108, 109–110, 111
Parasitic diseases, principal 271
Pasteur Institute 262
Pasteur 262, 263, 279, 294, 296
Pathological Society of Gt. Britain &
    Ireland 68, 70, 306, 311, 347
Pathological Society of London 48–50, 54,
    65, 68
Peninsular campaign 229
Physiological Society 249
Pitcairne, Archibald 130
Platt, Sir Robert 342
Postgraduate Education 338, 340
Power, William Henry 217–218
Pringle, Sir John 3, 227
Provisional Council and Officers of College
    360
Public Health Bacteriology 322
Public Health Laboratory Service 317
Pulvertaft, R.J.V. 332
Purkinje, Johannes Evangelista 90, 91
Purser, John Mallet 191
Pyaemia 221–222, 285, 287, 289

Queckett, John T. 53, 98
Queen's University of Ireland 118

Rabies treatment 262, 263, 264
Rabies prevention 245

Redi, Francisco 271–272
Religious restrictions 122
Reymond, Du Bois 242
Ritchie, James 102–103
Roberts, William 298
Rokitansky, Carl 59, 81, 83
Ross, Ronald 235
Royal College of Physicians, London 11,
    324, 325, 328–329
Royal College of Surgeons, Dublin 119
Royal College of Surgeons, England 11
Roy, Charles Smart 112, 179, 254
Rudolphi, K.A. 273
Ruffer, Armand 263, 264, 265, 299

Sanderson, John Burden 54, 101–103, 200,
    219–220, 252, 254, 284, 286, 287, 290, 293
Schleiden & Swann, Cellular theory 83, 90
Seaton, Edward C. 215–216, 284
Semmelweiss 281
Shaftesbury, Earl of 56
Sharpey, William 135, 247–248
Sheffield Memorandum to Hadfield
    Committee 336
Sibbald, Robert 129
Signy, C. Gordon 332
Simon, John 57, 62–64, 204, 211–223, 322
Smith, Southwood 55, 204, 205–206
Smith, Theobald 297
Snow, John 57, 210
Societies, pathological 47–48, 67
Splenic fever organisms 280
Spontaneous generation 279
Standing Committee on Pathology (RCP)
    326–327, 330
Standing Committee on Training (ACP)
    325, 329, 330
Steering Committee (ACP & Path. Soc.) to
    found College 359
Sternberg, George M. 300
Stokes, William 42, 45–46
St. Andrew's University and medical school
    122–123, 188
Subcommittee on Training and
    Qualifications (Allott Committee, ACP)
    325
Surgical infections 281, 285
Sutherland, Lewis Robertson 188
Symmers, William St. Clair 190–191

Taylor, A.S. 44
Thomson, John 42, 59, 60
Training & qualifications 313, 328, 325,
    330
Transfusions 21
Trinity College, Dublin 116–117, 191–192

Tubercles 286, 287, 291, 292
Tunnelling and ankylostomiasis 274–275
Türkheim, Ludwig von 82
Twort, F.W. 256
Tyndall, John 298–299

Vaccination 215–216
Vienna, New School 79–84
Vienna, Old School 76–78
Villemin 220, 222
Virchow, Rudolf 83, 84, 91–94
Viruses 299–300
Voit, Carl von 245
Von Swieten, Gerhard 76
Voting on College or Faculty 346–347, 348, 354, 356, 358

Wakley, Thomas 10–24
Waterloo campaign 229

Ways & Means Committee (ACP) (Cunningham) 350
Whewell, William 108–109
Whitby, Lionel 327– 328
White, Arthur Hamilton 189
White, C. Powell 306, 308, 309, 311–312
Wilks, Samueal 43, 44, 67
Williams, D.J. 47, 48
Woodhead, Sims 69, 113, 258, 260
Woodhouse, Stuart 189
Working Party on College (Cunningham), (ACP) 343, 345
World Federation of Associations of Clinical Pathology 332
World War II 316–319
Wright, Almroth 233, 234
Wucherer, Otto Edward Henry 272–273

Yale medical school 72